Antibacterial Therapy and Newer Agents

Guest Editors

KEITH S. KAYE, MD, MPH
DONALD KAYE, MD

INFECTIOUS DISEASE CLINICS OF NORTH AMERICA

www.id.theclinics.com

Consulting Editor
ROBERT C. MOELLERING, Jr, MD

December 2009 • Volume 23 • Number 4

SAUNDERS an imprint of ELSEVIER, Inc.

W.B. SAUNDERS COMPANY

A Division of Elsevier Inc.

1600 John F. Kennedy Blvd., Suite 1800, Philadelphia, PA 19103-2899.

http://www.theclinics.com

INFECTIOUS DISEASE CLINICS OF NORTH AMERICA Volume 23, Number 4

December 2009 ISSN 0891-5520, ISBN-10: 1-4377-1232-0, ISBN-13: 978-1-4377-1232-2

Editor: Barbara Cohen-Kligerman

Developmental Editor: Donald Mumford

Infectious Disease Clinics of North America (ISSN 0891-5520) is published in March, June, September, and December by Elsevier Inc., 360 Park Avenue South, New York, NY 10010-1710. Periodicals postage paid at New York, NY and additional mailing offices. Subscription prices are $235.00 per year for US individuals, $395.00 per year for US institutions, $118.00 per year for US students, $278.00 per year for Canadian individuals, $489.00 per year for Canadian institutions, $332.00 per year for international individuals, $489.00 per year for international institutions, and $163.00 per year for Canadian and international students. To receive student rate, orders must be accompanied by name of affiliated institution, date of term, and the *signature* of program/residency coordinator on institution letterhead. Orders will be billed at individual rate until proof of status is received. Foreign air speed delivery is included in all *Clinics* subscription prices. All prices are subject to change without notice. **POSTMASTER**: Send address changes to *Infectious Disease Clinics of North America*, Elsevier Health Sciences Division, Subcription Customer Service, 3251 Riverport Lane, Maryland Heights, MO 63043. **Customer Service: 1-800-654-2452 (US). From outside of the US and Canada, call 1-314-447-8871. Fax: 1-314-447-8029. E-mail: JournalsCustomerService-usa@elsevier.com (print support) or JournalsOnlineSupport-usa@elsevier.com (online support).**

Infectious Disease Clinics of North America is also published in Spanish by Editorial Inter-Médica, Junin 917, 1er A 1113, Buenos Aires, Argentina.

Reprints. For copies of 100 or more, of articles in this publication, please contact the Commercial Reprints Department, Elsevier Inc., 360 Park Avenue South, New York, New York 10010-1710. Tel. (212) 633-3812, Fax: (212) 462-1935, E-mail: reprints@elsevier.com.

Infectious Disease Clinics of North America is covered in *MEDLINE/PubMed (Index Medicus), Current Contents/Clinical Medicine, Science Citation Alert, SCISEARCH,* and *Research Alert.*

Printed and bound in the United Kingdom

Transferred to Digital Print 2011

Contributors

CONSULTING EDITOR

ROBERT C. MOELLERING, Jr, MD
Shields Warren-Mallinckrodt Professor of Medical Research, Harvard Medical School;
Department of Medicine, Beth Israel Deaconess Medical Center, Boston, Massachusetts

GUEST EDITORS

KEITH S. KAYE, MD, MPH
Professor of Medicine, Corporate Director, Infection Prevention, Epidemiology and
Antimicrobial Stewardship, Department of Medicine, Division of Infectious Diseases,
Detroit Medical Center and Wayne State University, Detroit, Michigan

DONALD KAYE, MD
Professor of Medicine, Drexel University College of Medicine, Philadelphia, Pennsylvania

AUTHORS

DEVERICK J. ANDERSON, MD, MPH
Assistant Professor, Department of Medicine, Duke University Medical Center, Durham,
North Carolina

JOSE A. BAZAN, DO
Clinical and Research Fellow, Division of Infectious Diseases, The Ohio State University
Medical Center, Columbus, Ohio

MAUREEN K. BOLON, MD, MS
Assistant Professor of Medicine, Division of Infectious Diseases, Northwestern University
Feinberg School of Medicine, Chicago, Illinois

BARTHOLOMEW R. BONO, MD
Assistant Professor of Medicine, Jefferson Medical College, Philadelphia, Pennsylvania;
Attending Physician, Division of Infectious Diseases, Department of Medicine, Albert
Einstein Medical Center, Philadelphia, Pennsylvania

SUSANA CHAVEZ-BUENO, MD
Assistant Professor, Department of Pediatrics, Section of Pediatric Infectious Diseases,
University of Oklahoma Health Sciences Center, Oklahoma City, Oklahoma

TEENA CHOPRA, MD
Fellow, Department of Medicine, Division of Infectious Diseases, Harper Hospital, Detroit
Medical Center and Wayne State University, Detroit, Michigan

LUKE F. CHEN, MBBS (Hons), CIC, FRACP
Assistant Professor of Medicine, Department of Medicine, Division of Infectious Diseases
and International Health, Duke University Medical Center, Durham, North Carolina

BRETT GILBERT, DO, FACOI
Clinical Instructor of Medicine, Thomas Jefferson University Hospital, Philadelphia; Division of Infectious Diseases, Lankenau Hospital, Wynnewood, Pennsylvania

THOMAS L. HOLLAND, MD
Fellow, Infectious Diseases, Duke University Medical Center, Durham, North Carolina

MARIA JOYCE, MD, DTM&H
Chief, Clinical Microbiology, Durham VAMC; Assistant Professor of Medicine and Pathology, Duke University Medical Center, Durham, North Carolina

DONALD KAYE, MD, MACP
Professor of Medicine, Drexel University College of Medicine, Philadelphia, Pennsylvania

ELAINE T. KAYE, MD
Clinical Assistant Professor in Dermatology, Department of Dermatology, Harvard Medical School, Children's Hospital Medical Center, Boston, Massachusetts

KEITH S. KAYE, MD, MPH
Professor of Medicine, Corporate Director, Infection Prevention, Epidemiology and Antimicrobial Stewardship, Department of Medicine, Division of Infectious Diseases, Detroit Medical Center and Wayne State University, Detroit, Michigan

KENNETH M. KAYE, MD
Associate Professor, Division of Infectious Diseases, Harvard Medical School, Channing Laboratory, Brigham and Women's Hospital, Boston, Massachusetts

JULIE H. LEVISON, MD, MPhil
Fellow, Division of Infectious Diseases, Brigham and Women's Hospital; Division of Infectious Diseases, Program in HIV Epidemiology and Outcomes Research, Massachusetts General Hospital, Boston, Massachusetts

MATTHEW E. LEVISON, MD
Adjunct Professor of Medicine and Professor of Public Health, Drexel University, Bryn Mawr, Philadelphia, Pennsylvania

PETER A. LIO, MD
Assistant Professor in Pediatrics and Dermatology, Department of Dermatology, Northwestern University Feinberg School of Medicine, Chicago, Illinois

LAWRENCE L. LIVORNESE, Jr, MD, FACP,FIDSA
Clinical Assistant Professor of Medicine, Drexel University College of Medicine, Philadelphia; Chief, Division of Infectious Diseases, Lankenau Hospital, Wynnewood, Pennsylvania

EMILY MAWDSLEY, MD
Fellow, Section of Infectious Diseases and Global Health, University of Chicago Medical Center, Chicago, Illinois

STANLEY I. MARTIN, MD
Assistant Professor of Clinical Internal Medicine, Division of Infectious Diseases, The Ohio State University Medical Center, Columbus, Ohio

JUSTINE MIRANDA, MD
Fellow, Division of Infectious Diseases, Baystate Medical Center, Springfield, Massachusetts

MICHAEL D. NAILOR, PharmD
Clinical Assistant Professor, University of Connecticut School of Pharmacy, Storrs, Connecticut; Formerly, Clinical Assistant Professor, Division of Infectious Diseases, Department of Internal Medicine, Wayne State University School of Medicine, Detroit, Michigan

FOZIA QAMAR, MD
Fellow, Division of Infectious Diseases, Department of Medicine, Albert Einstein Medical Center, Philadelphia, Pennsylvania

PAUL ROBBINS, DO
Division of Nephrology, Department of Medicine, Lankenau Hospital, Wynnewood, Pennsylvania

JACK D. SOBEL, MD
Chief, Division of Infectious Diseases, Department of Internal Medicine, Wayne State University, Detroit, Michigan

TERRENCE L. STULL, MD
Patricia Price Browne Distinguished Professor and Chair, Department of Pediatrics, University of Oklahoma Health Sciences Center, Oklahoma City, Oklahoma

ALLAN R. TUNKEL, MD, PhD
Department of Internal Medicine, Monmouth Medical Center, Long Branch, New Jersey

STEPHEN WEBER, MD, MS
Associate Professor, Section of Infectious Diseases and Global Health; Chief Healthcare Epidemiologist and Medical Director of Infection Control, University of Chicago Medical Center, Chicago, Illinois

CHRISTOPHER W. WOODS, MD, MPH
Chief, Infectious Diseases, Durham VAMC; Associate Professor of Medicine and Pathology, Duke University Medical Center, Durham, North Carolina

JERRY M. ZUCKERMAN, MD
Assistant Professor of Medicine, Jefferson Medical College; Attending Physician, Division of Infectious Diseases, Department of Medicine, Albert Einstein Medical Center, Philadelphia, Pennsylvania

Contents

This article familiarizes the clinician with the principles of bacterial susceptibility testing and reporting to facilitate communication with the clinical microbiology laboratory. As resistance continues to emerge among a wide
range of clinically relevant bacteria, the complexity of this communication
increases. This updated version provides an overview of the important
susceptibility concerns for most commonly isolated bacterial pathogens.

This article reviews pharmacodynamics of antibacterial drugs, which can
be used to optimize treatment strategies, prevent emergence of resistance
and rationalize the determination of antimicrobial susceptibility. Important
pharmacodynamic concepts include the requirements for bactericidal
therapy for endocarditis and meningitis, for synergistic combinations to
treat enterococcal endocarditis or to shorten the course of antimicrobial
therapy, for obtaining maximal plasma concentration/minimal inhibitory
concentration (MIC) ratios that are greater than 10 or 24 hour-area under
the plasma concentration curve (AUC)/MIC ratios that are greater than
100-125 for concentration-dependent agents against gram-negative
bacilli and 25-35 against *Streptococcus pneumoniae*, and for obtaining
percent of time that drug levels are greater than the MIC that is at least
40% to 50% of the dosing interval for time-dependent agents.

Resistance to antimicrobial drugs is increasing at an alarming rate among
both gram-positive and gram-negative bacteria. Traditionally, bacteria resistant to multiple antimicrobial agents have been restricted to the nosocomial environment. A disturbing trend has been the recent emergence and
spread of resistant pathogens in nursing homes, in the community, and in
the hospital. This article reviews the epidemiology, molecular mechanisms
of resistance, and treatment options for pathogens resistant to antimicrobial drugs.

Most evidence-based methods to control the spread of antimicrobial resistance have been developed and applied to the hospital setting.

Strategies to control the emergence and spread of antimicrobial resistance in hospitals can be categorized as either infection control or antibiotic stewardship strategies. Infection control is the discipline focused on preventing the spread of infections within the health care setting; antibiotic stewardship can help minimize the emergence of multidrug-resistant organisms by promoting prudent use of antibiotics. This article describes different infection control and antibiotic management strategies that can be used to control antimicrobial resistance in hospital settings.

Antibiotics are among the most frequently used drugs in children. Although antibacterials have been available for decades, many agents have not been studied to assess their safety and efficacy in the pediatric population. This article describes the pharmacologic characteristics and therapeutic use of the most commonly prescribed antibacterials for pediatric patients. Newer agents currently under clinical investigation are discussed as well.

Older patients disproportionately suffer the burden of infection in the community and in health care facilities. The rational approach to antimicrobial therapy for older patients with infection requires an appreciation and understanding of the complex immunologic, epidemiologic, pharmacologic, and microbiologic factors that influence the manifestations and consequences of infection in this group. Specific recommendations for common infectious syndromes must take into account the unique needs of older patients and should be tailored for each individual case.

This article provides background information on the pharmacokinetics of antibacterial agents in patients who have normal and impaired renal function. Tables are provided to allow quick determination of appropriate dosages for varying degrees of renal failure. The use of serum levels; newer strategies for cefazolin, vancomycin and aminoglycoside dosing; methods of dialysis and associated antibiotics dosage adjustments, and antibiotic toxicity in renal failure are reviewed.

The principles of antimicrobial therapy for acute bacterial meningitis include use of agents that penetrate well into cerebrospinal fluid and attain appropriate cerebrospinal fluid concentrations, are active in purulent cerebrospinal fluid, and are bactericidal against the infecting pathogen.

Recommendations for treatment of bacterial meningitis have undergone significant evolution in recent years, given the emergence of pneumococcal strains that are resistant to penicillin. Clinical experience with use of newer agents is limited to case reports, but these agents may be necessary to consider in patients who are failing standard therapy.

Peter A. Lio and Elaine T. Kaye

Decreased systemic toxicity, ease of application, and increased concentrations at the target site are some of the important advantages topical antibacterial agents offer. This article reviews the literature on selected indications for these agents and provides in-depth examination of specific agents for the prophylaxis and treatment of skin and wound infections.

Michael D. Nailor and Jack D. Sobel

An overview of the mechanism of action, dosing, clinical indications, and toxicities of the glycopeptide vancomycin is provided. The emerging gram-positive bacterial resistance to antimicrobials and its mechanisms are reviewed. Strategies to control this emergence of resistance are expected to be proposed. Newer antimicrobial agents that have activity against vancomycin-resistant organisms are now available and play a critical role in the treatment of life-threatening infections.

Jose A. Bazan, Stanley I. Martin, and Kenneth M. Kaye

This article reviews the new beta-lactam (β-lactam) antibiotics doripenem, ceftobiprole, and ceftaroline. It covers pharmacokinetic and pharmacodynamic properties, dosing, in vitro activities, safety, and clinical trial results. Doripenem (Doribax) has been approved by the US Food and Drug Administration (FDA) for the treatment of complicated intra-abdominal and urinary tract infections. At this writing, ceftobiprole is under review by the FDA for approval based on results of phase 3 clinical trials, whereas at least one phase 3 clinical trial of ceftaroline has been completed. The article also reviews recent data suggesting increased overall mortality with Cefepime (Maxipime) use compared with other beta-lactam antibiotics and the potential risk for neurotoxicity in the setting of renal failure.

Jerry M. Zuckerman, Fozia Qamar, and Bartholomew R. Bono

The advanced macrolides, azithromycin and clarithromycin, and the ketolide, telithromycin, are structural analogs of erythromycin. They have several distinct advantages when compared with erythromycin, including enhanced spectrum of activity, more favorable pharmacokinetics and pharmacodynamics, once-daily administration, and improved tolerability. Clarithromycin and azithromycin are used extensively for the treatment of respiratory tract infections, sexually transmitted diseases, and *Helicobacter pylori*–associated peptic ulcer disease. Telithromycin is approved for the treatment of community-acquired pneumonia. Severe hepatotoxicity has been reported with the use of telithromycin.

VISIT THE CLINICS ONLINE!

Access your subscription at:
www.theclinics.com

Preface

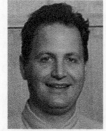 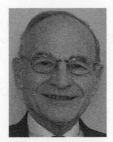

Keith S. Kaye, MD, MPH   Donald Kaye, MD
Guest Editors

The discipline of infectious diseases is one of the most rapidly changing fields in medicine. In most specialties of medicine, diseases remain relatively stable, and diagnostic and therapeutic approaches change slowly. In infectious diseases, the syndromes change with the emergence of new organisms, development of resistant pathogens, and resurgence of infections that have virtually disappeared. Clearly, the diagnostic and therapeutic approaches must change rapidly. In no area of medicine does the knowledge and art of clinical practice change as rapidly as in the use of antimicrobial agents.

In this issue of *Infectious Disease Clinics of North America*, we deal with antibacterial agents and their use, with concentration on newer agents and recent changes in the use of some older antibacterial agents. Pneumococci, enterococci, and gram-negative bacilli have continued to become increasingly resistant to existing antimicrobial agents, and in addition, community-acquired methicillin-resistant *Staphylococcus aureus* has spread dramatically. Criteria for susceptibility of pneumococci and enterococci to various antibacterial agents have changed. New β-lactam, antistaphylococcal, and glycylcycline antibiotics have been developed or are in development.

This issue reviews various aspects of in vitro testing of antibacterial agents, their pharmacodynamics and pharmacokinetics, and their clinical use and management. Problems with resistant bacteria as well as specific use of antibacterial agents in pediatrics, the elderly, and renal insufficiency are covered. The current status of important older antibiotics is summarized. Newer antibiotics are described, as well as the use of topical agents.

In choosing authors to address the different topics, an effort was made to select individuals who are experts in the areas assigned. The end result of their efforts is

Infect Dis Clin N Am 23 (2009) xiii–xiv
doi:10.1016/j.idc.2009.08.001
0891-5520/09/$ – see front matter   **id.theclinics.com**

a state-of-the-art review on the subject of the use of antibacterial agents and their interactions with bacteria.

Keith S. Kaye, MD, MPH
University Health Center
4201 Saint Antoine Boulevard, Suite 2B, Box 331
Detroit, MI 48201, USA

Donald Kaye, MD
Department of Medicine
Drexel University
College of Medicine
Philadelphia, PA
1535 Sweet Briar Road
Gladwyne, PA 19035, USA

E-mail addresses:
KKaye@dmc.org (K.S. Kaye)
donjank@aol.com (D. Kaye)

Antibacterial Susceptibility Testing in the Clinical Laboratory

Thomas L. Holland, MD[a,*], Christopher W. Woods, MD, MPH[b,d],
Maria Joyce, MD, DTM&H[c,d]

KEYWORDS

- Bacteria • Antibiotic • Susceptibility • Resistance
- Gram-negative • Gram-positive

The clinical microbiology laboratory has a mandate to provide reliable, accurate susceptibility data in a time frame that is useful to the clinicians requesting the information to optimize clinical outcomes and, when possible, to reduce the emergence of resistance. This mandate is served by selective reporting of results to the ordering clinician from isolates obtained from individual patients and by providing collective data on local prevalence of resistance to be used for empiric therapy. To meet these challenges and responsibilities, clinical microbiologists must continuously assess and update susceptibility testing and reporting strategies. Although classical methods remain the workhorse of susceptibility testing, molecular methods are on the cusp of challenging their primacy.

INDICATIONS FOR SUSCEPTIBILITY TESTING

Routine susceptibility testing should be reserved for clinically significant isolates retrieved from appropriately collected specimens that have a well-described capacity for resistance to primary therapeutic agents and for which standardized performance methodology and interpretive criteria are available. Testing is not routinely indicated for organisms with predictable responses to antimicrobial agents. Patient allergy, intolerance, or epidemiologic studies are alternative reasons, however, for susceptibility testing for these organisms. Susceptibility testing of isolates known or believed to be contaminants is actively discouraged, because provision of results may

[a] Infectious Diseases, Duke University Medical Center, Durham, NC 27710, USA
[b] Infectious Diseases, Service 113, Durham VAMC, Durham, NC 27710, USA
[c] Clinical Microbiology, Service 113, Durham VAMC, Durham, NC 27710, USA
[d] Department of Medicine and Pathology, Duke University Medical Center, Durham, NC 27710, USA
* Corresponding author.
E-mail address: thomas.holland@duke.edu (T.L. Holland).

Infect Dis Clin N Am 23 (2009) 757–790
doi:10.1016/j.idc.2009.06.001
0891-5520/09/$ – see front matter © 2009 Elsevier Inc. All rights reserved.

encourage inappropriate antibiotic use.[1] Special consideration should also be given to isolates retrieved from patients with bacterial meningitis, infective endocarditis, osteomyelitis, infections of the eye or other protected sites, and isolates with normally predictable susceptibility collected from patients with compromised immune systems.

METHODS: PHENOTYPIC (CONVENTIONAL)

Conventional inhibitory methods rely on the detection of in vitro phenotypic expression of resistance. The mean inhibitory concentration (MIC) is defined as the lowest concentration of an antimicrobial agent that inhibits the growth of an organism over a defined interval and is typically expressed in microgram per milliliter. Measuring the MIC involves exposing the organism to a series of twofold dilutions of the antimicrobial agent in a suitable culture media (broth or agar). This phenotypic resistance can be quantitatively reported as the MIC for dilution methods or qualitatively (sensitive, intermediate, resistant) as provided by either dilution or diffusion methods. These qualitative interpretations are based on MIC distributions, pharmacokinetics and pharmacodynamics, and clinical and bacteriologic response rates.[2]

Regardless of the organism-antimicrobial combination and the method used, the results of in vitro diagnostic tests can vary dramatically depending on the type of growth media used (nutritional supplements, cation content, pH); the amount of organism tested (inoculum effect); and the conditions of incubation (duration, temperature, atmosphere). For each test run, controls for viability (growth control), purity (purity plate), and methodology (quality control organisms) should be performed in parallel with the test organism. The Clinical and Laboratory Standards Institute (CLSI) provides standards for these performance variables, for quality control practices, and for the interpretation of the results of reference methods for antibacterial susceptibility testing. The organization publishes consensus standards for the reference methods of antibacterial susceptibility testing. The M2 standard covers disk diffusion, the M7 standard includes minimal inhibitory concentration techniques, and the M11 standard is for anaerobic methods. These standards are published every 3 years and supplemental tables (M100) are updated annually. A guideline for the analysis and presentation of cumulative susceptibility test data (M-39-A) is also available, as is a guideline for testing of infrequently isolated or fastidious bacteria (M45-A). Although these guidelines are available globally, different methods and interpretive criteria may be used outside of North America.[3]

Broth Dilution

For all broth methods, cation-adjusted Mueller-Hinton broth (CAMHB) is recommended for the routine testing of commonly encountered nonfastidious organisms. Cation adjustment (calcium and magnesium) is required to ensure acceptable results when aminoglycosides are tested against *Pseudomonas* isolates (and when tetracycline is tested against other bacteria).[4,5] Insufficient cation concentrations result in increased aminoglycoside activity and vice versa.[6] A standardized inoculum may be prepared by growing organisms to log phase (exponential growth) or by direct suspension of organisms to the turbidity of the 0.5 McFarland standard. Direct suspension is preferred for fastidious organisms (eg, *Haemophilus influenzae*, *Streptococcus pneumoniae*, *Neisseria meningitidis*) and for detection of methicillin resistance in staphylococci. In broth macrodilution, 13 mm × 100 mm tubes are inoculated with a minimum volume of 1 mL (usually 2 mL) and are evaluated macroscopically for growth. Microdilution methods typically use 96-well trays containing 0.1 mL of broth and viewing devices may be used for reading and recording. For either method, the inoculum should be adjusted to achieve a concentration of approximately 5×10^5 CFU/mL. Incubation is typically in air at 35°C for 16 to 20 hours and increased CO_2 is not required. Detection of low-level or inducible resistance in certain organisms requires longer incubation times, however, and additional supplementation (see later). Growth is best determined by comparison with that in the growth control well and is generally indicated by turbidity throughout the well or by buttons in the well bottom. To ensure that the method is testing a single organism, a purity plate should also be planted. Trailing end points may be seen when bacteriostatic antibiotics are tested, and the concentration at which 80% of growth is inhibited compared with the growth control is recorded as the MIC.[7]

Agar Dilution

Agar dilution is a well-established technique for obtaining quantitative susceptibility results and is the reference method commonly performed in Europe.[8] Mueller-Hinton agar (MHA) is the recommended medium for the testing of most commonly encountered aerobic and facultative anaerobic bacteria and is standardized such that calcium and magnesium supplementation is not indicated.[9] For predictable diffusion, the depth of the agar should be between 3 and 4 mm. The recommended final inoculum is 10^4 CFU per spot. The method is labor-intensive and costly, but is recommended for fastidious organisms that do not grow well in broth media (*Neisseria gonorrhoeae*, anaerobes).[10,11]

Disk Diffusion

The disk diffusion method has been standardized for the testing of common, rapidly growing organisms and allows for a qualitative categorization of isolates as susceptible, intermediate, or resistant.[12] An antibiotic-impregnated filter paper disk is placed on the surface of an agar plate (MHA) inoculated with a "lawn" of organism at a known turbidity (0.5 McFarland). The inoculum may be prepared by either log phase growth or direct suspension from colonies on the agar plate. As with dilution methods, direct suspension is preferred for fastidious organisms and for detection of methicillin resistance in staphylococci. The antibiotic diffuses through the agar almost instantaneously after placement on the agar and creates a zone of inhibition that can be measured in millimeters (edge to edge, including the disk).[13] Interpretation of the test is based on the inverse correlation of the zone diameter with MIC for each combination of antimicrobial and organism.[7]

Because interpretation is dependant on the rate of antibiotic diffusion versus bacterial growth, this method should not be used to evaluate the antimicrobial susceptibilities of bacteria that show marked variability in growth rates (eg, some glucose nonfermenting gram-negative bacilli and anaerobic bacteria). It has been modified for some fastidious organisms, however, when special media and interpretive breakpoints are used.[7,13]

SCREENING AND BREAKPOINT METHODS

In some instances, testing of a single drug concentration may be the most reliable and convenient method for the detection of resistance (eg, screen for high level aminoglycoside resistance in enterococci). In addition to single concentration screens, breakpoint susceptibility testing of antimicrobial agents only at the specific concentrations necessary for differentiating between the interpretive categories rather than the full range is often used. In particular, commercial methods with limited room on their panels frequently use breakpoint testing to permit a greater number of agents to be tested.[14]

AUTOMATED, SHORT INCUBATION, AND RAPID METHODS

Commercial microdilution accounts for two thirds of susceptibility testing in the United States.[15] When commercial systems are used, the manufacturer's recommendations concerning storage, inoculation, incubation, and interpretations should be followed precisely. An error rate for these systems has to be determined by comparison with the reference CLSI broth dilution method using at least 100 clinical isolates of a single genus or species. The detection rate for very major errors (false susceptibility) should be less than 1.5% and major errors (false resistance) less than 3% of isolates.[16] At present, there are at least five automated broth dilution antimicrobial susceptibility testing systems currently approved for use in the United States including the Vitek and Vitek 2 (bioMerieux, St. Louis, Missouri); the Microscan WalkAway and Microscan Walkaway Plus (Siemens Healthcare Diagnostics, Deerfield, Illinois); the Sensititre ARIS (Trek Diagnostic Systems, Westlake, Ohio); and the BD Phoenix (BD Diagnostic Systems, Sparks, Maryland). These systems vary in the extent of automation; the method of detection (turbidity, fluorometric); the speed of detection; data management; and interpretation packages to help verify reporting of results and provision of antibiograms.[15] The flexibility of commercially prepared broth microdilution trays is limited compared with in-house preparations. Special instrumentation is also available for reading, storing, and interpreting zone diameters from disk diffusion tests and this may reduce interobserver variability.[17–19]

In addition to labor savings resulting from decreased media preparation time and automated identification and susceptibility, most systems reduce the time to reporting. Several studies have addressed the clinical and economic benefits derived from the use of rapid susceptibility testing and reporting,[20–22] although others have failed to demonstrate improved outcomes with rapid results.[23] In addition, shortcomings of rapid methods include difficulty in detecting some inducible or subtle resistance mechanisms.[24–26]

One of the simplest and fastest susceptibility tests uses a chromogenic cephalosporin (nitrocefin) that changes color when hydrolyzed by β-lactamase. The test does not detect resistance to β-lactams from other mechanisms, but has been useful in evaluating *H influenzae*, *N gonorrhoeae*, *Moraxella catarrhalis*, enterococci, and some anaerobes.[4]

Conventional methods have also been adjusted to achieve more rapid reporting of results, including direct inoculation of positive blood cultures onto disk diffusion plates[27,28] or microdilution panels.[29] These methods need to be standardized and validated, however, with the emerging resistant organisms and fastidious organisms.

Other phenotypic methods for determining resistance primarily used for infection control purposes are selective agar plates with antibiotic (eg, oxacillin or cefoxitin for methicillin-resistant *Staphylococcus aureus* [MRSA] resistance determination, and vancomycin for resistance in staphylococci and enterococci).[30] The addition of chromogenic substances to the agar aids in the visual diagnosis of certain antibiotic-resistant bacteria and commercial versions are available for a number of resistant pathogens including MRSA, vancomycin-resistant enterococci, and extended-spectrum β-lactamases (ESBL).

NONREFERENCE QUANTITATIVE METHODS

The epsilometer test (E test, bioMerieux, Durham, North Carolina) uses a plastic-coated strip that releases an antimicrobial gradient into agar media. The MIC is read where the ellipse of growth inhibition intercepts the scale on the strip. Strips containing different antimicrobials can be placed in a radial fashion on the surface of a large MHA plate. The method is comparable with reference dilution methods for staphylococci, enterococci, anaerobes, and various gram-negative organisms.[31–33] Although very simple to perform and flexible, this method is relatively expensive. It is most commonly used for infrequent drug requests or for fastidious or anaerobic organisms because the strip may be placed onto enriched media to enhance growth. Strips may also be supplemented for detection of certain resistance mechanisms (ethylenediaminetetraacetic acid for metallo-β-lactamase)[34] or for effective use with certain agents (calcium for daptomycin).[35]

The spiral gradient end point method (Spiral Systems Instruments, Bethesda, Maryland; Spiral Biotech, Norwood, Massachusetts) uses increasing concentrations of an antibiotic in a radial fashion from the center of an agar plate.[36] The organism is streaked from the center and the end point is measured as the distance of growth to the center of the plate. This method is expensive, inefficient, and not widely used, but has been valuable in detecting heteroresistance to vancomycin in S aureus in population studies.[37]

METHOD SELECTION

The choice of methodology to be used in individual laboratories is usually based on financial and labor resources and the volume of tests to be performed. Variables to be considered include relative ease of performance, cost of equipment and contract arrangements, cost of media and supplemental materials, flexibility in selection of drugs for testing, use of automated or semiautomated devices to facilitate testing, and the perceived accuracy of the methodology.[4] The traditional macrodilution procedure is laborious and rarely performed in modern clinical microbiology laboratories, whereas some version of microdilution (particularly commercial methodology) is now standard in virtually all clinical laboratories. Despite the popularity of commercial microdilution systems, the disk method is flexible, technically simple, inexpensive, and its results are reproducible. In general, clinicians prefer categorical or qualitative results in most situations. The rising incidence of "MIC creep" in some organisms, such as S aureus with vancomycin, has renewed interest in the specific MIC value for an isolate. In situations where MICs are used clinically (eg, endocarditis and meningitis),[38] alternative methods that provide an MIC are available when quantitative results are indicated.

SELECTION OF AGENTS FOR ROUTINE TESTING AND REPORTING

The battery of agents to be tested depends on the species, the formulary, and demography of patients in the institution, and the likelihood of encountering highly resistant organisms.[39] Many compounds exhibit similar if not identical activities in vitro to other agents in their same class, so that in some cases, one compound may be chosen as a surrogate for an antimicrobial class because of a greater ability to detect resistance.

To discourage the indiscriminate use of broad-spectrum antimicrobials, the laboratory should establish a reporting cascade in which a few, narrow-spectrum, less-expensive antimicrobials are reported whereas other results are suppressed and released as needed. A restricted reporting policy can have a strong influence on prescribing patterns and ultimately on resistance.[40] Decisions regarding testing and reporting algorithms should be made in consultation with local infectious disease practitioners; pharmacists; and relevant committees (pharmacy and therapeutics, infection control).

BACTERICIDAL METHODS AND COMBINATION THERAPY

The methods described previously are measures of the inhibitory capacity of an anti-bacterial. In the absence of a robust immune system or when infection occurs in relatively protected sites, however, cure often depends on the killing capacity of a drug. Although most experts agree that every new drug should undergo testing to determine its bactericidal capacity, the benefit of testing isolates from individual patients with meningitis, endocarditis, or osteomyelitis remains controversial.[41]

Bactericidal activity can be measured by one of three methods: (1) calculation of the minimum bactericidal concentration; (2) performance of time-kill studies; or (3) serum bactericidal assay (Schlichter test). The minimum bactericidal concentration is obtained by subculturing the tubes (macrodilution) or wells (microdilution) that do not demonstrate growth at 24 hours and is defined as the lowest concentration of antibiotic at which a 99.9% reduction of viable organisms occurs.[42] A bactericidal drug achieves this within two dilutions of the MIC. A number of biologic and technical issues limit the clinical value of this information. Time-kill bactericidal tests plot the proportion of bacteria killed over time when exposed to a specific concentration of antimicrobial. The concentrations chosen for testing are based on achievable serum levels. The serum bactericidal test is a modified broth dilution test, in which serial dilutions of serum are tested rather than specific antimicrobial concentrations.[43] A correlation between specific bactericidal titers and outcome of antimicrobial therapy has been difficult to establish.

Synergy is usually defined by a 2 $\log_{10}$ drop (or greater) in CFU/mL between the combination of each of two antimicrobials (at one fourth of their respective minimum bactericidal concentration) compared with the more active drug alone at a concentration of one half its minimum bactericidal concentration.[44] The effects of these drug combinations may be additive, synergistic, or antagonistic. The clinical importance of assessing synergy in the treatment of endocarditis is well established, but is controversial for other infections. The test most frequently used is the two-dimensional checkerboard titration, which involves testing serial twofold dilutions of two agents, alone and in combination. Multiple combination bactericidal antibiotic testing can also be used to test targeted antibiotic combinations.[45] A randomized trial of synergy testing for multiresistant gram-negative rod infections in cystic fibrosis patients, however, did not demonstrate improved outcomes when applying the results of multiple combination bactericidal antibiotic testing.[46]

GENOTYPIC METHODS

In addition to rapid phenotypic methods, molecular methods targeting mutations responsible for antimicrobial resistance are increasingly available to the clinical laboratory. The genotypic approach is primarily attractive because these assays may facilitate real-time detection directly from patient specimens before culture results are available, they can arbitrate MIC results at or near breakpoints, they make excellent epidemiologic tools, and they can be used in the evaluation of new susceptibility tests.[47] A great number of different probes and primers have been developed targeting genes associated with resistance to most antimicrobial categories. Newer methods, including real-time polymerase chain reaction (PCR), ligase chain reaction, cleavage-based assays, and DNA sequence analysis, are often more rapid and more flexible.

Development of molecular assays has focused on resistance mechanisms in common organisms that are limited to a few, well-characterized genetic mechanisms (eg, *mecA* in MRSA; *vanA* in vancomycin-resistant enterococci).[48] Additionally, sequence analysis methodology is useful for point mutations associated with fluoro-quinolone resistance[49] and ESBL in reference laboratories.[50,51] Lack of consensus sequences among acetyltransferases and adenyltransferase genes makes the detection of multiple determinants of aminoglycoside resistance difficult, however, with a single primer set. Although many laboratories use in-house methods, only a few targets (eg, *mecA*, *vanA*) have been made commercially available.[52]

The expectation that molecular techniques would replace phenotypic susceptibility testing has not yet been realized. DNA microarray technology offers some hope for handling the large number of analyses required to pursue multiple resistance mechanisms.[53] Implementation of this technology awaits the successful handling of several technical impediments, and routine susceptibility testing will still need to be performed to look for new mechanisms.

PATHOGEN-SPECIFIC ISSUES
Gram-positive Organisms

Staphylococcus aureus

Among gram-positive pathogens, *S aureus* is the leading cause of morbidity and mortality among nosocomial infections.[54,55] *S aureus* is inherently very susceptible to antibiotics[56] but is also adept at developing resistance. Nearly all clinical isolates of *S aureus* produce a penicillinase[56]; however, if the organism tests susceptible to penicillin, it is the drug of choice. If the penicillin disk zone is greater than or equal to 29 mm or the MIC is between 0.03 and 0.25 μg/mL, then a β-lactamase test performed on growth from the margin around the oxacillin disk (induced β-lactamase test) is indicated.[12] If the isolate is β-lactamase negative and oxacillin susceptible, it can be reported as susceptible to all penicillins, cephalosporins, carbapenems, and monobactams.[12] MRSA is responsible for over 50% of *S aureus* infections, ranging from bacteremias to community-acquired skin and soft tissue infections.[57,58] Methicillin resistance in staphylococci is caused by an altered penicillin binding protein (PBP2a), which has a markedly low affinity for all β-lactam antibiotics, including penicillins, cephalosporins, and carbapenems. PBP2a is encoded by the *mecA* gene, which is carried by a large mobile genetic element designated "staphylococcal cassette chromosome mec" (SCCmec) and integrated into the chromosome of MRSA.[59] This large cassette frequently carries additional genes encoding resistance to aminoglycosides, macrolides, and fluoroquinolones.[60-62] In many cases, however, MRSA isolates are susceptible to clindamycin, trimethoprim-sulfamethoxazole, aminoglycosides, and tetracyclines. This more susceptible phenotype is associated with the smaller SCCmecIV and community-acquired *S aureus*.[63]

Phenotypic detection of methicillin resistance in *S aureus* is not straightforward because not all subpopulations express methicillin resistance. When phenotypic expression of resistance is 1 in 10^4 to 1 in 10^8 of *mecA* positive cells, the isolate is referred to as "heterogeneous" or "heteroresistant" and detection by standard methods is difficult.[13] The expression of heteroresistant populations is enhanced by higher salt concentrations and lower temperatures.[64] For broth dilution reference methods, CAMHB must be supplemented with 2% NaCl and incubation must complete a full 24 hours[10]; this method is cumbersome and rarely used in clinical practice. For routine disk diffusion, MHA is not supplemented with 2% NaCl because it may adversely affect the testing of other antimicrobial agents.[12] This reduces the chance of detecting heteroresistant colonies, however, around the oxacillin disk. The oxacillin-salt agar screen plate has traditionally been a practical and reliable method for MRSA detection in the clinical laboratory. MHA with oxacillin (6 μg/mL) and NaCl (4%) is spot inoculated with a direct growth suspension and incubated at 35°C for a full 24 hours. The oxacillin E test on MHA supplemented with 2% NaCl has also been found to give reliable results.[65]

Commercial panels are constantly being updated and their accuracy has improved with more discriminating tests. Rapid testing with certain commercial panels has achieved a sensitivity for MRSA versus *mecA* PCR of 98% to 100% with a specificity of 100% with results available in 8 hours.[14,66] The oxacillin salt screen plate in the same study by Yamazumi and coworkers[66] for MRSA was compared with PCR with a sensitivity of 98% and specificity of 100%.

The use of a cefoxitin disk (30 µg) for diffusion testing is now well-established as a better indicator of methicillin resistance than oxacillin because of *mecA*-mediated resistance,[67,68] making the salt screen plate unnecessary. In addition, to correlate better with the presence of the *mecA* gene, the zone size is easier to read because of crisper zone margins than with oxacillin (**Fig. 1**). These findings were first incorporated into the CLSI guidelines in 2004.

Other susceptibility testing issues for *S aureus* include small colony variants (<10x the size of the parent colony) or CO_2-dependant isolates. Small colony variants are fastidious organisms that are deficient in electron transport and are auxotrophs for thiamine, hemin, and menadione.[69] The colonies grow to a normal size when these nutrients are replaced. The CO_2-dependent isolates require enhanced CO_2 conditions for growth.

Molecular diagnostics for *S aureus* are now available in real-time to the clinical microbiology laboratory to identify *S aureus* and methicillin resistance.[30,70] Currently available MRSA screening tests include BD GeneOhm MRSA assay (BD Diagnostics-Gene-ohm, San Diego, California) and GeneXpert MRSA assay (Cepheid, Sunnyvale, California). The sensitivity and specificity of the GeneOhm MRSA assay and the GeneXpert are similar for MRSA detection from nasal swabs.[71] The GeneXpert PCR assay is fully automated requiring minimal hands-on time and expertise for operation, making PCR technology available to the small-to-medium sized laboratory. In addition, the GeneXpert has Food and Drug Administration (FDA) approval for distinguishing *S aureus* and MRSA by PCR directly from positive blood cultures showing gram-positive cocci in clusters and direct from wound swabs to determine the

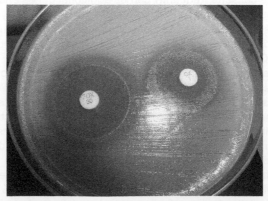

Fig. 1. Disk diffusion testing of a hyper β-lactamase producing *Staphylococcus aureus*. The zone of inhibition (clear halo) around the cefoxitin disk (FOX) is sharp. In contrast, the zone of inhibition around the oxacillin disk (OX) is blurred by the presence of individual colonies.

presence or absence of *S aureus* and MRSA a minimum of 48 hours earlier than with conventional culture and susceptibility. The BD GeneOhm assay is also FDA approved for *S aureus* and methicillin detection from positive blood cultures. For both these assays, subculture of positive blood cultures is necessary for identification of all isolates present and further susceptibility testing. Other commercial companies are in the process of pursuing FDA approval for methods of rapid detection of both methicillin-sensitive *S aureus* and MRSA.

There is growing concern for reduced susceptibility of *S aureus* to vancomycin. Fully vancomycin-resistant *S aureus* (MIC ≥ 16 µg/mL) isolates containing the *vanA* resistance gene from enterococci have been identified in the United States[72] but remain uncommon. Of more widespread concern is "MIC creep" and vancomycin heteroresistance (heteroresistant vancomycin-intermediate *S aureus*), a phenomenon in which groups of *S aureus* isolates seem susceptible to vancomycin by traditional broth dilution techniques but contain subpopulations of cells with higher vancomycin MICs.[73] Although disk diffusion testing seems to be accurate in detection of vancomycin-resistant *S aureus* isolates, detection of vancomycin-intermediate *S aureus* in the clinical laboratory can be difficult with conventional methods. Spiral plating to generate population analysis profiles is considered the gold standard and is used in the research setting,[37] but is impractical in the clinical laboratory because it is labor intensive and expensive (**Fig. 2**). E test screening has been suggested for detection of heteroresistant vancomycin-intermediate *S aureus*,[74] but the sensitivity of this method has been questioned.[75]

Higher vancomycin MICs have been linked to treatment failure.[76] Based on these and other data, the MIC breakpoints for vancomycin were lowered in 2006 to less than or equal to 2 µg/mL for "susceptible," 4 to 8 µg/mL for "intermediate," and greater than or equal to 16 µg/mL for "resistant." New CLSI guidelines are expected

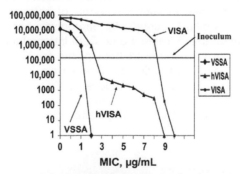

Fig. 2. Population analysis of a *Staphylococcus aureus* isolate. The horizontal line at 100,000 colony-forming units represents the limit of detection of the standard broth microdilution MIC reference method. The curve on the left side of the figure represents a vancomycin-susceptible organism. The curve on the right represents a vancomycin-intermediate *S aureus* (VISA) strain. The middle curve is a vancomycin-heteroresistant *S aureus* (hVISA) isolate that demonstrates the presence of a subpopulation of cells for which the vancomycin MICs are 3–8 mg/mL. This resistant subpopulation is unlikely to be detected by the broth microdilution reference method, because the number of colony-forming units demonstrating the elevated vancomycin MICs (ie, 3–8 mg/mL) are present in ~1 of every 100,000 colony-forming units. VSSA, vancomycin-susceptible *S aureus*. (*From* Tenover FC, Moellering RC. The rationale for revising the clinical and laboratory standards institute vancomycin minimal inhibitory concentration interpretive criteria for *Staphylococcus aureus*. Clin Infect Dis 2007;44:1208–15; with permission.)

to recommend that all staphylococcal isolates be tested for susceptibility to vancomycin by an MIC method.[73] For the clinical laboratory, however, the most appropriate MIC-generating method is under debate. A recent study suggests that E test MICs are consistently onefold or twofold higher than CLSI broth or agar dilution results. The authors recommend that therapeutic guidelines should specify the MIC methods on which the recommendations are based.[73]

Non–cell wall active agents/D test

Most macrolide-lincosamide-streptogramin b resistance in *S aureus* is coded for by *ermA* and *ermC* genes.[77,78] Macrolide-lincosamide-streptogramin b resistance may be inducible (in vitro susceptible to clindamycin) or constitutive (in vitro resistant to all macrolide-lincosamide-streptogramin b).[79] Treatment of inducible macrolide-lincosamide-streptogramin b resistant isolates with clindamycin may lead to clinical failure.[80–83] For isolates that are erythromycin resistant and clindamycin susceptible, the D test or D diffusion zone test can be used to detect the presence of the inducible phenotype. An erythromycin disk (15 µg) is placed between 15 and 26 mm away from a clindamycin disk (2 µg) and observed for blunting or formation of a D-shape around the clindamycin zone resulting from induced resistance (**Fig. 3**). The streptogramin combination quinupristin-dalfopristin is bactericidal for *S aureus*, but becomes bacteriostatic for those with constitutive expression of macrolide-lincosamide-streptogramin b. Clinical data suggest, however, that it does not impair the clinical efficacy so long as an adequate dose is given.[84]

Other drugs reported selectively

Resistance to linezolid, the first oxazolidinone, is rare but has been documented.[85–87] Accurate susceptibility testing requires an experienced technologist because interpreting results can be difficult because the drug is bacteriostatic; however, there are now approved CLSI interpretative criteria for linezolid.[7] For daptomycin, MIC testing requires supplementation with 50 µg/mL of calcium to cation adjusted MHB[13]; there are no disk diffusion criteria for daptomycin because they have been demonstrated to be unreliable.[88] There are no CLSI interpretative criteria for tigecycline; however, there are FDA-approved breakpoints for MIC results.[89] Trimethoprim-sulfamethoxazole is an alternative to vancomycin in uncomplicated MRSA infections.[90–93] Susceptibility testing can be done by MIC or disk diffusion. All seven vancomycin-resistant *S aureus* isolates reported in the United States from 2002 to 2006 were susceptible to trimethoprim-sulfamethoxazole.[94] Novel anti-MRSA

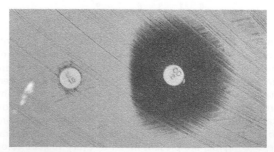

Fig. 3. Disk diffusion "D test" to detect the presence of the macrolide lincosamide streptogramin b (MLSb) phenotype with inducible clindamycin resistance in a *Staphylococcus aureus* isolate that was found to be resistant to erythromycin and sensitive to clindamycin on routine susceptibility testing.

cephalosporins are in development (eg, ceftibiprole); these agents inhibit the PBP2a in staphylococci and early clinical data suggest that these agents are effective against MRSA,[95] but guidelines are not yet available.

Several agents are used in various combinations to achieve synergy with cell wall active agents or other bactericidal agents. Aminoglycosides are widely used in prosthetic valve endocarditis.[96-99] In these situations, high-level aminoglycoside resistance implies that synergy is not achieved. As with aminoglycosides, fluoroquinolone resistance is more common in MRSA than methicillin-sensitive S aureus and resistance develops quickly. Rifampin should not routinely be reported on S aureus isolates because resistance develops quickly when used as monotherapy.[100,101]

Coagulase-negative staphylococci

The mechanisms of resistance in coagulase-negative staphylococci are the same as those of S aureus; however, resistance is usually expressed at a lower level. To enhance detection of methicillin-resistant strains, the MIC breakpoint with oxacillin for coagulase-negative staphylococci except S lugdunensis is less than or equal to 0.25 µg/mL instead of less than or equal to 2 µg/mL, three dilutions lower than that for S aureus. For disk diffusion, the susceptible breakpoint is greater than or equal to 18 mm instead of greater than or equal to 13 mm with oxacillin, and greater than 25 mm instead of greater than 22 mm with cefoxitin.[7] S lugdunensis mecA mediated resistance is more accurately detected with cefoxitin disk diffusion and interpretative breakpoint criteria are the same as for S aureus. Cefoxitin disk testing has been shown to have higher specificity than oxacillin.[102] The oxacillin result should be reported as susceptible or resistant based on cefoxitin result because cefoxitin is a surrogate for oxacillin. Most S lugdunensis are β-lactamase negative and oxacillin susceptible.[7] For more serious infections with coagulase-negative staphylococci other than S epidermidis, CLSI recommends testing for the mecA gene or the gene product PBP2a, when results are in the intermediate or resistant category.[7] Vancomycin resistance has been recognized and described in coagulase-negative staphylococci.[103] Linezolid and daptomycin resistance among coagulase-negative staphylococci are rare.[104]

Enterococcus spp

Enterococcus spp are part of the normal gastrointestinal flora; however, they are an increasingly important cause of invasive disease including bacteremia, meningitis, and endocarditis. Resistance in enterococci has evolved over the past 30 years to become the prototype of multiresistant bacteria, carrying with it an independent risk of mortality.[105] Enterococci are intrinsically resistant to a large number of antibiotics including carboxypenicillins, cephalosporins, trimethoprim-sulfamethoxazole, and clindamycin.[106] These agents can seem active in vitro, but do not work in clinical situations. Ampicillin is the drug of choice for susceptible enterococcal infections. Reduced affinity for penicillin-binding proteins (PBP) mediates resistance to penicillin, ampicillin, and other β-lactams used in therapy including the ureidopenicillins and imipenem. Testing for PBP-mediated resistance can be done by either broth dilution or disk diffusion. Another mechanism of resistance to penicillin in Enterococcus faecalis is β-lactamase production; this is much less common and the need for routine testing is questionable.[107,108] CLSI recommends routinely testing sterile site isolates. A positive β-lactamase test implies resistance to penicillin and ureidopenicillins, but susceptibility to imipenem and β-lactam–β-lactamase inhibitor combinations.[109] At present there are no CLSI criteria for testing susceptibility to imipenem; however, studies have supported the notion that ampicillin or penicillin may be used to predict susceptibility to imipenem,[109,110] although this practice has been questioned, especially for Enterococcus faecium.[111]

Vancomycin resistance was first reported in Europe in 1988[112] and since that time has spread worldwide. The gene clusters responsible for high-level vancomycin resistance in E faecium and E faecalis are predominantly vanA and vanB. Other genes associated with vancomycin resistance include vanD; moderate level (MIC 16–256 μg/mL) vanC; vanE; and vanG (intrinsic, low-level).[113–116] The vanA and vanB phenotypes are highly transmissible, but vanC, found predominantly in Enterococcus gallinarum, Enterococcus flavescens, or Enterococcus casseliflavus, is intrinsic and low level (MIC 8–16 μg/mL) and does not seem to carry an infection control risk.[117]

Most laboratories readily detect high-level vancomycin resistance. Surveys have shown that reporting laboratories that purportedly followed CLSI guidelines were, in practice, noncompliant.[118,119] The main area of difficulty was with isolates that were intermediately resistant to vancomycin (MIC 8–16, vanC phenotype).[119] CLSI recommends testing by MIC and further speciation of the isolate with a pigment and motility test to look for the vanC phenotype. Other problem areas noted in these studies were with failure to use the correct medium (MHA or CAMHB) and failure to incubate for a complete 24 hours.[118] A comparison of agar dilution, broth microdilution, E test, disk diffusion, and automated Vitek Methods for Enterococcus spp to vancomycin with the vancomycin resistance genotype found major errors primarily with the commercial method (Vitek) and with disk diffusion. BHI medium performed better than Mueller-Hinton.[120]

Aminoglycosides are not clinically active for enterococci except when used in conjunction with an active cell-wall agent (eg, ampicillin or vancomycin). For serious infections, particularly endocarditis, achieving a bactericidal effect is essential. Synergy between aminoglycosides and a cell-wall agent is predicted by using a high-level aminoglycoside screening test. For E faecium and E faecalis, resistance to gentamicin and streptomycin can be tested by using high concentrations in a brain-heart infusion broth or agar for 24 hours. Any growth in broth is considered resistant. Streptomycin should be incubated 48 hours if susceptible at 24 hours. A comparison was made of three CLSI-approved screening methods for high-level aminoglycoside resistance: (1) Microscan broth microdilution, (2) synergy quad plate agar dilution, and (3) disk diffusion. Screening methods showed an agreement of 99% for all three methods for high-level gentamicin and 96% for high-level streptomycin.[121]

For clinically significant isolates that are ampicillin and vancomycin resistant, additional testing is required. Linezolid is bacteriostatic for both E faecalis and E faecium. Resistance has been described but is rare.[104] Quinupristin-dalfopristin is bactericidal (erm gene negative), but testing and reporting is recommended for E faecium only (less than 2% of E faecalis are susceptible). Daptomycin seems to be equally effective against vancomycin-resistant enterococci and vancomycin-susceptible enterococci; however, these data were interpreted with a tentative MIC of less than or equal to 2 μg/mL considered to be susceptible. CLSI has since established an MIC of less than or equal to 1 as susceptible. There are no resistant criteria established.[122,123] Other drugs that should be tested and are effective for all enterococci if susceptible are tetracycline and rifampin. Tigecycline is another agent that seems to have activity against enterococci; CLSI breakpoints are not established.

Streptococcus pneumoniae

Streptococcus pneumoniae is the leading bacterial cause of community-acquired pneumonia and bacterial meningitis.[124] Subsequently, the emergence of penicillin resistance in the pneumococcus has become a worldwide problem.[125–128] After introduction of the seven-valent pneumococcal vaccine in 2000, there was an initial decrease in rates of nonsusceptibility.[129] There have since been shifts, however, in the dominant serotypes; serotype 19A, which has higher rates of antibiotic resistance, is now the most prevalent cause of invasive pneumococcal disease in the United States.[130,131] Resistance results from complex alterations in PBPs caused by formation of mosaic genes that affect binding affinity for all β-lactam antibiotics.[132] The extended-spectrum cephalosporins and carbapenems retain more activity than penicillin.[133] To complicate therapeutic issues further, isolates have often acquired the transposon Tn1546 that possesses ermB, tetM, and aphA3 resulting in resistance to macrolides, tetracyclines, and aminoglycosides.[134] Other therapeutic options for multidrug-resistant isolates include the newer fluoroquinolones (levofloxacin, moxifloxacin, gemifloxacin) and vancomycin. Resistance has begun to emerge among the fluoroquinolones, with ciprofloxacin retaining less activity than levofloxacin or moxifloxacin.[128] Of particular concern is a small population of highly resistant clones that dominate multidrug-resistant S pneumoniae (eg, Spain 23F), which has disseminated to many parts of the world.[135–137] Resistance to trimethoprim-sulfamethoxazole and macrolides is also increasing, particularly among penicillin-resistant isolates.[132]

Accurate susceptibility testing of S pneumoniae requires special conditions. MHB or MHA is supplemented with 5% sheep blood (SBMHA) and incubated at 35°C for 20 to 24 hours in ambient air for broth dilution or 5% CO_2 for agar dilution. Broth or agar dilution may be used to test all antimicrobial agents recommended by CLSI. No reliable interpretative criteria exist, however, for disk diffusion testing of β-lactam antibiotics on SBMHA except for oxacillin.[7] Non–β-lactam antibiotics may be tested by disk diffusion. The E test for penicillin, ceftriaxone, and vancomycin was found to be greater than 98% accurate when compared with CLSI methods on SBMHA, but for other antimicrobials is unreliable.[138] PCR has been evaluated for detection of the mefA and ermB in S pneumoniae and seems reliable.[139] S pneumoniae poses a challenge to commercial methods because of special nutritional and incubation requirements. Commercial microdilution methods have been studied extensively and most current panels (frozen and dried) were found to be comparable with CLSI reference broth dilution in 2% to 5% lysed horse blood.[13,140]

MIC values are reported based on sources using either meningitis criteria or nonmeningitis criteria. For cerebrospinal fluid (CSF) isolates, only penicillin, ceftriaxone or cefotaxime, meropenem, and vancomycin are reported. The β-lactam antimicrobials are tested by MIC for CSF isolates. Interpretative criteria are different for penicillin, ceftriaxone, and cefotaxime based on source site: a CSF isolate is interpreted as susceptible at a lower dilution range that those from non-CSF site. Vancomycin may be tested by either MIC (broth, agar, or E test) or disk diffusion. Laboratories may choose to report only the MIC values or the MIC values with interpretations specific to the source of the isolate.

For non-CSF source sites, β-lactams are reported, and macrolides and fluoroquinolones. Disk diffusion using a 1-μg oxacillin disk has been advocated as a screen for penicillin susceptibility in pneumococci recovered from nonsterile sites, such as the respiratory tract. A zone diameter of greater than or equal to 20 mm is considered susceptible to all β-lactam antibiotics including cephalosporins and carbapenems and no further testing is required. Isolates with a zone diameter of less than or equal to 19 mm to oxacillin do not reliably predict resistance to penicillin. For these isolates, MICs should be used to determine susceptibility to penicillin, ceftriaxone or cefotaxime, and meropenem when clinically indicated.[7] The laboratory should bypass the oxacillin screen test on CSF isolates and an MIC determination should be made available for penicillin, ceftriaxone or cefotaxime, and meropenem on these isolates.

Vancomycin susceptibility may be determined by MIC or disk diffusion. Although isolates recovered from CSF should receive an MIC test, a survey by the Centers for Disease Control and Prevention showed that 53% of laboratories performed the oxacillin-screening test inappropriately on isolates from sterile sites, delaying MIC results by greater than 24 hours.[125]

Viridans group and other streptococci

Viridans group streptococci refer to a group of streptococcal species that are part of the normal flora in healthy humans: they are found on the mucosa, gastrointestinal tract, and upper respiratory tract and as transient commensals of skin. Viridans streptococci are divided into small colony β-hemolytic strains with A, C, F, and G antigens and viridans groups. Viridans species are frequent contaminants and only clinically significant isolates from a normally sterile site should be routinely tested for susceptibility.

When performing susceptibility testing for viridans group streptococci, either disk diffusion or MIC methods may be used for non–β-lactams. As with S pneumoniae, viridans group streptococci require SBMHA, direct colony inoculum preparation, and incubation in 5% CO_2 for 20 to 24 hours. Penicillin, ampicillin, and oxacillin disk diffusion testing is considered unreliable and testing should be performed by an MIC method. For broth dilution, the CAMHB must be supplemented with lysed horse blood (2%–5%). SBMHA is used for agar dilution and disk diffusion. The sheep blood should be replaced with lysed horse blood when testing a sulfonamide.[7] The E test for β-lactam testing is convenient and reliable when compared with the reference agar dilution method, which can be time consuming and cumbersome.[141]

For nutritionally deficient streptococci (Abiotrophia defectiva or adaciens) susceptibility testing requires SBMHA supplemented with pyridoxine (Vit B6) or cysteine. E test is comparable with the agar dilution reference method.[142]

Other than the small colony variants, β-hemolytic streptococci (Groups A, B, C, and G) should be considered separately from viridans group streptococci. Penicillin is considered uniformly active against Streptococcus pyogenes (Group A) and Streptococcus agalactiae (Group B) and no susceptibility testing to penicillin is recommended. For the penicillin allergic patient, testing is recommended for the non–β-lactam antibiotics. As in S aureus, inducible resistance to clindamycin is found in β-hemolytic streptococci; the erythromycin-clindamycin D test has been found to be accurate in identifying this inducible resistance.[143]

Other fastidious organisms

Clinically important drug resistance has been described in a number of fastidious organisms, prompting new CLSI guidelines for testing these organisms.[144] For all of the organisms covered in this guideline, MIC testing is recommended by MHB or CAMHB supplemented with 2.5% to 5% lysed horse blood. Listeria monocytogenes is an opportunistic pathogen that is empirically treated with ampicillin and gentamicin. Listeria spp have remained stable in susceptibility to antimicrobials over the past 50 years and most drugs remain active.[145] Susceptibility to ampicillin may be determined by MIC in broth microdilution, CAMHB with lysed horse blood (2%–5%) at 35°C for 16 to 20 hours.[144] Aminoglycosides may be added for synergy.[146] Cephems may test susceptible, but are not effective clinically.[144] Corynebacterium spp are frequent laboratory contaminants; however, multidrug resistance has been described in Corynebacterium jeikeium and Corynebacterium urealyticum.[147] Vancomycin is traditionally the drug of choice for serious C jeikeium infections.[148] Like corynebacterium, Bacillus spp (not anthracis) are frequent environmental contaminants, but do manifest clinically important resistance. *Bacillus cereus* produces a broad-spectrum β-lactamase and is frequently resistant to penicillin, ampicillin, and cephalosporins. It is also frequently resistant to trimethoprim-sulfamethoxazole, but usually susceptible to carbapenems, clindamycin, gentamicin, chloramphenicol, and vancomycin.[149] Other more infrequently encountered gram-positive organisms covered in this recent CLSI guideline include *Abiotrophia* and *Granulicatella* spp, *Erysipelothrix rhusiopathiae*, *Lactobacillus* spp, *Leuconostoc* spp, and *Pediococcus* spp.[147]

Gram-negative Organisms

Enterobacteriaceae

The family Enterobacteriaceae includes many species of aerobic or facultatively anaerobic, gram-negative, non–spore-forming bacilli. Although these organisms are endogenous flora, several cause disease including outpatient urinary tract infections and outbreaks of multidrug-resistant nosocomial infections. Twenty species are responsible for approximately 50% of all organisms isolated in the clinical microbiology laboratory. Resistant phenotypes for most antibiotic classes have been described and are increasingly common. Susceptibility testing should be performed on all clinically significant isolates in this group of organisms. CLSI has specific standards for all Enterobacteriaceae. Either disk diffusion or MIC-obtaining dilution methods may be performed using reference procedures or comparable commercial products.[7,12]

Resistance to β-lactams in Enterobacteriaceae is primarily mediated by an everincreasing number of β-lactamases.[150,151] The presence of Class A (Bush 2b) β-lactamases that confer resistance to penicillin and aminopenicillins is commonly detected among enteric gram-negative bacilli in clinical laboratories. In addition, there is an increasing number of ESBL that confer resistance to penicillins; first-, second-, and third-generation cephalosporins; and aztreonam. ESBL production in Enterobacteriaceae is associated with increased mortality and delay to appropriate therapy,[152] highlighting the need for reliable identification. Detection of these Bush 2be ESBLs, AmpC (Bush 1, chromosomal or plasmid-mediated), metallo-β-lactamases, carbapenemases, and other resistance mechanisms creates a vexing problem for laboratories.

For the most part, ESBLs result from simple-point mutations in the genes generally responsible for ampicillin resistance in *Escherichia coli* (TEM-1, TEM-2); *Klebsiella* spp (SHV-1); and *Proteus mirabilis* (TEM-type). At least 200 different ESBLs have been detected in different species and present with a variety of susceptibility profiles.[151] In vitro results for these isolates often do not follow the standard "hierarchy" rules for cephalosporins. In particular, the cephamycins (cefoxitin and cefotetan) often seem active. Traditional breakpoints of extended-spectrum cephalosporins for Enterobacteriaceae do not reliably detect the presence of these β-lactamases.[25,153] CLSI recommends the use of lower screening breakpoints for certain extended-spectrum cephalosporins or aztreonam for *E coli* and *Klebsiella* spp.[13,151] Even so, lower inoculum size has been shown to cause false-negative ESBL screening results.[154] Confirmation relies on the susceptibility of ESBLs to clavulanic acid (CA). Cefotaxime and ceftazidime are tested with and without CA (4 μg/mL in broth, 10 μg in disk). A decrease of three dilutions or more in the MIC or a 5 mm or greater increase in the zone size with CA compared with the cephalosporin alone is indicative of ESBL production (**Fig. 4**). Automated systems have had variable sensitivity and specificity for detection of ESBL-producing organisms; manual confirmatory testing is recommended for isolates testing positive by automated systems.[155]

Confirmed ESBL producers should be reported as resistant to penicillins (not including β-lactam–β-lactamase inhibitor combinations); cephalosporins (excluding

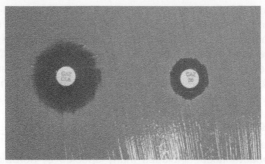

Fig. 4. ESBL confirmation test on *Klebsiella pneumoniae* ATCC strain 700,603, a known ESBL producer (SHV-18). The zone of inhibition surrounding the disk impregnated with both ceftazidime and clavulanic acid is more than 5 mm larger than the zone around ceftazidime alone, demonstrating susceptibility to the β-lactamase inhibitor.

the cephamycins); and aztreonam.[151] Reporting the cephamycins and β-lactam–β-lactamase inhibitor combinations is controversial, because very limited clinical data exist to support their use in these patients.[156] With the paucity of such data, however, some laboratories choose to report these agents as resistant. Although resistance factors for other antibiotic classes are often found in these organisms, the results of in vitro tests should not be altered outside of routine CLSI reporting guidelines. Those isolates that are not confirmed to have ESBLs despite positive screening tests highlight the limitations of phenotypic testing. In addition to an ESBL, this heterogeneous group of organisms may contain alterations in porin production; hyperproduction of CA-susceptible β-lactamase (including ESBLs); production of a class I β-lactamase (AmpC) that is not CA susceptible; or a combination of these resulting in the CA-resistant phenotype.[157] Use of the CLSI criteria for detecting ESBL production among Enterobacteriaceae other than *E coli*, *Klebsiella* spp, and *P mirabilis* as routine practice in the United States is discouraged as a result of poor specificity.[158]

Chromosomally mediated inducible AmpC is present in essentially all *Enterobacter*, *Serratia*, *Providencia*, *Morganella morganii*, *Citrobacter freundii*, *Hafnia alvei*, and *Aeromonas* spp (in addition to *Pseudomonas aeruginosa*). Current CLSI guidelines encourage reporting in vitro susceptibility patterns obtained in routine testing with a comment that these organisms may develop resistance during prolonged treatment with third-generation cephalosporins and that repeat testing may be warranted 3 to 4 days after initiation of therapy. Detection of ESBLs is particularly difficult among species or strains that coproduce an inhibitor-resistant β-lactamase, such as AmpC. For organisms that possess chromosomal AmpC and *E coli* or *Klebsiella* spp that contain plasmid-mediated AmpC, clavulanate may act as an inducer of high-level AmpC expression resulting in a false-negative ESBL test. Methods that use either tazobactam or sulbactam as inhibitors have been considered for these organisms[159]; boronic acid has also been proposed for this purpose.[155] Also, high-level AmpC is much less active on cefepime, so inclusion of cefepime as a screening agent or as part of confirmatory testing coupled with an inhibitor has improved sensitivity for ESBLs, but is not widely accepted as a standard method.[160]

Carbapenem resistance is a growing threat, especially with emergence of plasmid-encoded *Klebsiella pneumoniae* carbapenemases (KPCs) on a global scale.[161] Initially described in *Klebsiella pneumoniae*, they have now been found in a range of Enterobacteriaceae, including *E coli*, *Enterobacter* spp, *Citrobacter* spp, *Salmonella* spp, *Serratia marcescens*, and *P mirabilis*,[162,163] and in *P aeruginosa*. Presence of a carbapenemase is suggested by elevated carbapenem MICs; however, failure of automated systems to detect KPC-producing isolates has been described.[164] Reference broth microdilution, ertapenem disk diffusion, and the modified Hodge test[165] have all been proposed as more sensitive methods to detect KPC-mediated resistance.[166] For the modified Hodge test a 10-μg ertapenem disk is placed in the center of a MHA plate inoculated with a 1:10 dilution of a 0.5 McFarland suspension of E coli ATCC 25,922. The test strain is streaked from the center of the plate to the periphery; a distorted inhibition zone indicates the presence of a carbapenemase (**Fig. 5**).[165]

Klebsiella spp, *Providencia* spp, *Proteus vulgaris*, *C freundii*, *Enterobacter* spp, or *S marcescens* susceptible to ampicillin or first-generation cephalosporins require verification. Enterobacteriaceae may also possess numerous resistance factors for aminoglycosides, fluoroquinolones, tetracyclines, chloramphenicol, and trimethoprim-sulfamethoxazole. Fortunately, the reference methods for susceptibility testing are generally accurate for the detection of these phenotypes. Tigecycline seems to be active against most multidrug-resistant Enterobacteriaceae.[167]

Special consideration should be given to the enteric pathogens *Salmonella* and *Shigella*. For these pathogens, susceptibility results for first- and second-generation cephalosporins and aminoglycosides can be misleading and should not be reported. CLSI guidelines recommend testing nalidixic acid against invasive *Salmonella* isolates, acknowledging evidence that nalidixic acid resistance in *Salmonella* spp is associated with higher ciprofloxacin MICs and possibly an association with worse outcome.[7,168–170]

Non-Enterobacteriaceae

Like the Enterobacteriaceae, most of the fast-growing, nonfermenting, gram-negative bacilli can be tested using the published reference methods or a wide variety of approved commercial methods. In addition to *P aeruginosa*, CLSI provides specific interpretive guidelines for *Stenotrophomonas maltophilia*, *Burkholderia cepacia* genomovars, *Acinetobacter* spp, and other non-Enterobacteriaceae.

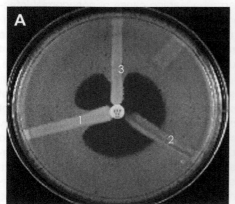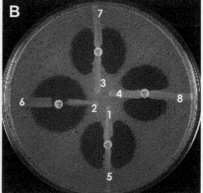

Fig. 5. (*A*) Modified Hodge test. Background is a lawn of a susceptible *Escherichia coli* ATCC 25,922 and an ertapenem disk with streaks of (1) *K pneumoniae* ATCC BAA-1705, positive result; (2) *K pneumonia* ATCC BAA-1706, negative result; and (3) a clinical isolate, positive result. (*B*) The modified Hodge test performed on a large MHA plate showing (1) *K pneumoniae* ATCC BAA-1705, positive result; (2) *K pneumoniae* ATCC BAA-1706, negative result; (3–8) clinical isolates; (6) negative result; and (4, 5, 7, 8) positive result.

Pseudomonas aeruginosa

Pseudomonas aeruginosa is infrequently part of the normal human flora; however, hospitalization may greatly increase rates of colonization. This colonization often precedes nosocomial infection. P aeruginosa possesses a number of resistance mechanisms for all major antibiotic groups requiring that most severe infections have to be treated by more than one effective antibiotic.[171] P aeruginosa isolates are intrinsically resistant to narrow-spectrum penicillins, first- and second-generation cephalosporins, and trimethoprim-sulfamethoxazole. P aeruginosa is usually fast growing, so susceptibility testing may be accomplished by any of the reference methods (agar dilution, broth dilution, or disk diffusion) or approved commercial systems. Because of the large number of inducible resistance characteristics, repeat isolates after 3 or 4 days should be considered for retesting. For multidrug-resistant specimens, colistin and polymyxin B are often considered. For these agents disk diffusion is not recommended and MIC interpretive criteria are not yet available.[172] Recent data on poorer outcomes in bacteremic patients with reduced susceptibility to piperacillin-tazobactam have called into question the CLSI breakpoints.[173]

Isolates of P aeruginosa obtained from patients with cystic fibrosis pose a special problem for susceptibility testing and usually require separate testing protocols. Multiple isolates are often obtained from single specimens, but mixed morphotype susceptibility should be discouraged.[174–176] These isolates often grow slowly, produce a mucoid exopolysaccharide, and are multiply resistant after many years of antibiotic exposure.[177] Commercial microdilution systems have not performed well with these isolates and their use is discouraged in favor of the reference disk diffusion, broth microdilution, or E test.[178,179] Incubation should be increased to 24 hours for the slow-growing isolates, but little is gained from extended incubation to 48 hours.[180] Although not generally available in clinical laboratories, synergy testing may be performed in a reference laboratory on a variety of antimicrobial combinations for particularly resistant isolates. The clinical value of this testing has not been established[46] despite in vitro testing that has identified occasional synergistic and additive effects.[181,182]

Stenotrophomonas maltophilia

Stenotrophomonas maltophilia is emerging as a leading cause of nosocomial infections.[183] The organism is not part of the normal flora and usually affects immunocompromised or debilitated patients.[184] Trimethoprim-sulfamethoxazole remains the treatment of choice despite increasing resistance.[185,186] Treatment is a significant challenge secondary to inherent multidrug resistance that affects many β-lactams, aminoglycosides, and other drug classes through β-lactamase, decreased outer membrane permeability, or multidrug resistance efflux pumps.[187] Notably, most of these isolates produce L1 (a zinc-dependent metallo-β-lactamase that does not respond to CA) or L2 (an extended-spectrum cephalosporinase that is inhibited by CA). Independent studies have demonstrated methodologic problems associated with susceptibility testing of S maltophilia.[188] Disk diffusion particularly was problematic with ciprofloxacin and trimethoprim-sulfamethoxazole. Specific MIC breakpoints and new disk diffusion recommendations were added, however, to the CLSI guidelines.[7] E test has been shown to be comparable with broth microdilution. Many studies have demonstrated in vitro susceptibility of the organism to newer fluoroquinolones, including levofloxacin, gatifloxacin, and moxifloxacin,[189] but few clinical data are available. Testing a newer fluoroquinolone in addition to minocycline should be considered for primary reporting. In vitro evidence of synergy has been demonstrated with certain combinations including ticarcillin-clavulanate with aztreonam.[190] Carbapenem-susceptible isolates should be verified before reporting.

Burkholderia cepacia

Organisms belonging to the *Burkholderia cepacia* complex are problematic for patients with cystic fibrosis and are emerging as a nosocomial problem. The organism is very resistant to many agents commonly used in patients with cystic fibrosis. Commercial identification methods have not performed well with this group of organisms. Broth microdilution or E test are the methods most frequently used, although new breakpoints for disk diffusion have been available since 2004. As with the mucoid *Pseudomonas*, tests for synergy are often performed, but the usefulness of the data is controversial. Although tests of combinations of two and three agents have been performed using different methodologies, consistent in vitro synergy has not been observed and the patient response to therapy when synergy is observed has not been confirmed.[191]

Acinetobacter spp

This genus consists of strictly aerobic, gram-negative coccobacillary rods that can be difficult to decolorize and may be mistaken for gram-positive cocci in blood culture media. *Acinetobacter baumannii* has emerged as an important pathogen, implicated in 7% of ICU-acquired pneumonias in one review.[192] *Acinetobacter* spp can acquire a wide array of resistance mechanisms, including β-lactamases, altered membrane proteins, and multidrug efflux pumps,[193] and resistance to all known antibiotics has been described.[194] CLSI guidelines advocate MIC testing by CAMHB or on agar; disk diffusion can also be done.[195] Discrepancies have been noted, however, between broth microdilution and disk diffusion methods when testing β-lactams; it has been recommended that piperacillin-tazobactam and ticarcillin-clavulanate not be at all tested.[193,196] Although tigecycline is often used for multidrug-resistant *Acinetobacter* infections, there are no CLSI-established breakpoints for susceptibility. There are, however, breakpoints for colistin and polymyxin B.

Fastidious Gram-negative Organisms

Haemophilus influenzae

Globally, 5% to 40% of *H influenzae* isolates produce β-lactamase (plasmid-mediated TEM-1) resulting in resistance to ampicillin and amoxicillin.[197,198] Occasionally, resistant strains do not produce β-lactamase, but have altered PBP. These isolates are referred to as "β-lactamase negative, ampicillin resistant." Resistance to extended-spectrum cephalosporins has not been reported and resistance to new macrolides and fluoroquinolones is rare; any of these phenotypes should be verified. Trimethoprim-sulfamethoxazole testing may be warranted because of resistance rates of 10% to 45%.[199,200] Because resistance is predominantly mediated by a predictable β-lactamase, most facilities continue only to screen. When indicated and requested, broth dilution or disk diffusion can be performed using a hematin, NAD (thymidine phosphorylase-for dilution tests only), and yeast extract supplemented MHB or MHA (*Haemophilus* test medium), inoculated directly from a chocolate plate. Growth on solid media requires 5% CO_2. Agar dilution techniques have not been studied. Alternatively, FDA-approved commercial methods, including E test, are available.

Neisseria spp

Like *H influenzae*, *N gonorrhoeae* can either produce a plasmid-mediated β-lactamase or develop β-lactam resistance by altered PBP encoded on the chromosome. Tetracycline resistance is also common and fluoroquinolone resistance has emerged in the United States[201]; at this point quinolones are no longer recommended for treatment of gonorrhea. Resistance to extended-spectrum cephalosporins has not been reported in the United States and should be confirmed if identified in the laboratory. Agar dilution or disk diffusion on a supplemented GC agar base inoculated from direct growth and incubated in 5% CO_2 for 20 to 24 hours is the reference method.[7,202] When testing carbapenems or clavulanate containing compounds, cysteine should be left out of the GC supplement. E test is the only nonreference method to demonstrate comparable results.[203] With the introduction of molecular diagnostics, however, N gonorrhoeae susceptibility testing is not recommended and not practical, and is usually only performed as part of surveillance programs.

Breakpoints exist for N meningitidis tested by either broth dilution using CAMHB supplemented with 2% to 5% lysed horse blood or agar dilution on MHA with 5% sheep blood incubated in 5% CO_2. E test results with meningococci have demonstrated variable performance to reference methods.[204–206] Fluoroquinolone resistance has been reported in N meningitidis; the use of single-dose ciprofloxacin as chemoprophylaxis has been called into question.[207]

Other testing issues

More than 90% of M catarrhalis produce β-lactamase. Reporting of the presence of β-lactamase may be useful by reinforcing that ampicillin is not appropriate therapy. Sulfonamide and tetracycline resistance has also been reported.[147]

For research purposes, the CLSI has provided reference agar dilution method for testing Helicobacter pylori.[7] In clinical situations, however, an E test on SBMHA incubated in a microaerophilic atmosphere for 3 to 5 days is a simpler approach[208] but may sacrifice accuracy with metronidazole.[209]

The recent CLSI guidelines for testing of fastidious organisms also include breakpoints for clinically important fastidious gram-negatives, including Aeromonas; Plesiomonas; Campylobacter jejuni and Campylobacter coli; HACEK organisms (Haemophilus, Actinobacillus, Cardiobacterium, Eikenella, and Kingella); Pasteurella; and Vibrio spp excluding V cholerae.[147]

Anaerobes

Anaerobes, both strict and aerotolerant, are part of the normal human flora. Over 100 different species have been identified in clinical specimens. Approximately one third of those isolates are of the Bacteroides fragilis group; another third are Peptostreptococcus; and the last third are usually Prevotella, Fusobacterium, or Clostridia spp. Resistance, primarily caused by β-lactamases, is increasing.[210] Although appropriate therapy for anaerobic infections has been associated with significant reductions in mortality,[211] most clinical laboratories still do not perform routine anaerobic susceptibility testing. Reference methods are labor-intensive and interpretation may be complicated. CLSI recommends that isolates obtained from patients with brain abscess, endocarditis, osteomyelitis, joint infection, grafts and prosthetic material, and bacteremia should be considered for testing.[212] Virulent organisms with unpredictable susceptibility include Bacteroides, Prevotella, Fusobacterium, Clostridium, Bilophila, and Sutterella. Agar dilution using Brucella blood agar supplemented with hemin and vitamin K_1 is the reference method. Microdilution (Brucella broth) is now recognized, however, as a reference method for B fragilis.[213] Gradient methods, including both E test[214] and spiral gradient, has been shown to be effective for certain anaerobes. Disk diffusion is not an alternative. Testing for β-lactamase activity is a reasonable approach for non–B fragilis group organisms before susceptibility testing. It may not always predict hydrolysis of imipenem and cephamycins, however, and other mechanisms for β-lactam resistance may be present. For example, reviews of anaerobic susceptibilities have found rates of carbapenem resistance ranging from 1% to 10% among B fragilis.[210,215]

Resistance to metronidazole in *Clostridium difficile* has garnered recent attention,[216] although it has not been established that treatment failure in the epidemic strain NAP1 is related to antibiotic resistance.[217]

Agents Associated with Bioterrorism

Public health authorities should be notified immediately on the preliminary identification of any pathogen potentially related to a deliberate release. The three Centers for Disease Control and Prevention class "A" bacterial agents (*Bacillus anthracis*, *Yersinia pestis*, and *Francisella tularensis*), although infrequent, are endemic to the United States and may be routinely isolated in a clinical laboratory. Biosafety level 2 with biosafety level 3 personnel precautions is appropriate for diagnostic quantities of infectious cultures, but ideally any subsequent confirmation or susceptibility work should take place in an approved reference or public health facility. Despite precautions, recent exposures of laboratory workers to agents associated with biologic terrorism have been documented, including some resulting in clinical disease.[218,219]

CLSI guidelines contain interpretive standards and recommendations for performance variables and quality control organisms for broth microdilution with *B anthracis* and *Y pestis*.[7] A comparison of 50 historical and 15 recent *B anthracis* isolates demonstrated that although the E test was comparable with broth microdilution, the MICs were one to nine dilutions lower and reading the results through biosafety cabinets was difficult.[220] One of these isolates was β-lactamase positive and resistant to penicillin, but resistance to fluoroquinolones, tetracyclines, clindamycin, and vancomycin was not identified. In broth microdilution, *Y pestis* requires 24 hours incubation and potentially 48 hours if growth is inadequate.[7] Although *Y pestis* may seem susceptible to β-lactam agents in vitro, these agents lack efficacy in animal models and should not be reported.[221]

SUMMARY

Despite increasing attention to antimicrobial stewardship and infection control, resistant pathogens have continued to emerge at a pace that outstrips the development of new antibiotics. Now more than ever, clinicians and the clinical microbiology laboratory must work together to detect and report clinically important resistance, and to use that information to improve clinical outcomes and reduce emergence of resistance. Phenotypic susceptibility testing maintains its central role in the laboratory, but as genotypic methods continue to advance, they will increasingly augment and replace traditional methods.

REFERENCES

1. Bates DW, Goldman L, Lee TH. Contaminant blood cultures and resource utilization: the true consequences of false-positive results. JAMA 1991;265:365–9.
2. Ferraro MJ. Should we reevaluate antibiotic breakpoints? Clin Infect Dis 2001; 33(Suppl 3):S227–9.
3. Gould IM, MacKenzie FM, Struelens MJ, et al. Towards a European strategy for controlling antibiotic resistance Nijmegen, Holland August 29–31, 1999. Clin Microbiol Infect 2000;6:670–4.
4. Jorgensen JH, Ferraro MJ. Antimicrobial susceptibility testing: general principles and contemporary practices. Clin Infect Dis 1998;26:973–80.
5. Reller LB, Schoenknecht FD, Kenny MA, et al. Antibiotic susceptibility testing of *Pseudomonas aeruginosa*: selection of a control strain and criteria for magnesium and calcium content in media. J Infect Dis 1974;130:454–63.

6. D'Amato RF, Thornsberry C, Baker CN, et al. Effect of calcium and magnesium ions on the susceptibility of *Pseudomonas* species to tetracycline, gentamicin polymyxin B, and carbenicillin. Antimicrob Agents Chemother 1975;7:596–600.

7. CLSI. Performance standards for antimicrobial susceptibility testing; eighteenth informational supplement. Wayne (PA): CLSI; 2008.

8. European Committee for Antimicrobial Susceptibility Testing (EUCAST) of the European Society of Clinical Microbiology and Infectious Diseases (ESCMID). EUCAST Definitive Document E.DEF 2.1, August 2000: determination of antimicrobial susceptibility test breakpoints. Clin Microbiol Infect 2000;6:570–2.

9. CLSI. Quality control for commercially prepared microbiological culture media. 3rd edition. Wayne (PA): CLSI; 2004.

10. Jorgensen JH, Turnidge JD. Susceptibility test methods: dilution and disk diffusion methods. In: Murray PR, Baron EJ, Jorgensen JH, et al, editors. Manual of clinical microbiology. 9th edition. Washington (DC): American Society for Microbiology; 2007. p. 1152–72.

11. Labbe AC, Bourgault AM, Vincelette J, et al. Trends in antimicrobial resistance among clinical isolates of the *Bacteroides fragilis* group from 1992 to 1997 in Montreal, Canada. Antimicrob Agents Chemother 1999;43:2517–9.

12. Bauer AW, Kirby WM, Sherris JC, et al. Antibiotic susceptibility testing by a standardized single disk method. Am J Clin Pathol 1966;45:493–6.

13. Jorgensen JH, Ferraro MJ. Antimicrobial susceptibility testing: special needs for fastidious organisms and difficult-to-detect resistance mechanisms. Clin Infect Dis 2000;30:799–808.

14. Evangelista AT, Truant AL. Rapid systems and instruments for antimicrobial susceptibility testing of bacteria. In: Truant AL, editor. Manual of commercial methods in medical microbiology. Washington (DC): American Society of Microbiology; 2002. p. 413–29.

15. Richter SS, Ferraro MJ. Susceptibility testing instrumentation and computerized expert systems for data analysis and interpretation. In: Murray PR, Baron EJ, Jorgensen JH, editors. Manual of clinical microbiology. 9th edition. Washington (DC): American Society for Microbiology; 2007. p. 245–56.

16. Food and Drug Administration. Review criteria for assessment of antimicrobial susceptibility. Rockville (MD): Food and Drug Administration; 1991.

17. Korgenski EK, Daly JA. Evaluation of the BIOMIC video reader system for determining interpretive categories of isolates on the basis of disk diffusion susceptibility results. J Clin Microbiol 1998;36:302–4.

18. Medeiros AA, Crellin J. Evaluation of the Sirscan automated zone reader in a clinical microbiology laboratory. J Clin Microbiol 2000;38:1688–93.

19. Nijs A, Cartuyvels R, Mewis A, et al. Comparison and evaluation of Osiris and Sirscan 2000 antimicrobial susceptibility systems in the clinical microbiology laboratory. J Clin Microbiol 2003;41:3627–30.

20. Barenfanger J, Drake C, Kacich G. Clinical and financial benefits of rapid bacterial identification and antimicrobial susceptibility testing. J Clin Microbiol 1999; 37:1415–8.

21. Doern GV, Vautour R, Gaudet M, et al. Clinical impact of rapid in vitro susceptibility testing and bacterial identification. J Clin Microbiol 1994;32:1757–62.

22. Kerremans JJ, Verboom P, Stijnen T, et al. Rapid identification and antimicrobial susceptibility testing reduce antibiotic use and accelerate pathogen-directed antibiotic use. J Antimicrob Chemother 2008;61(2):428–35.

23. Bruins M, Oord H, Bloembergen P, et al. Lack of effect of shorter turnaround time of microbiological procedures on clinical outcomes: a randomised controlled trial among hospitalised patients in the Netherlands. Eur J Clin Microbiol Infect Dis 2005;24(5):305–13.

24. Jett B, Free L, Sahm DF. Factors influencing the Vitek gram-positive susceptibility system's detection of vanB-encoded vancomycin resistance among enterococci. J Clin Microbiol 1996;34:701–6.

25. Katsanis GP, Spargo J, Ferraro MJ, et al. Detection of *Klebsiella pneumoniae* and *Escherichia coli* strains producing extended-spectrum beta-lactamases. J Clin Microbiol 1994;32:691–6.

26. Tenover FC, Swenson JM, O'Hara CM, et al. Ability of commercial and reference antimicrobial susceptibility testing methods to detect vancomycin resistance in enterococci. J Clin Microbiol 1995;33:1524–7.

27. Doern GV, Scott DR, Rashad AL, et al. Evaluation of a direct blood culture disk diffusion antimicrobial susceptibility test. Antimicrob Agents Chemother 1981; 20:696–8.

28. Mirrett S, Reller LB. Comparison of direct and standard antimicrobial disk susceptibility testing for bacteria isolated from blood. J Clin Microbiol 1979; 10:482–7.

29. Ling TK, Liu ZK, Cheng AF. Evaluation of the VITEK 2 system for rapid direct identification and susceptibility testing of gram-negative bacilli from positive blood cultures. J Clin Microbiol 2003;41:4705–7.

30. Malhotra-Kumar S, Haccuria K, Michiels M, et al. Current trends in rapid diagnostics for methicillin-resistant *Staphylococcus aureus* and glycopeptide-resistant enterococcus species. J Clin Microbiol 2008;46(5):1577–87.

31. Baker CN, Stocker SA, Culver DH, et al. Comparison of the E test to agar dilution, broth microdilution, and agar diffusion susceptibility testing techniques by using a special challenge set of bacteria. J Clin Microbiol 1991;29:533–8.

32. Huang MB, Baker CN, Banerjee S, et al. Accuracy of the E test for determining antimicrobial susceptibilities of staphylococci, enterococci, *Campylobacter jejuni*, and gram-negative bacteria resistant to antimicrobial agents. J Clin Microbiol 1992;30:3243–8.

33. Schulz JE, Sahm DF. Reliability of the E test for detection of ampicillin, vancomycin, and high-level aminoglycoside resistance in *Enterococcus* spp. J Clin Microbiol 1993;31:3336–9.

34. Walsh TR, Bolmstrom A, Qwarnstrom A, et al. Evaluation of a new E test for detecting metallo-beta-lactamases in routine clinical testing. J Clin Microbiol 2002; 40:2755–9.

35. Fuchs PC, Barry AL, Brown SD. Evaluation of daptomycin susceptibility testing by E test and the effect of different batches of media. J Antimicrob Chemother 2001;48:557–61.

36. Hill GB. Spiral gradient endpoint: a new method of susceptibility testing. Hosp Pract (Off Ed) 1990;25(Suppl 4):31–7.

37. Wootton M, Howe RA, Hillman R, et al. A modified population analysis profile (PAP) method to detect hetero-resistance to vancomycin in *Staphylococcus aureus* in a UK hospital. J Antimicrob Chemother 2001;47(4):399–403.

38. Craig WA. Qualitative susceptibility tests versus quantitative MIC tests. Diagn Microbiol Infect Dis 1993;16:231–6.

39. Jorgensen JH. Selection of antimicrobial agents for routine testing in a clinical microbiology laboratory. Diagn Microbiol Infect Dis 1993;16:245–9.

40. Greenwood D. Detection of antibiotic resistance in vitro. Int J Antimicrob Agents 2000;14:303–6.
41. Peterson LR, Shanholtzer CJ. Tests for bactericidal effects of antimicrobial agents: technical performance and clinical relevance. Clin Microbiol Rev 1992;5:420–32.
42. Shanholtzer CJ, Peterson LR, Mohn ML, et al. MBCs for *Staphylococcus aureus* as determined by macrodilution and microdilution techniques. Antimicrob Agents Chemother 1984;26:214–9.
43. Wolfson JS, Swartz MN. Drug therapy: serum bactericidal activity as a monitor of antibiotic therapy. N Engl J Med 1985;312:968–75.
44. Hallander HO, Dornbusch K, Gezelius L, et al. Synergism between aminoglyco-sides and cephalosporins with antipseudomonal activity: interaction index and killing curve method. Antimicrob Agents Chemother 1982;22:743–52.
45. Aaron SD, Ferris W, Henry DA, et al. multiple combination bactericidal antibiotic testing for patients with cystic fibrosis infected with *Burkholderia cepacia*. Am J Respir Crit Care Med 2000;161:1206–12.
46. Aaron SD, Vandemheen KL, Ferris W, et al. Combination antibiotic susceptibility testing to treat exacerbations of cystic fibrosis associated with multiresistant bacteria: a randomised, double-blind, controlled clinical trial. Lancet 2005; 366(9484):463–71.
47. Rasheed JK, Tenover FC. Detection and characterization of antimicrobial resistance genes in bacteria. In: Murray PR, Baron EJ, Pfaller MA, editors. Manual of clinical microbiology. Washington (DC): American Society of Microbiology; 2003. p. 1196–212.
48. Tenover FC. Rapid detection and identification of bacterial pathogens using novel molecular technologies: infection control and beyond. Clin Infect Dis 2007;44(3):418–23.
49. Deguchi T, Yasuda M, Asano M, et al. DNA gyrase mutations in quinolone-resis-tant clinical isolates of *Neisseria* gonorrhoeae. Antimicrob Agents Chemother 1995;39:561–3.
50. Rasheed JK, Jay C, Metchock B, et al. Evolution of extended-spectrum beta-lac-tam resistance (SHV-8) in a strain of *Escherichia coli* during multiple episodes of bacteremia. Antimicrob Agents Chemother 1997;41:647–53.
51. Rasheed JK, Anderson GJ, Yigit H, et al. Characterization of the extended-spec-trum beta-lactamase reference strain, *Klebsiella pneumoniae* K6 (ATCC 700603), which produces the novel enzyme SHV-18. Antimicrob Agents Chemo-ther 2000;44:2382–8.
52. Arbique J, Forward K, Haldane D, et al. Comparison of the Velogene rapid MRSA identification assay, Denka MRSA-screen assay, and BBL crystal MRSA ID system for rapid identification of methicillin-resistant *Staphylococcus aureus*. Diagn Microbiol Infect Dis 2001;40:5–10.
53. Marshall A, Hodgson J. DNA chips: an array of possibilities. Nat Biotechnol 1998;16:27–31.
54. Hope R, Livermore DM, Brick G, et al. Non-susceptibility trends among staphy-lococci from bacteraemias in the UK and Ireland, 2001–06. J Antimicrob Chemo-ther 2008;62(Suppl 2):ii65–74.
55. Klevens RM, Morrison MA, Nadle J, et al. Invasive methicillin resistant *Staphylo-coccus aureus* infections in the United States. JAMA 2007;298:1763–71.
56. Livermore DM. Antibiotic resistance in staphylococci. Int J Antimicrob Agents 2000;16(Suppl 1):S3–10.

57. King MD, Humphrey BJ, Wang YF, et al. Emergence of community-acquired methicillin-resistant *Staphylococcus aureus* USA 300 clone as the predominant cause of skin and soft-tissue infections. Ann Intern Med 2006;144(5):309–17.
58. Corey GR, Boucher HW. Epidemiology of methicillin-resistant *Staphylococcus aureus*. Clin Infect Dis. 2008;46(Suppl 5):S344–9.
59. Katayama Y, Ito T, Hiramatsu K. A new class of genetic element, staphylococcus cassette chromosome mec, encodes methicillin resistance in *Staphylococcus aureus*. Antimicrob Agents Chemother 2000;44:1549–55.
60. Crisostomo MI, Westh H, Tomasz A, et al. The evolution of methicillin resistance in *Staphylococcus aureus*: similarity of genetic backgrounds in historically early methicillin-susceptible and -resistant isolates and contemporary epidemic clones. Proc Natl Acad Sci U S A 2001;98:9865–70.
61. Schmitz FJ, Fluit AC, Gondolf M, et al. The prevalence of aminoglycoside resistance and corresponding resistance genes in clinical isolates of staphylococci from 19 European hospitals. J Antimicrob Chemother 1999;43:253–9.
62. Ito T, Katayama Y, Asada K, et al. Structural comparison of three types of staphylococcal cassette chromosome mec integrated in the chromosome in methicillin-resistant *Staphylococcus aureus*. Antimicrob Agents Chemother 2001;45: 1323–36.
63. Ma XX, Ito T, Tiensasitorn C, et al. Novel type of staphylococcal cassette chromosome mec identified in community-acquired methicillin-resistant *Staphylococcus aureus* strains. Antimicrob Agents Chemother 2002;46:1147–52.
64. Finan JE, Rosato AE, Dickinson TM, et al. Conversion of oxacillin resistant staphylococci from heterotypic to homotypic resistance expression. Antimicrob Agents Chemother 2002;46:24–30.
65. Huang MB, Gay TE, Baker CN, et al. Two percent sodium chloride is required for susceptibility testing of staphylococci with oxacillin when using agar-based dilution methods. J Clin Microbiol 1993;31:2683–8.
66. Yamazumi T, Marshall SA, Wilke WW, et al. Comparison of the Vitek gram-positive susceptibility 106 card and the MRSAscreen latex agglutination test for determining oxacillin resistance in clinical bloodstream isolates of *Staphylococcus aureus*. J Clin Microbiol 2001;39:53–6.
67. Swenson JM, Tenover FC. Results of disk diffusion testing with cefoxitin correlate with presence of *mecA* in *Staphylococcus* spp. J Clin Microbiol 2005;43(8): 3818–23.
68. Velasco D, del Mar Tomas M, Cartelle M, et al. Evaluation of different methods for detecting methicillin (oxacillin) resistance in *Staphylococcus aureus*. J Antimicrob Chemother 2005;55:379–82.
69. Proctor RA, Kahl B, Von Eiff C, et al. Staphylococcal small colony variants have novel mechanisms for antibiotic resistance. Clin Infect Dis 1998;27(Suppl 1):S68–74.
70. Baron EJ. Implications of new technology for infectious diseases practice. Clin Infect Dis 2006;43:1318–23.
71. Rossney AS, Herra CM, Brennan GI, et al. Evaluation of the xpert methicillin-resistant *Staphylococcus aureus* (MRSA) assay using the genexpert real-time PCR platform for rapid detection of MRSA from screening specimens. J Clin Microbiol 2008;46(10):3285–90.
72. Hiramatsu K, Hanaki H, Ino T, et al. Methicillin-resistant *Staphylococcus aureus* clinical strain with reduced vancomycin susceptibility. J Antimicrob Chemother 1997;40:135–6.

73. Tenover FC, Moellering RC. The rationale for revising the clinical and laboratory standards institute vancomycin minimal inhibitory concentration interpretive criteria for *Staphylococcus aureus*. Clin Infect Dis 2007;44(9):1208–15.
74. Maor Y, Rahav G, Belausov N, et al. Prevalence and characteristics of heteroresistant vancomycin-intermediate *Staphylococcus aureus* bacteremia in a tertiary care center. J Clin Microbiol 2007;45(5):1511–4.
75. Sader HS, Jones RN, Rybak MJ. Evaluation of the accuracy of the Etest Macromethod for the detection of heterogeneous vancomycin-intermediate Staphylococcus aureus (hVISA) strains. Poster session presented at 48th Annual ICAAC/IDSA 46th Annual Meeting; October 25–28, 2008; Washington DC.
76. Soriano A, Marco F, Martinez JA, et al. Influence of vancomycin minimum inhibitory concentration on the treatment of methicillin-resistant *Staphylococcus aureus* bacteremia. Clin Infect Dis 2008;46(2):193–200.
77. Lina G, Quaglia A, Reverdy ME, et al. Distribution of genes encoding resistance to macrolides, lincosamides, and streptogramins among staphylococci. Antimicrob Agents Chemother 1999;43:1062–6.
78. Roberts MC, Sutcliffe J, Courvalin P, et al. Nomenclature for macrolide and macrolide-lincosamide-streptogramin B resistance determinants. Antimicrob Agents Chemother 1999;43:2823–30.
79. Zelazny AM, Ferraro MJ, Glennen A, et al. Selection of strains for quality assessment of the disk induction method for detection of inducible clindamycin resistance in staphylococci: a CLSI collaborative study. J Clin Microbiol 2005; 43(6):2613–5.
80. Frank AL, Marcinak JF, Mangat PD, et al. Clindamycin treatment of methicillin-resistant *Staphylococcus aureus* infections in children. Pediatr Infect Dis J 2002;21:530–4.
81. Panagea S, Perry JD, Gould FK. Should clindamycin be used as treatment of patients with infections caused by erythromycin-resistant staphylococci? J Antimicrob Chemother 1999;44:581–2.
82. Rao GG. Should clindamycin be used in treatment of patients with infections caused by erythromycin-resistant staphylococci? J Antimicrob Chemother 2000;45:715.
83. Siberry GK, Tekle T, Carroll K, et al. Failure of clindamycin treatment of methicillin resistant *Staphylococcus aureus* expressing inducible clindamycin resistance in vitro. Clin Infect Dis 2003;37:1257–60.
84. Johnson AP, Livermore DM. Quinupristin/dalfopristin, a new addition to the antimicrobial arsenal. Lancet 1999;354:2012–3.
85. Pillai SK, Sakoulas G, Wennersten C, et al. Linezolid resistance in *Staphylococcus aureus*: characterization and stability of resistant phenotype. J Infect Dis 2002;186:1603–7.
86. Tsiodras S, Gold HS, Sakoulas G, et al. Linezolid resistance in a clinical isolate of *Staphylococcus aureus*. Lancet 2001;358:207–8.
87. Brauers J, Kresken M, Hafner D, et al. Surveillance of linezolid resistance in Germany, 2001–2002. Clin Microbiol Infect 2005;11:39–46.
88. Jevitt LA, Thorne M, Traczewski MM, et al. Multicenter evaluation of the E test and disk diffusion methods for differentiating daptomycin-susceptible from non-daptomycin-susceptible *Staphylococcus aureus* Isolates. J Clin Microbiol 2006;44(9):3098–104.
89. Pankey GA. Tigecycline. J Antimicrob Chemother 2005;56(3):470–80.
90. Bishara J, Pitlik S, Samra Z, et al. Co-trimoxazole-sensitive, methicillin-resistant *Staphylococcus aureus*, Israel, 1988–1997. Emerg Infect Dis 2003;9:1168–9.

91. Markowitz N, Quinn EL, Saravolatz LD. Trimethoprim-sulfamethoxazole compared with vancomycin for the treatment of *Staphylococcus aureus* infection. Ann Intern Med 1992;117:390–8.

92. Schmitz FJ, Verhoef J, Fluit A, et al. Stability of the MICs of various antibiotics in different clonal populations of methicillin-resistant *Staphylococcus aureus*. J Antimicrob Chemother 1998;41:311–3.

93. Yeldandi V, Strodtman R, Lentino JR. In-vitro and in-vivo studies of trimethoprim-sulphamethoxazole against multiple resistant *Staphylococcus aureus*. J Antimicrob Chemother 1988;22:873–80.

94. Sievert DM, Rudrik JT, Patel JB, et al. Vancomycin-resistant *Staphylococcus aureus* in the United States, 2002–2006. Clin Infect Dis 2008;46(5):668–74.

95. Bogdanovich T, Ednie LM, et al. Antistaphylococcal activity of ceftobiprole, a new broad-spectrum cephalosporin. Antimicrob Agents Chemother 2005;4210–9.

96. Graham JC, Gould FK. Role of aminoglycosides in the treatment of bacterial endocarditis. J Antimicrob Chemother 2002;49:437–44.

97. Mulazimoglu L, Drenning SD, Muder RR. Vancomycin-gentamicin synergism revisited: effect of gentamicin susceptibility of methicillin-resistant *Staphylococcus aureus*. Antimicrob Agents Chemother 1996;40:1534–5.

98. Mulligan ME, Murray-Leisure KA, Ribner BS, et al. Methicillin-resistant *Staphylococcus aureus*: a consensus review of the microbiology, pathogenesis, and epidemiology with implications for prevention and management. Am J Med 1993;94:313–28.

99. Watanakunakorn C, Tisone JC. Synergism between vancomycin and gentamicin or tobramycin for methicillin-susceptible and methicillin-resistant *Staphylococcus aureus* strains. Antimicrob Agents Chemother 1982;22:903–5.

100. O'Neill AJ, Cove JH, Chopra I. Mutation frequencies for resistance to fusidic acid and rifampicin in *Staphylococcus aureus*. J Antimicrob Chemother 2001; 47:647–50.

101. Wichelhaus TA, Boddinghaus B, Besier S, et al. Biological cost of rifampin resistance from the perspective of *Staphylococcus aureus*. Antimicrob Agents Chemother 2002;46:3381–5.

102. Perazzi B, Fermepin MR, Malimovka A, et al. Accuracy of cefoxitin disk testing for characterization of oxacillin resistance mediated by penicillin-binding protein 2a in coagulase-negative staphylococci. J Clin Microbiol 2006;44(10):3634–9.

103. Schwalbe RS, Stapleton JT, Gilligan PH. Emergence of vancomycin resistance in coagulase-negative staphylococci. N Engl J Med 1987;316:927–31.

104. Jones RN, Ross JE, Castanheira M, et al. United States resistance surveillance results for linezolid (LEADER Program for 2007). Diagn Microbiol Infect Dis 2008;62(4):416–26.

105. Vergis EN, Hayden MK, Chow JW, et al. Determinants of vancomycin resistance and mortality rates in enterococcal bacteremia: a prospective multicenter study. Ann Intern Med 2001;135:484–92.

106. Fontana R, Canepari P, Lleo MM, et al. Mechanisms of resistance of enterococci to beta-lactam antibiotics. Eur J Clin Microbiol Infect Dis 1990;9:103–5.

107. Murdoch DR, Mirrett S, Harrell LJ, et al. Sequential emergence of antibiotic resistance in enterococcal bloodstream isolates over 25 years. Antimicrob Agents Chemother 2002;46:3676–8.

108. Okhuysen PC, Singh KV, Murray BE. Susceptibility of beta-lactamase-producing enterococci to piperacillin with tazobactam. Diagn Microbiol Infect Dis 1993;17: 219–24.

109. Weinstein MP. Comparative evaluation of penicillin, ampicillin, and imipenem MICs and susceptibility breakpoints for vancomycin-susceptible and vancomycin-resistant *Enterococcus faecalis* and *Enterococcus faecium*. J Clin Microbiol 2001;39:2729–31.
110. Weinstein MP, Mirrett S, Kannangara S, et al. Multicenter evaluation of use of penicillin and ampicillin as surrogates for in vitro testing of susceptibility of enterococci to imipenem. J Clin Microbiol 2004;42(8):3747–51.
111. El Amin N, Wretlind B, Wenger A, et al. Ampicillin-sensitive, imipenem resistant strains of *Enterococcus faecium*. J Clin Microbiol 2002;40:738.
112. Leclercq R, Derlot E, Duval J, et al. Plasmid-mediated resistance to vancomycin and teicoplanin in *Enterococcus faecium*. N Engl J Med 1988;319:157–61.
113. Boyd DA, Cabral T, Van Caeseele P, et al. Molecular characterization of the vanE gene cluster in vancomycin-resistant *Enterococcus faecalis* N00–410 isolated in Canada. Antimicrob Agents Chemother 2002;46:1977–9.
114. Depardieu F, Reynolds PE, Courvalin P. VanD-type vancomycin-resistant *Enterococcus faecium*. Antimicrob Agents Chemother 2003;47:7–18.
115. Dutta I, Reynolds PE. Biochemical and genetic characterization of the vanC-2 vancomycin resistance gene cluster of *Enterococcus casseliflavus* ATCC 25788. Antimicrob Agents Chemother 2002;46:3125–32.
116. Malani PN, Thal L, Donabedian SM, et al. Molecular analysis of vancomycin-resistant *Enterococcus faecalis* from Michigan hospitals during a 10 year period. J Antimicrob Chemother 2002;49:841–3.
117. Nelson RR. Intrinsically vancomycin-resistant gram-positive organisms: clinical relevance and implications for infection control. J Hosp Infect 1999;42:275–82.
118. Kiehlbauch JA, Hannett GE, Salfinger M, et al. Use of the national committee for clinical laboratory standards guidelines for disk diffusion susceptibility testing in New York State laboratories. J Clin Microbiol 2000;38:3341–8.
119. Rosenberg J, Tenover FC, Wong J, et al. Are clinical laboratories in California accurately reporting vancomycin-resistant enterococci? J Clin Microbiol 1997;35:2526–30.
120. Kohner PC, Patel R, Uhl JR, et al. Comparison of agar dilution, broth microdilution, E-test, disk diffusion, and automated Vitek methods for testing susceptibilities of *Enterococcus* spp. to vancomycin. J Clin Microbiol 1997;35:3258–63.
121. Murdoch DR, Mirrett S, Harrell LJ, et al. Comparison of microscan broth microdilution, synergy quad plate agar dilution, and disk diffusion screening methods for detection of high-level aminoglycoside resistance in enterococcus species. J Clin Microbiol 2003;41:2703–5.
122. Jorgensen JH, Crawford SA, Kelly CC, et al. In vitro activity of daptomycin against vancomycin-resistant enterococci of various Van types and comparison of susceptibility testing methods. Antimicrob Agents Chemother 2003;47:3760–3.
123. Richter SS, Kealey DE, Murray CT, et al. The in vitro activity of daptomycin against *Staphylococcus aureus* and *Enterococcus* species. J Antimicrob Chemother 2003;52:123–7.
124. Centers for Disease Control. Preventing pneumococcal disease among infants and young children. MMWR Recomm Rep 2000;49(RR09):1–38.
125. Centers for Disease Control and Prevention. Assessment of susceptibility testing practices for *Streptococcus pneumoniae*—United States, February 2000. MMWR Morb Mortal Wkly Rep 2002;51:392–4.
126. Breiman RF, Butler JC, Tenover FC, et al. Emergence of drug resistant pneumococcal infections in the United States. JAMA 1994;271:1831–5.

127. Doern GV, Heilmann KP, Huynh HK, et al. Antimicrobial resistance among clinical isolates of *Streptococcus pneumoniae* in the United States during 1999–2000, including a comparison of resistance rates since 1994–1995. Antimicrob Agents Chemother 2001;45:1721–9.

128. Doern GV, Richter SS, Miller A, et al. Antimicrobial resistance among *Streptococcus pneumoniae* in the United States: have we begun to turn the corner on resistance to certain antimicrobial classes? Clin Infect Dis 2005;41(2):139–48.

129. Whitney CG, Farley MM, Hadler J, et al. Decline in invasive pneumococcal disease following the introduction of protein-polysaccharide conjugate vaccine. N Engl J Med 2003;348:1737–46.

130. Moore MR, Gertz RE, Woodbury RL, et al. Population snapshot of emergent *Streptococcus pneumoniae* serotype 19A in the United States, 2005. J Infect Dis 2008;197(7):1016–27.

131. Hanage WP, Huang SS, Lipsitch M, et al. Diversity and antibiotic resistance among nonvaccine serotypes of *Streptococcus pneumoniae* carriage isolates in the post-heptavalent conjugate vaccine era. J Infect Dis 2007;195(3):347–52.

132. Appelbaum PC. Resistance among *Streptococcus pneumoniae*: implications for drug selection. Clin Infect Dis 2002;34:1613–20.

133. Ward JI, Moellering RC Jr. Susceptibility of pneumococci to 14 beta-lactam agents: comparison of strains resistant, intermediate-resistant, and susceptible to penicillin. Antimicrob Agents Chemother 1981;20:204–7.

134. Witte W. Antibiotic resistance in gram-positive bacteria: epidemiological aspects. J Antimicrob Chemother 1999;44(Suppl A):1–9.

135. Klugman KP. The successful clone: the vector of dissemination of resistance in *Streptococcus pneumoniae*. J Antimicrob Chemother 2002;50(Suppl S2):1–5.

136. Perez-Trallero E, Marimon JM, Gonzalez A, et al. Spain14-5 international multiresistant *Streptococcus pneumoniae* clone resistant to fluoroquinolones and other families of antibiotics. J Antimicrob Chemother 2003;51:715–9.

137. Zhanel GG, Palatnick L, Nichol KA, et al. Antimicrobial resistance in respiratory tract *Streptococcus pneumoniae* isolates: results of the Canadian respiratory organism susceptibility study, 1997 to 2002. Antimicrob Agents Chemother 2003;47:1867–74.

138. Tenover FC, Baker CN, Swenson JM. Evaluation of commercial methods for determining antimicrobial susceptibility of *Streptococcus pneumoniae*. J Clin Microbiol 1996;34:10–4.

139. Fukushima KY, Yanagihara K, Hirakata Y, et al. Rapid identification of penicillin and macrolide resistance genes and simultaneous quantification of *Streptococcus pneumoniae* in purulent sputum samples by use of a novel real-time multiplex PCR assay. J Clin Microbiol 2008;46(7):2384–8.

140. Jorgensen JH, Barry AL, Traczewski MM, et al. Rapid automated antimicrobial susceptibility testing of *Streptococcus pneumoniae* by use of the bioMerieux VITEK 2. J Clin Microbiol 2000;38:2814–8.

141. Rosser SJ, Alfa MJ, Hoban S, et al. E test versus agar dilution for antimicrobial susceptibility testing of viridans group streptococci. J Clin Microbiol 1999;37:26–30.

142. Douglas CP, Siarakas S, Gottlieb T. Evaluation of E test as a rapid method for determining MICs for nutritionally variant streptococci. J Clin Microbiol 1994;32:2318–20.

143. Raney PM, Tenover FC, Carey RB, et al. Investigation of inducible clindamyinc and telithromycin resistance in isolates of β-hemolytic streptococci. Diagn Microbiol Infect Dis 2006;55(3):213–8.

144. CLSI. Methods for antimicrobial dilution and disk susceptibility testing of infrequently isolated or fastidious bacteria. Approved standard M45-A. Wayne (PA): CLSI; 2006.

145. Safdar A, Armstrong D. Antimicrobial activities against 84 *Listeria monocytogenes* isolates from patients with systemic listeriosis at a comprehensive cancer center (1955–1997). J Clin Microbiol 2003;41:483–5.

146. Moellering RC Jr, Medoff G, Leech I, et al. Antibiotic synergism against *Listeria monocytogenes*. Antimicrob Agents Chemother 1972;1:30–4.

147. Jorgensen JH, Hindler JE. New consensus guidelines from the clinical and laboratory standards institute for antimicrobial susceptibility testing of infrequently isolated or fastidious bacteria. Clin Infect Dis 2007;44(2):280–6.

148. Soriano F, Zapardiel J, Nieto E. Antimicrobial susceptibilities of corynebacterium species and other non-spore-forming gram-positive bacilli to 18 antimicrobial agents. Antimicrob Agents Chemother 1995;39:208–14.

149. Logan NA, Popovic T, Hoffmaster A. Bacillus and other aerobic endospore-forming bacteria. In: Murray PR, Baron EJ, Jorgensen JH, editors. Manual of clinical microbiology. 9th edition. Washington (DC): American Society for Microbiology; 2007. p. 455–73.

150. Medeiros AA. Evolution and dissemination of beta-lactamases accelerated by generations of beta-lactam antibiotics. Clin Infect Dis 1997;24(Suppl 1):S19–45.

151. Paterson DL, Bonomo RA. Extended-spectrum beta-lactamases: a clinical update. Clin Microbiol Rev 2005;18(4):657–86.

152. Schwaber MJ, Carmeli Y. Mortality and delay in effective therapy associated with extended-spectrum beta-lactamase production in Enterobacteriaceae bacteraemia: a systematic review and meta-analysis. J Antimicrob Chemother 2007; 60(5):913–20.

153. Moland ES, Sanders CC, Thomson KS. Can results obtained with commercially available MicroScan microdilution panels serve as an indicator of beta-lactamase production among *Escherichia coli* and *Klebsiella* isolates with hidden resistance to expanded spectrum cephalosporins and aztreonam? J Clin Microbiol 1998;36:2575–9.

154. Queena AM, Foleno B, Gownley C, et al. Effects of inoculum and ß-lactamase activity in AmpC- and Extended-Spectrum ß-Lactamase (ESBL)-producing *Escherichia coli* and *Klebsiella pneumoniae* clinical isolates tested by using NCCLS ESBL methodology. J Clin Microbiol 2004;42(1):269–75.

155. Wiegand I, Geiss HK, Mack D, et al. Detection of extended-spectrum beta-lactamases among Enterobacteriaceae by use of semiautomated microbiology systems and manual detection procedures. J Clin Microbiol 2007;45(4): 1167–74.

156. Gavin PJ, Suseno MT, et al. Clinical correlation of the CLSI susceptibility breakpoint for piperacillin-tazobactam against extended-spectrum-β-lactamase-producing *Escherichia coli* and *Klebsiella* species. Antimicrob Agents Chemother 2006;50:2244–7.

157. Thomson KS, Smith ME. Version 2000: the new beta-lactamases of gram-negative bacteria at the dawn of the new millennium. Microbes Infect 2000;2: 1225–35.

158. Schwaber MJ, Raney PM, Rasheed JK, et al. Utility of NCCLS guidelines for identifying extended-spectrum b-lactamases in non- *Escherichia coli* and non- *Klebsiella* spp. of Enterobacteriaceae. J Clin Microbiol 2004;42:294–8.

159. Thomson KS, Sanders CC, Moland ES. Use of microdilution panels with and without beta-lactamase inhibitors as a phenotypic test for beta-lactamase

production among *Escherichia coli*, *Klebsiella spp.*, *Enterobacter spp.*, *Citrobacter freundii*, and *Serratia marcescens*. Antimicrob Agents Chemother 1999;43:1393–400.

160. Steward CD, Mohammed JM, Swenson JM, et al. Antimicrobial susceptibility testing of carbapenems: multicenter validity testing and accuracy levels of five antimicrobial test methods for detecting resistance in Enterobacteriaceae and *Pseudomonas aeruginosa* isolates. J Clin Microbiol 2003;41:351–8.

161. Bush K, Queenan AM. Carbapenemases: the versatile beta-lactamases. Clin Microbiol Rev 20:440–458.

162. Tibbetts R, Frye JG, Marschall J, et al. Detection of KPC-2 in a clinical isolate of *Proteus mirabilis* and first reported description of carbapenemase resistance caused by a KPC beta-lactamase in *P. mirabilis*. J Clin Microbiol 2008;46(9): 3080–3.

163. Marchaim D, Navon-Venezia S, Schwaber MJ, et al. Isolation of imipenem-resistant *Enterobacter* species: emergence of kpc-2 carbapenemase, molecular characterization, epidemiology, and outcomes. Antimicrob Agents Chemother. 2008;52(4):1413–8.

164. Tenover FC, Kalsi RK, Williams PP, et al. Carbapenem resistance in *Klebsiella pneumoniae* not detected by automated susceptibility testing. Emerg Infect Dis 2006;12(8):1209–13.

165. Lee K, Chong Y, Shin HB, et al. Modified Hodge and EDTA-disk synergy tests to screen metallo-beta-lactamase-producing strains of *Pseudomonas* and *Acinetobacter* species. Clin Microbiol Infect 2001;7(2):88–91.

166. Anderson KF, Lonsway DR, Rasheed JK, et al. Evaluation of methods to identify the *Klebsiella pneumoniae* carbapenemase in Enterobacteriaceae. J Clin Microbiol 2007;45(8):2723–5.

167. Kelsidis T, Karageorgopoulos DE, Kelesidis J, et al. Tigecycline for the treatment of multidrug-resistant Enterobacteriaceae: a systematic review of the evidence from microbiological and clinical studies. J Antimicrob Chemother 2008;62(5):895–904.

168. Crump JA, Barrett TJ, Nelson JT, et al. Reevaluating fluoroquinolone breakpoints for *Salmonella enterica* serotype *typhi* and for non-*typhi* salmonellae. Clin Infect Dis 2003;37:75–81.

169. Gupta SK, Medella F, Omondi MW, et al. Laboratory-based surveillance of paratyphoid fever in the United States: travel and antimicrobial resistance. Clin Infect Dis 2008;46(11):1656–63.

170. Kadhiravan T, Wig N, Kapil A, et al. Clinical outcomes in typhoid fever: adverse impact of infection with nalidixic acid-resistant *Salmonella typhi*. BMC Infect Dis 2005;5(1):37.

171. Livermore DM. Multiple mechanisms of antimicrobial resistance in *Pseudomonas aeruginosa*: our worst nightmare? Clin Infect Dis 2002;34:634–40.

172. Gales AC, Reis AO, Jones RN. Contemporary assessment of antimicrobial susceptibility testing methods for polymyxin B and colistin: review of available interpretative criteria and quality control guidelines. J Clin Microbiol 2001;39: 183–90.

173. Tam VH, Gamez EZ, Weston JS, et al. Outcomes of bacteremia due to *Pseudomonas aeruginosa* with reduced susceptibility to piperacillin-tazobactam: implications on the appropriateness of the resistance breakpoint. Clin Infect Dis 2008;46(6):862–7.

174. Morlin GL, Hedges DL, Smith AL, et al. Accuracy and cost of antibiotic susceptibility testing of mixed morphotypes of *Pseudomonas aeruginosa*. J Clin Microbiol 1994;32:1027–30.

175. Thomassen MJ, Demko CA, Boxerbaum B, et al. Multiple of isolates of *Pseudomonas aeruginosa* with differing antimicrobial susceptibility patterns from patients with cystic fibrosis. J Infect Dis 1979;140:873–80.
176. Fowerakeri JE, Laughton CR, Brown DFJ, et al. Phenotypic variability of *Pseudomonas aeruginosa* in sputa from patients with acute infective exacerbation of cystic fibrosis and its impact on the validity of antimicrobial susceptibility testing. J Antimicrob Chemother 2005;55(6):921–7.
177. Govan JR, Deretic V. Microbial pathogenesis in cystic fibrosis: mucoid *Pseudomonas aeruginosa* and *Burkholderia cepacia*. Microbiol Rev 1996;60:539–74.
178. Burns JL, Saiman L, Whittier S, et al. Comparison of two commercial systems (Vitek and MicroScan-WalkAway) for antimicrobial susceptibility testing of *Pseudomonas aeruginosa* isolates from cystic fibrosis patients. Diagn Microbiol Infect Dis 2001;39:257–60.
179. Marley EF, Mohla C, Campos JM. Evaluation of E-Test for determination of antimicrobial MICs for *Pseudomonas aeruginosa* isolates from cystic fibrosis patients. J Clin Microbiol 1995;33:3191–3.
180. Burns JL, Saiman L, Whittier S, et al. Comparison of agar diffusion methodologies for antimicrobial susceptibility testing of *Pseudomonas aeruginosa* isolates from cystic fibrosis patients. J Clin Microbiol 2000;38:1818–22.
181. Neu HC, Niu WW, Chin NX. Tazobactam prevention of emergence of resistance. Diagn Microbiol Infect Dis 1989;12:477–80.
182. Saiman L, Mehar F, Niu WW, et al. Antibiotic susceptibility of multiply resistant *Pseudomonas aeruginosa* isolated from patients with cystic fibrosis, including candidates for transplantation. Clin Infect Dis 1996;23:532–7.
183. Rolston KV, Safdar A. *Stenotrophomonas maltophilia*: changing spectrum of a serious bacterial pathogen in patients with cancer. Clin Infect Dis 2007;45(12):1602–9.
184. Denton M, Kerr KG. Molecular epidemiology of *Stenotrophomonas maltophilia* isolated from cystic fibrosis patients. J Clin Microbiol 2002;40:1884.
185. Tsiodras S, Pittet D, Carmeli Y, et al. Clinical implications of *Stenotrophomonas maltophilia* resistant to trimethoprim-sulfamethoxazole: a study of 69 patients at 2 university hospitals. Scand J Infect Dis 2000;32:651–6.
186. Jones RN, Sader HS. Antimicrobial susceptibility of uncommonly isolated non-enteric gram-negative bacilli. Int J Antimicrob Agents 2005;25(2):95–109.
187. Zhang L, Li XZ, Poole K. SmeDEF multidrug efflux pump contributes to intrinsic multidrug resistance in *Stenotrophomonas maltophilia*. Antimicrob Agents Chemother 2001;45:3497–503.
188. Carroll KC, Cohen S, Nelson R, et al. Comparison of various in vitro susceptibility methods for testing *Stenotrophomonas maltophilia*. Diagn Microbiol Infect Dis 1998;32:229–35.
189. Nicodemo AC, Araujo MRE, Ruiz AS, et al. In vitro susceptibility of *Stenotrophomonas maltophilia* isolates: comparison of disc diffusion, E test and agar dilution methods. J Antimicrob Chemother 2004;53(4):604–8.
190. Krueger TS, Clark EA, Nix DE. In vitro susceptibility of *Stenotrophomonas maltophilia* to various antimicrobial combinations. Diagn Microbiol Infect Dis 2001;41:71–8.
191. Zhou J, Chen Y, Tabibi S, et al. Antimicrobial susceptibility and synergy studies of *Burkholderia cepacia* complex isolated from patients with cystic fibrosis. Antimicrob Agents Chemother 2007;51(3):1085–8.
192. Gaynes R, Edwards JR. Overview of nosocomial infections caused by gram-negative bacilli. Clin Infect Dis 2005;41:848–54.

193. Peleg AY, Seifert H, Paterson DL. *Acinetobacter baumannii*: emergence of a successful pathogen. Clin Microbiol Rev 2008;21(3):538–82.
194. Landman D, Quale JM, Mayorga D, et al. Citywide clonal outbreak of multiresistant *Acinetobacter baumannii* and *Pseudomonas aeruginosa* in Brooklyn, N.Y.: the preantibiotic era has returned. Arch Intern Med 2002;162:1515–20.
195. M7-A7 CLSI. Dilution antimicrobial susceptibility tests for bacteria that grow aerobically. Wayne (PA): CLSI; 2007.
196. Swenson JM, Killgore GE, Tenover FC. Antimicrobial susceptibility testing of *Acinetobacter* spp. by NCCLS broth microdilution and disk diffusion methods. J Clin Microbiol 2004;42:5102–8.
197. Hoban DJ, Doern GV, Fluit AC, et al. Worldwide prevalence of antimicrobial resistance in *Streptococcus pneumoniae, Haemophilus influenzae*, and *Moraxella catarrhalis* in the SENTRY antimicrobial surveillance program, 1997–1999. Clin Infect Dis 2001;32(Suppl 2):S81–93.
198. Sahm DF, Jones ME, Hickey ML, et al. Resistance surveillance of *Streptococcus pneumoniae, Haemophilus influenzae* and *Moraxella catarrhalis* isolated in Asia and Europe, 1997–1998. J Antimicrob Chemother 2000;45:457–66.
199. Sahm DF, Brown NP, Thornsberry C, et al. Antimicrobial susceptibility profiles among common respiratory tract pathogens: a GLOBAL perspective. Postgrad Med 2008;120(3 Suppl 1):16–24.
200. Critchley IA, Brown SD, Traczewski MM, et al. National and regional assessment of antimicrobial resistance among community-acquired respiratory tract pathogens identified in a 2005–2006 U.S. faropenem surveillance study. Antimicrob Agents Chemother 2007;51(12):4382–9.
201. Wang SA, Harvey AB, Conner SM, et al. Antimicrobial resistance for *Neisseria gonorrhoeae* in the United States, 1988 to 2003: the spread of fluoroquinolone resistance. Ann Intern Med 2007;147(2):81–8.
202. Jorgensen JH, Crawford SA, Fulcher LC, et al. Multilaboratory evaluation of disk diffusion antimicrobial susceptibility testing of *Neisseria meningitidis* isolates. J Clin Microbio 2006;44(5):1744–54.
203. Biedenbach DJ, Jones RN. Comparative assessment of E test for testing susceptibilities of *Neisseria gonorrhoeae* to penicillin, tetracycline, ceftriaxone, cefotaxime, and ciprofloxacin: investigation using 510(k) review criteria, recommended by the food and drug administration. J Clin Microbiol 1996;34:3214–7.
204. Daher O, Lopardo HA, Rubeglio EA. Value of E test penicillin V and penicillin G strips for penicillin susceptibility testing of *Neisseria meningitidis*. Diagn Microbiol Infect Dis 2002;43:119–21.
205. Gomez-Herruz P, Gonzalez-Palacios R, Romanyk J, et al. Evaluation of the E test for penicillin susceptibility testing of *Neisseria meningitidis*. Diagn Microbiol Infect Dis 1995;21:115–7.
206. Vazquez JA, Arreaza L, Block C, et al. Interlaboratory comparison of agar dilution and E test methods for determining the MICs of antibiotics used in management of *Neisseria meningitidis* infections. Antimicrob Agents Chemother 2003;47:3430–4.
207. Emergence of fluoroquinolone-resistant *Neisseria meningitidis*—Minnesota and North Dakota, 2007-2008. MMWR Morb Mortal Wkly Rep 2008;57(7):173–5.
208. Hachem CY, Clarridge JE, Reddy R, et al. Antimicrobial susceptibility testing of *Helicobacter pylori*: comparison of E-test, broth microdilution, and disk diffusion for ampicillin, clarithromycin, and metronidazole. Diagn Microbiol Infect Dis 1996;24:37–41.

209. Osato MS, Reddy R, Reddy SG, et al. Comparison of the Etest and the NCCLS-approved agar dilution method to detect metronidazole and clarithromycin resistant *Helicobacter pylori*. Int J Antimicrob Agents 2001;17:39–44.

210. Liu CY, Huang YT, Liao CH, et al. Increasing trends in antimicrobial resistance among clinically important anaerobes and *Bacteroides fragilis* isolates causing nosocomial infections: emerging resistance to carbapenems. Antimicrob Agents Chemother 2008;52(9):3161–8.

211. Nguyen MH, Yu VL, Morris AJ, et al. Antimicrobial resistance and clinical outcome of *Bacteroides* bacteremia: findings of a multicenter prospective observational trial. Clin Infect Dis 2000;30:870–6.

212. CLSI. Methods for antimicrobial susceptibility testing of anaerobic bacteria; approved standard. 7th edition. Wayne (PA): CLSI; 2007.

213. Roe DE, Finegold SM, Citron DM, et al. Multilaboratory comparison of anaerobe susceptibility results using 3 different agar media. Clin Infect Dis 2002; 35(Suppl 1):S40–6.

214. Citron DM, Ostovari MI, Karlsson A, et al. Evaluation of the E test for susceptibility testing of anaerobic bacteria. J Clin Microbiol 1991;29:2197–203.

215. Hecht DW. Anaerobes: antibiotic resistance, clinical significance, and the role of susceptibility testing. Anaerobe 2006;12(3):115–21.

216. Baines SD, O'Connor R, Freeman J, et al. Emergence of reduced susceptibility to metronidazole in *Clostridium difficile*. J Antimicrob Chemother 2008;62(5): 1046–52.

217. Al-Nassir WN, Sethi AK, Nerandzic MM, et al. Comparison of clinical and microbiological response to treatment of *Clostridium difficile*-associated disease with metronidazole and vancomycin. Clin Infect Dis 2008;47(1):56–62.

218. Shapiro DS, Schwartz DR. Exposure of laboratory workers to *Francisella tularensis* despite a bioterrorism procedure. J Clin Microbiol 2002;40:2278–81.

219. Centers for Disease Control and Prevention. Suspected cutaneous anthrax in a laboratory worker—Texas, 2002. JAMA 2002;287:2356–8.

220. Mohammed MJ, Marston CK, Popovic T, et al. Antimicrobial susceptibility testing of *Bacillus anthracis*: comparison of results obtained by using the National Committee for Clinical Laboratory Standards both microdilution reference and E test agar gradient diffusion methods. J Clin Microbiol 2002;40: 1902–7.

221. Perry RD, Fetherston JD. *Yersinia pestis*: etiologic agent of plague. Clin Microbiol Rev 1997;10:35–66.

Pharmacokinetics and Pharmacodynamics of Antibacterial Agents

Matthew E. Levison, MD[a],*, Julie H. Levison, MD, MPhil[b,c]

KEYWORDS

- Pharmacokinetics • Pharmacodynamics
- Antimicrobial susceptibility
- Concentration-dependent antimicrobial activity
- Time-dependent antimicrobial activity

The pharmacodynamics of an antimicrobial drug relates its pharmacokinetics to the time course of the antimicrobial effects at the site of the infection. Knowledge of the drug's antimicrobial pharmacodynamic effects (eg, rate and extent of bactericidal action and postantibiotic effect) provides a more rational basis for determination of optimal dosing regimens in terms of the dose and the dosing interval than do the minimal inhibitory concentrations (MICs) and minimal bactericidal concentrations (MBCs) determined in vitro. This article reviews pharmacokinetics, antimicrobial pharmacodynamics, the effect of pharmacodynamics on the emergence of resistant bacterial subpopulations, and the development of pharmacodynamic breakpoints for use in the design of trials of these drugs and in the treatment of infected patients.

IN VITRO ANTIMICROBIAL ACTIVITY OF DRUGS
Minimal Inhibitory Concentrations and Minimal Bactericidal Concentrations

Despite acknowledged exceptions with certain drug–bacteria combinations, antibacterial drugs are usually divided into two groups: those that are primarily bacteriostatic (ie, that inhibit growth of the organism) and those that are primarily bactericidal (ie, that kill the organism). Bacteriostatic drugs require the aid of host defenses to clear tissues of the infecting microorganism; if the host defenses are systemically inadequate (eg, agranulocytosis) or the host defenses are impaired locally at the site of infection (eg, cardiac vegetation in left-sided endocarditis, cerebrospinal fluid in meningitis),

[a] Drexel University, 708 Mt. Pleasant Road, Bryn Mawr, Philadelphia, PA 19010, USA
[b] Division of Infectious Diseases, Brigham and Women's Hospital, 15 Francis Street, Boston, MA 02115, USA
[c] Division of Infectious Diseases, Program in HIV Epidemiology and Outcomes Research, Massachusetts General Hospital, 50 Staniford Street, Boston, MA 02114, USA
* Corresponding author.
E-mail address: ml46@drexel.edu (M.E. Levison).

Infect Dis Clin N Am 23 (2009) 791–815
doi:10.1016/j.idc.2009.06.008
0891-5520/09/$ – see front matter © 2009 Elsevier Inc. All rights reserved.

id.theclinics.com

the pathogen will resume growth after stopping the bacteriostatic drug, and the infection will relapse. Bacterial infection in these circumstances will require the use of bactericidal drugs. Bacteriostatic drugs are sufficient for most other infections.

The in vitro antimicrobial activity of drugs is usually assessed by determining of the MIC and MBC after overnight aerobic incubation of a standard and size inoculum of bacteria in a low protein liquid medium at pH 7.2. These in vitro conditions are likely very different from those expected at the site of infection, where the milieu is frequently acidic and anaerobic, and tissue protein may bind a variable amount of the drug. The MIC and MBC, which are determined at a fixed point in time after exposure to drug concentrations that remain constant throughout an overnight incubation period, do not provide information on the time course of the antimicrobial effect of the fluctuating antimicrobial drug levels that are present in a treated patient. In addition, the MIC and MBC are measured against a standard bacterial inoculum (about 10^5 colony-forming units/mL) that does not necessarily correspond to bacterial densities at the site of infection (10^{8-10} colony-forming units/g of tissue or pus). The in vitro inoculum is also in the exponential phase of growth, unlike the majority of organisms in an established infection, which are nongrowing.

The MIC is defined as the minimal concentration of antibiotic that prevents a clear suspension of 10^5 colony-forming units (CFUs) of bacteria/mL from becoming turbid after overnight incubation; turbidity usually connotes at least a 10-fold increase in bacterial density. Because clear bacterial suspensions may have bacterial densities that are 10^5 CFU/mL or less, the MIC may actually be bactericidal to some extent.

If the minimal concentration of the antibiotic that prevented turbidity lowered the bacterial density from 10^5 to at least 10^2 CFU/mL, that is, a 99.9% (3-$\log_{10}$) reduction in bacterial inoculum, the minimal concentration that prevented turbidity (ie, the MIC) is also the MBC. For bactericidal drugs, the MBC is usually the same as, and generally not more than fourfold greater than, the MIC. In contrast, the MBCs of bacteriostatic drugs are many-fold greater than their MICs. Bacteriostatic drugs include the macrolides, clindamycin, the tetracyclines, the sulfonamides, linezolid, and chloramphenicol. Bactericidal drugs include the beta-lactams, vancomycin, the aminoglycosides, the fluoroquinolones, daptomycin, and metronidazole.

Time-kill studies, which are used to determine the rate of bactericidal activity, involve sampling a bacterial suspension of 10^5 CFU/mL in broth at various time intervals, (eg, at 2, 4, 6, and 24 hours of incubation) after addition to a particular concentration of the antibiotic. This method is also used to assess the interaction of two antimicrobial drugs for synergy or antagonism.

The MIC is a measure of the potency of an antimicrobial drug. Isolates of a particular species will have varying MICs; sensitive strains will have relatively low MICs, and resistant strains will have relatively high MICs. The breakpoint MIC is the MIC that separates sensitive and resistant strains, and it was traditionally selected on its ability to distinguish two disparate populations: one population with MICs at less than the breakpoint (ie, susceptible) and one with MICs at more than the breakpoint (ie, resistant). Another attribute of the breakpoint MIC is correspondence to achievable serum drug levels using standard dosing. However, concentrations may be much higher than serum levels for drugs that concentrate at intracellular sites or at excretory sites, such as in urine or bile, or may be considerably lower than serum levels at secluded foci, such as the cerebrospinal fluid, the eye, the prostate, or centers of abscesses.

For example, the breakpoint concentration for susceptibility to azithromycin is 0.5 μg/mL or less, which may be barely higher than the usual peak serum level of 0.4 μg/mL. Because azithromycin in sequestered within phagocytes, this serum concentration may be fine for predicting its effectiveness against intracellular pathogens, such as legionella, mycoplasma, or chlamydia, but may be problematic for extracellular pathogens such as *Streptococcus pneumoniae*. In addition, drugs that are highly bound to serum protein may have reduced antibacterial activity in serum and will not penetrate tissues as well as drugs that are less protein bound. In these cases, the results of in vitro testing may not predict the in vivo effect.

PHARMACOKINETICS

Pharmacokinetics describes the time course of drug levels in body fluids as a result of absorption, distribution, and elimination of a drug after administration.

Absorption

Most antimicrobial drugs are administered either by the intravenous (IV) or oral administration (PO) routes. Absorption is best described by the drug's bioavailability, which is defined as the percentage of a drug's dose that reaches the systemic circulation.

Intravenous Administration

When the entire dose is administered by the IV route, 100% of that dose is bioavailable. Rates of IV administration can vary from a bolus infusion (in which the total IV dose is given over a very short interval of time, eg, a minute or less) to a very slow infusion over many hours. Delivery of drugs by the IV route is complete by the end of the infusion, when a peak plasma level is achieved. The height of the peak plasma drug level is determined by the rate of IV infusion, the size of the dose, the size of the drug's volume of distribution, and its rate of elimination. Peak plasma drug levels will be the highest after bolus administration because the duration of infusion is too short for significant distribution or elimination of the drug to occur. For these reasons, relatively rapid IV administration is most often chosen for antimicrobial therapy of a patient who has severe infection, when an antimicrobial effect is sought as soon as possible. Slowing the rate of IV infusion allows distribution of the drug in the body and drug elimination to take place, and consequently, lower peak plasma drug levels occur.

Use of bolus administration, however, may be limited by concentration-dependent drug toxicities (eg, red-person's syndrome, which is related to rapid infusion of vancomycin). Also, because the drug will have to be diluted in a relative small volume, bolus infusion will expose the vein through which the drug is infused to high drug concentrations that may limit the use of bolus infusion because of venous irritation and pain. For example, because of its propensity for causing phlebitis when infused by way of a peripheral vein, quinupristin/dalfopristin must be infused using a central venous catheter, in which greater dilution of the drug will occur.

Oral Administration

A few antibacterial agents have excellent bioavailability after oral administration. For example, the fluoroquinolones, metronidazole, tetracycline, minocycline, doxycycline, linezolid, and trimethoprim-sulfamethoxazole are well-absorbed drugs, for which PO and IV doses are similar. Because absorption and distribution is taking place while a drug is being absorbed after oral administration, peak plasma levels can be delayed and usually are not as high as those achieved by IV infusion.

After oral administration, the bioavailability of penicillin G, which is destroyed by gastric acid, is low (< 30%). Penicillin V is more acid-stable, and its bioavailability (60%–70%) is better than that of penicillin G. Amoxicillin offers an advantage over penicillin V in that it has greater oral bioavailability (74%–92%). Only 30% to 55% of an oral ampicillin dose is absorbed.

Many of the oral cephalosporins, such as cefaclor, cefadroxil, cefprozil, cephalexin, ceftibuten, and loracarbef (technically a carbacephem) are acid-stable and have high bioavailability (80%–95%). The bioavailability of cefixime, however, is lower (40%–50%).

Effect of Food on Absorption

Generally, drugs are better absorbed in the small intestine (because of the larger surface area) than in the stomach; therefore, the quicker the stomach emptying, the earlier and higher are the plasma drug concentrations. Food, especially fatty food, delays gastric emptying, delays and lowers peak plasma levels, and may or may not lower a drug's bioavailability. Because eating stimulates production of gastric acid, penicillin G, which is unstable in gastric acid, is best administered in the fasting state (ie, $\frac{1}{2}$ hour before or 2 hours after eating). Penicillin V is also better absorbed in the fasting state. Amoxicillin is equally well absorbed with food or in the fasting state. However, when amoxicillin is combined with clavulanate, absorption of clavulanate potassium is enhanced when it is administered at the start of a meal.

The bioavailability of erythromycin and azithromycin is low (about 40%), and because their bioavailability is furthered lowered in the presence of food, these drugs should be administered in the fasting state, whereas clarithromycin has better bioavailability (50%) and can be administered with or without food.

Food has no effect on the bioavailability of the fluoroquinolones, metronidazole, minocycline, doxycycline, linezolid, and trimethoprim-sulfamethoxazole. Food lowers the bioavailability of the first-generation cephalosporin cefaclor, second-generation loracarbef, and third-generation ceftibuten, but not that of the first-generation cephalosporins cephalexin and cefadroxil, second-generation cefprozil, and third-generation cefixime.

Because most drugs are absorbed from the intestinal mucosa by passive diffusion, absorption across the intestinal epithelium is enhanced if the drug is lipophilic. To this end, some oral cephalosporins are esterified (eg, cefuroxime axetil, cefpodoxime proxetil, and cefditoren pivoxil) to increase lipid solubility and enhance absorption. These prodrugs are hydrolyzed after intestinal absorption by esterases in the intestinal epithelium to their active metabolites. Nevertheless, their bioavailability is relatively low (25%–50%) and is enhanced by concomitant food intake.

Drug interactions can also alter absorption after oral administration. For example, multivalent cations such as aluminum, magnesium, and calcium in antacids can chelate the fluoroquinolones and tetracyclines, which may decrease the intestinal absorption of these antimicrobials after concurrent oral administration.

Oral absorption, of even highly bioavailable agents, may be impaired by poor circulation associated with hypotension. Gastrointestinal absorption also may be altered by ileus, colitis, bowel ischemia, and changes in gastric pH. Many of these conditions may be present in sepsis.

After oral administration, at the time when the rate of the drug entering the plasma (through absorption) and the rate of the drug disappearing from the plasma (through distribution and elimination) are equal, or at completion of IV infusion, the maximal concentration (Cmax) is reached (**Fig. 1**). Thereafter, the rate of distribution or elimination of the drug exceeds the rate of drug absorption, and the plasma concentration starts to decline to a minimal concentration. The area under the plasma concentration versus time curve (AUC, for "area under the curve") is a pharmacokinetic measure that indicates the exposure to a drug during the full dosing interval.

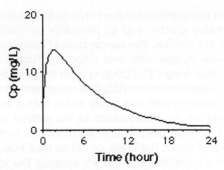

Fig. 1. A typical example of a plot of the log plasma concentration (Cp) curve over time that may be measured in plasma after administration of a single IV infusion or oral administration of an antimicrobial drug.

Distribution

Distribution is the process by which a drug diffuses from the intravascular fluid space to extravascular fluid spaces, and it is best described by the drug's volume of distribution. The volume of distribution, which is the volume of body fluid into which a drug's dose is dissolved, is an important determinant of drug concentration.

The central volume of distribution (Vc) is a hypothetical volume into which a drug initially distributes on administration. This compartment can be thought of as the plasma in blood vessels and the fluid in tissues that are highly perfused by blood. The Vc is defined mathematically as the dose administered divided by the peak plasma concentration at the end of a bolus IV infusion (Vc = dose/peak serum level). All drugs initially distribute into the smaller Vc before distributing into the more peripheral volume, referred to as the tissue volume of distribution (Vt). Together, the Vc and the Vt, in a two-compartment model, create the apparent volume of distribution (Vd). The Vd is a hypothetical parameter used to describe the volume of fluid that would be required to account for all of the drug in the body; its value may correspond to an anatomic body fluid compartment, but it does not actually represent a discrete anatomic compartment. Because the Vd is hypothetical in nature, it is referred to as an apparent volume. If the linear beta-phase elimination curve is extrapolated to the y-intercept, then the Vd equals the dose divided by this hypothetical zero-time drug concentration (see the Elimination section and **Fig. 2**).

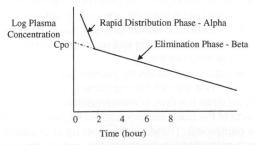

Fig. 2. A plot of the log plasma concentration (Cp) over time after rapid IV infusion. The linear beta-phase elimination curve has been extrapolated to the y-intercept to obtain the Cpo, which is the hypothetical zero-time drug concentration.

The largest body fluid compartment is the intracellular compartment. The extracellular compartment is mainly divided into an interstitial compartment (ie, the spaces between the cells) and the plasma. The percentage of body weight in each of these fluid compartments varies by age, sex, and adiposity. Total body water constitutes about 60% of the lean body weight (0.6 L/kg) in adult men and 50% (0.5 L/kg) in adult women. Fatty tissue contains proportionately less water than muscle tissue, so a more adipose person has proportionately less body water than a leaner person. A Vd of about 0.06 L/kg of body weight corresponds to the plasma compartment; a Vd of about 0.2 L/kg, or 1/3 of total body water, corresponds to the extracellular fluid compartment; and a Vd of about 0.4 L/kg, or 2/3 of total body water, corresponds to the intracellular fluid compartment. If the Vd exceeds the total body water (>0.6 L/kg), the drug is likely sequestered in the intracellular fluid of certain tissues.

For example, the Vd of daptomycin and the beta-lactam ceftriaxone, which are highly bound to plasma proteins, approximates the plasma volume because the drugs are part of a large molecular complex that does not diffuse easily out of capillaries. The Vd of most other beta-lactam antibiotics and aminoglycosides, which have lower plasma protein-binding, corresponds to the extracellular fluid compartment. Because the Vd of vancomycin varies widely (0.4–1 L/kg) as a result of highly variable distribution in the body, standard dosing of vancomycin is likely to be associated with a significant degree of variability in serum concentrations.

The Vd of quinupristin/dalfopristin, tigecycline,[1] rifampin, clindamycin, metronidazole, trimethoprim, erythromycin, clarithromycin, the tetracyclines, linezolid, and the fluoroquinolones is equal to or greater than that of total body water (≥0.6 L/kg), which suggests wide distribution of these drugs throughout the body. The Vd of azithromycin is greater than 32 L/kg, (ie, >50 times that of total body water), which suggests its sequestration within tissues.

In patients who have high total body water (eg, those who have cirrhosis or congestive heart failure, or are pregnant), the volume of distribution for a given drug may be larger than expected, and the plasma drug levels correspondingly low.[2] Sepsis and fever alone may increase the Vd of a drug.[3,4]

Most sites of infection are extravascular, and treatment of infections in these sites depends on movement of the antimicrobial agent out of the bloodstream and into interstitial and sometimes intracellular fluid. The ability of a drug to do so depends on tissue-related factors (such as perfusion to the tissues, the surface area of the tissue's vascular bed, and specialized vascular bed features, such as tight junctions or capillary pores) and drug-related factors (such as lipid solubility, molecular size, the drug's pKa, and plasma protein binding).

The perfusion rate is greatest for the brain, kidney, liver, and heart. It would be expected that drug concentrations would increase most rapidly in these organs. As the surface area of the capillary bed increases, the rate of diffusion also increases. Poor vascularity as a result of comorbid conditions (eg, large or small vessel peripheral vascular disease) results in impaired drug delivery and difficulty in achieving effective drug concentrations in the infected tissue.

Most drugs cross biologic membranes by passive diffusion. Diffusion occurs when the drug concentration on one side of the membrane is higher than that on the other side, in an attempt to equalize the drug concentration on both sides of the membrane. Capillaries in most parts of the body are fenestrated (ie, have pores between the endothelial cells lining the capillaries). These pores allow rapid diffusion of most drugs into the interstitial space. In some tissues, however, the endothelial cells are connected by "tight junctions," without the presence of capillary pores between the endothelial cells. The capillary membranes between the blood and the eye, prostate, and brain have effectively no pores. In these areas, drugs must pass through, rather than between, endothelial cells. Because biologic membranes are mainly lipid in nature, the ability of an antimicrobial drug to traverse nonfenestrated capillaries depends on its lipid solubility.

Lipid-soluble drugs, such as metronidazole and rifampin, penetrate nonfenestrated capillary beds better than drugs that are more water soluble, such as beta-lactams, aminoglycosides, and glycopeptides. In some circumstances, for example, in the use of beta-lactams to treat bacterial meningitis, this disadvantage can be overcome by increasing the dose of the drug. In other situations, such as the treatment of intra-ocular infections, topical or direct instillation is necessary to convey the drug to the site of infection.[5,6] Penetration of the antimicrobial agent into the eye and the central nervous system is further complicated by the presence of efflux pumps that actively transport some drugs, notably beta-lactams and the fluoroquinolones out of cerebro-spinal fluid and beta-lactams out of vitreous humor.[7,8] However, inflammation can partially overcome the exclusion of hydrophilic drugs into tissues that have nonfenes-trated capillary beds.

Drug levels in the interstitial fluid relate to the concentration of that portion of a drug that is not bound to plasma protein (ie, free). As an example, beta-lactams that have different percentages of plasma protein binding, when dosed to achieve similar free-plasma drug levels, will have similar interstitial fluid levels, despite having very different total plasma levels.[9] However, the penetration of vancomycin, which has serum protein binding levels of 50% or less, into epithelial lining fluid is variable, ranging from 0.4 to 8.1 mg/L after several hours, with an overall blood-to-epithelial-lining fluid penetration ratio of 6:1, and penetration is higher in the presence of lung inflammation.[10]

Only an unbound drug is considered active against microorganisms. Therefore, despite apparently adequate total plasma levels of highly protein-bound drugs, the concentration of free (ie, active) drug might be less than the MIC of the pathogen, which will necessitate the use of higher doses.[11] The clinical significance of this phenomenon was shown by the failure of cefonicid, an agent that is highly active against *Staphylococcus aureus* in vitro but is highly protein bound in vivo, to cure endocarditis caused by *S aureus*.[12]

When the drug ultimately reaches the site of infection, local factors may play a role in the effectiveness of its antibacterial activity. For example, the aminoglycosides and erythromycin have decreased activity at an acid pH, such as occurs in an abscess. The aminoglycosides are also less active against facultative organisms in an anaer-obic environment because the penetration of aminoglycosides into bacterial cells depends on an oxygen-dependent reaction.[13] Substances that inactivate or lessen the antibacterial activity of antimicrobial agents, such as beta-lactamases and other deactivating enzymes, may be present at the site.[14] As another example, aminoglyco-sides become less active as the concentration of calcium ions increases. Additionally, dense populations of organisms, such as occur in an abscess, tend to be slow growing, and antibiotics that are active against dividing cells, such as beta-lactams, may therefore be less effective in that setting.[15] Bacterial meningitis is another infec-tion in which bacterial growth rates tend to be slow, decreasing the effectiveness of beta-lactams.[16] The presence of a foreign body may also adversely influence the effectiveness of an antimicrobial agent. The foreign body acts as a nidus on which microorganisms may grow as a biofilm. A biofilm is a community of microorganisms embedded in a matrix secreted by the microorganisms, which helps them attach to other bacteria, host cells, or foreign objects and which shields them against host defenses and penetration by many antimicrobial drugs.[17,18]

For some microorganisms that are preferentially intracellular pathogens (eg, *Salmonella, Listeria, Chlamydia, Mycobacteria,* and *Mycoplasma*), the antimicrobial drugs that are effective against them must reach and be active in the intracellular space occupied by these pathogens. Clindamycin, the macrolides, and linezolid may be actively transported into cells.[8,19,20] However, drugs may be also actively transported out of cells, so the intracellular concentration reflects a balance between ingoing and outgoing processes.[21,22] Just as with interstitial fluid, local factors within the cell may affect the activity of a drug (eg, pH, enzymatic activity).

Drugs that are weak bases are un-ionized at the pH of extracellular fluid. The relatively lipid-soluble, un-ionized moiety is able to diffuse easily across the cell membrane into the cytoplasm and then into the lysosome. Within the lysosome, where the pH is relatively low, the weak base becomes ionized. The hydrophilic, ionized moiety is unable to diffuse out (ie, is "trapped" within the lysosome). This scenario is believed to explain the intracellular accumulation of azithromycin, the concentration of which can be 100-fold greater within the lysosome than within plasma. Ion trapping is also believed to explain the accumulation of drugs that are weak bases in prostatic fluid, which has a lower pH (pH 6.3) than plasma (pH 7.4). These drugs include clindamycin, erythromycin, and trimethoprim.

Elimination

Fig. 1 represents a typical example of a pharmacokinetic curve that may be seen in plasma after administration of a single IV infusion or oral administration of an antimicrobial drug. After a peak plasma drug level is attained, the plasma level declines as a consequence of drug distribution and elimination. Drugs may be eliminated by being converted to metabolites (mainly in the liver); unchanged drugs or their metabolites may be eliminated in feces or urine by the excretory organs, mainly the kidneys, liver, and gut. Some drugs or their metabolites that are excreted in bile may be reabsorbed into the bloodstream and recycled by a process called enterohepatic circulation.

Renal excretion of drugs and their metabolites is determined by three processes: glomerular filtration, tubular secretion, and passive tubular reabsorption. Most beta-lactams, the aminoglycosides, tetracycline, vancomycin, daptomycin, and the sulfonamides are excreted by the kidneys, either by glomerular filtration, tubular secretion, or both. The aminoglycosides, tetracycline, and vancomycin are excreted primarily by glomerular filtration. More than 80% to 90% of vancomycin is recovered unchanged in urine within 24 hours after administration of a single dose.[23] Only that portion of the drug that is not protein bound (ie, free) in the plasma can pass through the glomerular filter, so a high degree of protein binding can prolong the duration of highly protein-bound drugs, such as ceftriaxone, in the body. Most fluoroquinolones are eliminated primarily by renal mechanisms (eg, glomerular filtration and tubular secretion) and, to a lesser extent, by nonrenal mechanisms, such as hepatic metabolism and transepithelial intestinal elimination; the fluoroquinolone moxifloxacin, however, is eliminated mainly by nonrenal mechanisms. Tubular secretion occurs by way of two active transport mechanisms: one for anions (weak organic acids) and one for cations (weak organic bases). Competition between drugs for the carriers can occur within each transport system. The organic acid transport mechanism contributes to the elimination of many beta-lactam antibiotics, fluoroquinolones, and some sulfonamides. Competition between probenecid and these beta-lactams, fluoroquinolones, and sulfonamides for the organic acid transport carriers can prolong the duration that these antimicrobial drugs are in the body.

After filtration, polar substances are eliminated efficiently by the kidneys because they are not freely diffusible across the tubular membrane and so remain in the urine despite the concentration gradient that favors back-diffusion into interstitial fluid. Renal elimination of nonpolar drugs usually depends on metabolic conversion of the drugs in the liver to more polar metabolites, which cannot diffuse out of the tubular lumen and are then excreted in the urine. Erythromycin, azithromycin, moxifloxacin, clindamycin, rifampin, nafcillin, and cefoperazone are excreted mainly by the liver into bile; about 40% of a dose of ceftriaxone is eliminated by the liver in bile, but in the presence of renal failure, hepatic excretion increases. Doxycycline is eliminated by the gut. The streptogramin combination quinupristin/dalfopristin, the oxazolidinone linezolid, and the glycylcycline tigecycline are eliminated mainly by nonrenal mechanisms.

Colistin (also called polymyxin E) belongs to the polymyxin group of antibiotics. It is available for IV administration as colistin methanesulfonate (CMS), which is less toxic but also has less antimicrobial activity than colistin. CMS undergoes rapid hydrolysis in vivo to colistin, the bioactive drug. Notwithstanding that CMS has been used for more than 40 years, understanding of its pharmacokinetics has been problematic because previous pharmacokinetic data on CMS were obtained by using microbiological assays, which are unable to differentiate CMS from colistin. High-pressure liquid chromatography, which can distinguish both components, has shown rapid conversion of CMS to colistin in vivo. CMS is mainly eliminated in urine. The high urinary recovery of colistin after dosing with CMS, despite that fact that colistin is not itself excreted in urine, is likely the result conversion of CMS into colistin within the kidney or bladder, with the majority of the colistin formed in that way being excreted directly into urine.[24]

For most drugs, a plot of the log plasma concentration over time results in a straight line, the slope of which equals the elimination rate constant (−Kel) (**Fig. 3**). The half-life (T1/2) is the time it takes for the plasma drug concentration to decrease by half, and is equal to 0.693/Kel.

After rapid IV administration, the decline in plasma drug levels may follow a biphasic curve (see **Fig. 2**). The T1/2 of the initial phase (alpha-phase T1/2) mainly represents distribution of the drug, and the T1/2 of the second phase (beta-phase T1/2) mainly represents elimination of the drug from the body. For example, in patients who have normal creatinine clearance, vancomycin has an alpha-distribution phase of ~30 minutes to 1 hour and a beta-elimination T1/2 of 6 to 12 hours. The T1/2 that is usually reported is the beta-phase (bp) T1/2. Ninety-four percent of any drug's dose will have been eliminated after four bpT1/2s, and about 99% of the drug will have been eliminated after 6.6 bpT1/2s.

If the drug is dosed more than every 4 to 5 bpT1/2s, the drug concentration will have fallen to almost zero before the next dose, and there will then be little accumulation of

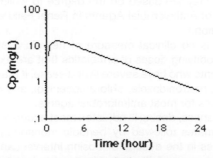

Fig. 3. A plot of the log plasma concentration (Cp) over time.

drug in the body. However, if the dosing interval is less than 4 bpT1/2s, the drug will start to accumulate, and steadily higher concentrations will occur with each subsequent dose until a steady state is achieved at about 4 bpT1/2s, when the amount of drug administered during each dosing interval exactly replaces the amount of the drug excreted. Similarly, during continuous IV infusion, plasma levels gradually increase until the steady state is achieved at about 4 bpT1/2s. When using continuous IV infusion, to ensure rapid onset of antimicrobial action, a loading dose is given. The loading dose equals the desired therapeutic plasma concentration multiplied by the Vd.

In people whose kidney or liver function has declined, the "normal" dosage of a drug may result in accumulation of the drug if the dosage or the dosing interval is not altered. Toxic side effects may occur as plasma and tissue drug concentrations increase. For example, high levels of imipenem, the penicillins, or the fluoroquinolones may cause seizures; high aminoglycoside levels may exacerbate renal failure or cause hearing impairment or vestibular damage; and high levels of vancomycin, especially in combination with aminoglycosides, may exacerbate renal failure. Therefore, the drug dosage must be adjusted based on the amount of decline in the person's kidney or liver function.

A reduction in the creatinine clearance to 30% of normal or less results in an exponential increase in the bpT1/2 of those drugs that are eliminated by the kidneys. The creatinine clearance can serve as a useful indicator of renal function. A quick estimate of the creatinine clearance can be made using this equation: creatinine clearance = [(140 − age) × ideal body weight in kg]/(serum creatinine × 72) (0.85 for females).

Males: ideal body weight = 50 kg + 2.3 kg for each inch more than 5 ft.

Females: ideal body weight = 45.5 kg + 2.3 kg for each inch more than 5 ft.

The initial dose should be the usual dose given to people with normal renal function. Subsequent doses may be reduced by a percentage based on the estimated creatinine clearance. (See "Use of Antimicrobial Agents in Renal Failure" on page 899 of this issue for details on the use of antibiotics in patients who have renal insufficiency.) An alternative measure is to lengthen the dosing interval. Lengthening the dosing interval results in a concentration versus time curve that approximates the situation in normal renal function, and therefore is preferred for drugs that exhibit concentration-dependent pharmacodynamics (see later discussion). On the other hand, using a longer dosing interval runs the risk for incurring longer periods during which the plasma level has dropped to less than the MIC of the organism, and for that reason, administration of smaller doses given at the regular interval would be preferred for drugs that exhibit time-dependent pharmacodynamics (see later discussion).[25,26]

The use of hemodialysis, peritoneal dialysis, and continuous arteriovenous hemofiltration further confounds calculations of dose modification. Guidelines for dosage modification in dialysis patients can usually be obtained from the manufacturer's product literature, and they are based on the degree to which the drug is removed by dialysis. (See "Use of Antimicrobial Agents in Renal Failure" on page 899 of this issue for more information.)

Unfortunately, there is no clinical measure of hepatic dysfunction that is easily adaptable for use in modifying doses of antibiotics that are excreted or metabolized by the liver.[27,28] In patients who have severe liver disease, it may be prudent to reduce doses of erythromycin, metronidazole, chloramphenicol, and clindamycin, but there are no specific guidelines for most antimicrobial agents.

Under ideal circumstances, dosing is adjusted most accurately by using a combination of calculated estimates followed by periodic monitoring of measured plasma concentrations. Changes in the dosage or dosing interval can be made in response to the measured levels, and follow-up plasma levels can be obtained at the appropriate time (4–5 dosing intervals), whereupon new adjustments can be made. This procedure is particularly helpful in patients whose renal (or hepatic) functioning is fluctuating. Although levels of almost any antimicrobial agent can be measured by using bioassays, radioimmunoassays, or high-pressure liquid chromatography, such laboratory studies are available only for the aminoglycosides and vancomycin, at least within a time-frame that is clinically useful.

PHARMACODYNAMICS

After a dose of a bactericidal drug, the bacterial count may decline in the early portion of the dosing interval, when levels of the portion of the drug not bound to protein exceed the MBC as a result of drug effects and host defenses (**Fig. 4**). When unbound drug levels decrease to less than the MBC but still exceed the MIC, the bacterial count may remain stable or continue to decline as a result of host defenses.[29] For a bacteriostatic drug, when drug levels are in excess of the MIC, the bacterial count declines as a result of host defenses alone. Eventually, unbound drug levels decrease to less than the MIC, at which point any persistent antibacterial effect can be due to several causes. First, persistent suppression of bacterial growth after a brief exposure of bacteria to an antibacterial agent may occur, even in the absence of host defenses; this is the postantibiotic effect (PAE). Second, after antibiotic exposure, organisms may be more susceptible than untreated bacteria to the antibacterial activity of phagocytes; this is called postantibiotic leukocyte enhancement (PALE). Third, drug concentrations that are less than the MIC have been shown to alter bacterial morphology, slow the rate of bacterial growth, and prolong the PAE. The minimal drug concentration that alters bacterial cell morphology has been termed the minimal antibacterial concentration (MAC).

Eventually, residual drug effects wane, and the remaining bacteria will begin to resume growth.[29] The extent of regrowth before the next dose is given will depend in part on the inherent doubling time of the organism, on available nutrients being present in the infected tissues, and on the adequacy of host defenses. For example,

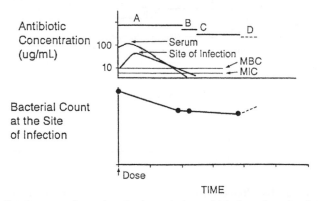

Fig. 4. Antibiotic pharmacodynamics. A, time during which free-drug levels at the site of infection exceed the MBC; B, time during which free-drug levels at the site of infection are less than the MBC but exceed the MIC; C, persistent antimicrobial effects (postantibiotic effect, postantibiotic leukocyte enhancement, and minimal antibacterial concentration) when free-drug levels at the site of infection are less than the MIC; D, regrowth of residual bacteria. (*From* Levison ME. Pharmacodynamics of antimicrobial agents: bactericidal and postantibiotic affects. Infect Dis Clin N Am 1995;9:483–95.)

in the absence of host defenses, such as occurs in early cardiac vegetation cases and in cerebrospinal fluid in cases of early meningitis, the number of microorganisms can double every 20 minutes, which is similar to the doubling time during the logarithmic phase of growth under optimal in vitro conditions (**Fig. 5**). In contrast, the numbers of *Mycobacterium tuberculosis* and *Treponema pallidum* double every 36 hours. Some regrowth may, in fact, restore susceptibility to beta-lactam antibiotics.[30]

The next dose ideally is given before clinically significant regrowth has occurred (**Fig. 6**), so that after multiple doses, the tissues are cleared of the pathogen. However, if the doses are spaced too far apart, the residual bacteria may resume growth in the later portion of each dosing interval, and the bacterial count may become equal to, or perhaps exceed, the count at the beginning of the dosing interval, which can compromise drug efficacy (**Fig. 7**).[29] The size of the residual bacterial population at the end of each dosing interval, and ultimately the efficacy of the antimicrobial regimen, thus will depend on the interplay of a variety of bacterial, drug, and host factors that includes (1) the size of the initial bacterial population, (2) the potency (MIC and MBC) and pharmacokinetic characteristics of the antimicrobial agent, (3) the rate and extent of any bactericidal effect, (4) the presence of a PAE, (5) the rate of regrowth of persistent organisms, and (6) the presence of host defenses.

Antimicrobial drugs can be divided into three main groups based on pharmacodynamic characteristics that affect bacterial clearance.[31] The first group consists of drugs that exhibit mainly time-dependent bactericidal action that has only a minimal relationship to drug concentrations that are greater than the MIC (eg, beta-lactam antibiotics and vancomycin). These drugs have relatively slow bactericidal action, and little increase in bactericidal activity is seen when concentrations are increased to more than a point of maximal killing action, which is approximately four times the MIC. These drugs have short PAEs for gram-positive cocci and no or short PAEs for gram-negative bacilli; the duration that drug levels exceed the MIC relative to the dosing interval and, consequently, the frequency of drug administration are important determinants of outcome for these drugs. A shorter dosing interval will increase the

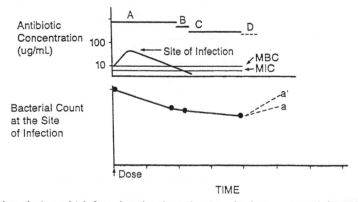

Fig. 5. A, time during which free-drug levels at the site of infection exceed the MBC; B, time during which free-drug levels at the site of infection are less than the MBC but exceed the MIC; C, persistent antimicrobial effects (PAE, MAC, and PALE) when free-drug levels at the site of infection are less than the MIC; D, regrowth of residual bacteria, with (a) and without (a') adequate host defenses. Inadequate host defenses at the site of infection may result in a higher residual bacteria population at the time the next dose is given (a'). (*From* Levison ME. Pharmacodynamics of antimicrobial agents: bactericidal and postantibiotic affects. Infect Dis Clin N Am 1995;9:483–95.)

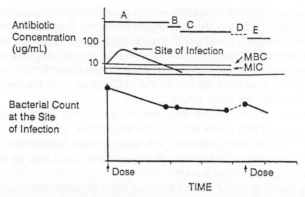

Fig. 6. A, time during which free-drug levels at the site of infection exceed the MBC; B, time during which free-drug levels at the site of infection are less than the MBC but exceed the MIC; C, persistent antimicrobial effects (PAE, MAC, and PALE) when free-drug levels at the site of infection are less than the MIC; D, regrowth of residual bacteria; E, bactericidal effect following the next dose. If the next dose is given before significant regrowth occurs, multiple doses can eventually clear bacteria from the site of infection. (*From* Levison ME. Pharmacodynamics of antimicrobial agents: bactericidal and postantibiotic affects. Infect Dis Clin N Am 1995;9:483–95.)

time that concentrations remain greater than the MIC of the infecting microorganism. (The only exceptions among the beta-lactam class are the carbapenems, which possess a PAE against a variety of gram-negative bacilli). Even a paradoxic pattern (the "Eagle effect") of bactericidal activity, which is characterized by a decreasing rate of killing at higher concentrations, has been reported. Consequently, there is no advantage to achieving high antibiotic concentrations, except that an increase in the dose will increase the duration that levels exceed the MIC and the maximal level (Cmax) in serum, which frequently results in a covariance of time and drug concentrations.

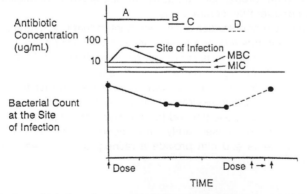

Fig. 7. A, time during which free drug levels at the site of infection exceed the MBC; B, time during which free drug levels at the site of infection are less then the MBC, but exceed the MIC; C, persistent antimicrobial effects (PAE, MAC, and PALE) when free drug levels at the site of infection are less than the MIC; D, regrowth of residual bacteria. Regrowth as a result of a longer dosing interval, which compromises drug efficacy. (*From* Levison ME. Pharmacodynamics of antimicrobial agents: bactericidal and postantibiotic affects. Infect Dis Clin N Am 1995;9:483–95.)

The second group includes drugs that exhibit concentration-dependent bactericidal action and prolonged PAEs (eg, the aminoglycosides, the fluoroquinolones, daptomycin, colistin, metronidazole, possibly the azalide azithromycin, and the ketolides). Both the rate of cidal action and the duration of the PAE for these drugs are concentration-dependent over a wide range of concentrations; consequently the amount of drug (based on the Cmax and AUC relative to the MIC) rather than the dosing frequency determines the efficacy for these drugs.

The third group includes drugs that are predominantly bacteriostatic and that produce moderate to prolonged PAEs (eg, the macrolides, clindamycin, the streptogramins such as quinupristin/dalfopristin, the tetracyclines, tigecycline, and linezolid). Because of their prolonged PAE, their efficacy is determined less by time and more by the AUC that is greater than the MIC.

Usually, drug concentrations in the blood are used to determine pharmacodynamic parameters because of the relative accessibility of this body fluid and the correlation of pharmacodynamic parameters that are based on serum levels. However, the use of serum levels to determine pharmacodynamic parameters may not always be appropriate.[31] Because infection usually occurs at extravascular sites, the use of drug concentrations in the blood will only be satisfactory if the blood levels are an adequate surrogate for levels at the site of infection. Theoretically, at equilibrium, free-drug levels in plasma and extracellular tissue fluid should be equal.[32] However, depending on the ratio of surface area of the capillary bed to the volume of the tissue compartment, the physico-chemical characteristics of the drug, and special anatomic barriers (eg, those in the brain, eye and prostate), drug levels at the site of certain infections can be much lower than free-drug levels in plasma. For cases of meningitis, the use of cerebrospinal fluid levels is appropriate for determination of pharmacodynamic parameters.[33] Recent studies also suggest that concentrations of epithelial lining fluid are important determinants of the efficacy of treatment of bacterial pneumonia, such that concentrations in epithelial lining fluid can be better predictors of outcome than serum levels for certain antibiotics (eg, vancomycin).[10] Serum drug levels are also poor predictors of intracellular concentrations, which is of major importance for the treatment of intracellular pathogens. Beta-lactams and vancomycin penetrate cells poorly, whereas other drugs, such as azithromycin, achieve intracellular concentrations many-fold greater than serum levels.

In vitro and animal model studies have documented that the magnitude of the pharmacodynamic parameters required to achieve a specific target (eg, bacteriostasis or various degrees of cidal action) is similar for different drugs within the same class.[31] For those drugs that are highly protein bound, efficacy is predicted when serum concentrations of the drug that are not bound to protein, rather than the total drug levels, are used.[31] Pharmacodynamics that are derived from in vitro and animal data are concordant with those derived from human data, with some exceptions, as detailed in a later section. Consequently, pharmacodynamics can be used to predict drug efficacy in patients and can provide a rational basis for establishing optimal dosing regimens.[34]

Time Course of Time-Dependent Bactericidal Action

Because the bactericidal action of beta-lactams is relatively slow,[29,31] there will be a relatively large residual population of microorganisms that remain when drug levels decrease to less than the MBC. After drug levels at the site of infection decrease to less than the MIC, the residual population can resume growth quickly because there are either no or short-lived PAEs for most beta-lactams.[29,31]

Beta-lactams exhibit an inoculum effect; that is, the lower the bacterial density, the lower the concentration of the beta-lactam that is required to inhibit growth.[35] The minimal concentration of these drugs that inhibits growth can progressively decrease to less than the standard MIC (determined by using an inoculum of 10^5 CFU/mL) because the bacterial count progressively falls during the time course of antimicrobial therapy, and thus the time during the dosing interval that levels exceed the MIC may progressively lengthen.

The efficacy for drugs such as the beta-lactams can be optimized by using dosing strategies that maximize the duration of drug exposure (ie, time-dependent bactericidal activity), such as using smaller fractions of the total daily dose given at frequent intervals, larger doses, beta-lactams with long serum T1/2s, such as ceftriaxone with a T1/2 of 6 to 8 hours, or longer IV infusions or even continuous IV infusion. However, there have been few trials of continuous versus intermittent infusions.[36–38]

Effective dosing regimens for time-dependent antibiotics require that serum drug concentrations exceed the MIC of the causative pathogen for at least 40% to 50% of the dosing interval. For beta-lactam drugs that have high serum protein binding (eg, ceftriaxone and ertapenem), when drug concentrations that are not bound to serum protein are used, the percentage of the dosing interval during which drug concentrations are greater than the MIC, can be used to predict efficacy; these percentages are similar for all beta-lactams within a class. The percentage of time that concentrations are greater than the MIC, which correlates with efficacy, varies among classes within the beta-lactams, and is greater for the cephalosporins and aztreonam than the penicillins, and greater for the penicillins than the carbapenems. Among bacterial species, the percentage is less for staphylococci, for which beta-lactams have a PAE, than for streptococci and gram-negative bacilli, for which beta-lactams do not have a PAE.[31] The percent of time that concentrations are greater than the MIC for a dosing interval can be used to compare the effectiveness of different time-dependent antibiotics within a class, and as a corollary, those drugs having the greater potency (ie, a lower MIC) can be anticipated to have a longer percentage of the dosing interval at which concentrations will be greater than the MIC, and therefore to have greater effectiveness.

For susceptible pathogens with MICs that are close to a particular beta-lactam's breakpoint, serum levels of the beta-lactam will be in excess of the MIC for a smaller percentage of the dosing interval than for strains that have lower MICs. For example, patients infected with borderline cephalosporin-sensitive ESBL-producing strains of gram-negative bacilli with MICs from 4 to 8 μg/mL did much worse when treated using cephalosporin monotherapy than did patients infected with strains having lower MICs.[39] Similarly, free-drug levels of ceftriaxone can not remain at concentrations greater than the MICs for more than 50% of the 24-hour dosing interval for strains of S aureus, which have MICs close to the breakpoint, especially with a 1-g dose. Also, extending the dosing interval of cefoperazone (which may be no longer available in the United States), which has relatively high serum-protein binding and a short bpT1/2 (2 hours), from 6 or 8 hours to 12 hours for susceptible strains of Pseudomonas aeruginosa that have MICs close to the breakpoint of 16 μg/mL may be similarly problematic.

The glycopeptides vancomycin and teicoplanin demonstrate concentration-independent (ie, time-dependent), slow bactericidal activity and a short PAE in vitro. However, there is conflicting data about which pharmacodynamic parameter best predicts bacterial eradication and clinical outcome. For example, studies that used an in vivo rabbit model of S aureus aortic valve endocarditis[40] and clinical studies of S aureus septicemia[41] and endocarditis[42] showed that the glycopeptides exhibit time-dependent action, with the trough plasma concentration of protein free vancomycin that is greater than the MIC being the therapeutically relevant pharmacodynamic parameter. In contrast, in a study of patients who had a S aureus lower respiratory tract infection, clinical and bacteriologic response to vancomycin therapy was correlated with the 24 hour AUC/MIC value, but no relationship was identified between outcome and vancomycin the percentage of time that concentrations were greater than the MIC.[43] In another study of patients who had S aureus bacteremia (MIC range 0.25–1.0 mg/L), no relationship was found between successful outcomes and a specific AUC/MIC value.[44] In clinical practice, maintenance of trough serum levels of free drug that are greater than the MIC is most commonly recommended.[45]

If the rate of cidal action of beta-lactams or vancomycin were increased, lower residual bacterial counts would occur during the dosing interval, when drug levels decrease to less than the MIC; this would prolong the intervals before significant regrowth occurs and either allow for more extended dosing intervals or allow for shorter durations of therapy as a consequence of accelerated clearance of bacteria from sites of infection (**Fig. 8**). Indeed, combinations of these antibiotics with aminoglycosides can enhance the relatively slow rate of bactericidal activity of beta-lactams and vancomycin. For example, a bacterial cell-wall-active agent alone, such as penicillin, ampicillin, or vancomycin, is at best only slowly bactericidal against enterococci, and an aminoglycoside alone at concentrations achieved in serum after standard dosing exhibits only inhibitory activity, but the combination of the cell-wall-active agent with an aminoglycoside results in rapid bactericidal activity. The synergy achieved by the combination has been shown to be due to the enhanced bacterial penetration of the aminoglycoside in the presence of the cell-wall-active agent.

Synergistic bactericidal activity, usually defined as achieving a $2\log_{10}$ or greater (ie, $\geq 99\%$) reduction in bacterial count after overnight incubation using a combination of antibiotics versus the outcome using each of the agents alone. Synergism has also been shown when using combinations of cell-wall-active agents and aminoglycosides against viridans streptococci, S aureus, and many gram-negative bacilli. Synergistic

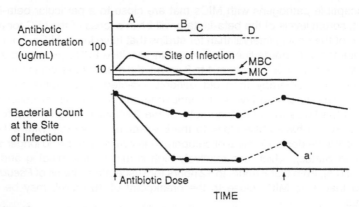

Fig. 8. A, time during which free drug levels at the site of infection exceed the MBC; B, time during which free drug levels at the site of infection are less than the MBC, but exceed the MIC; C, persistant antimicrobial effects (PAE, MAC, and PALE) when free drug levels at the site of infection are less than the MIC; D, regrowth of residual bacteria. The effect of more rapid and extensive bactericidal action (a') on the residual bacterial population despite prolongation of the dosing interval. (*From* Levison ME. Pharmacodynamics of antimicrobial agents: bactericidal and postbiotic affects. Infect Dis Clin N Am 1995;9:483–95.)

combinations that more rapidly clear the tissues of the infecting microorganism have been used to shorten the course of antimicrobial therapy for viridans streptococcal endocarditis (penicillin or ceftriaxone plus gentamicin for 2 weeks versus penicillin or ceftriaxone alone for 4 weeks) and for uncomplicated, methicillin-sensitive, S aureus, right-sided endocarditis (nafcillin plus gentamicin for 2 weeks versus nafcillin alone for 4 weeks).

Some combinations of antimicrobial agents have been found to be antagonistic (eg, penicillin plus a tetracycline). In such cases, the penicillin's bactericidal effect, which requires the presence of growing organisms, may be converted to a bacteriostatic effect when combined with a tetracycline that prevents microbial growth. This has been the explanation for the findings of Lepper and Dowling,[46] in which patients who had pneumococcal meningitis and were treated using penicillin combined with a tetracycline had 2.6-fold greater mortality than those patients treated using penicillin alone.

Time Course of Concentration-Dependent Bactericidal Action

For drugs that have concentration-dependent bactericidal action, such as aminoglycosides and fluoroquinolones, the rate of bactericidal activity will be maximum at the peak concentration (Cmax) in serum.[47–49] As the drug concentration decreases, the rate of bactericidal activity will decrease. Higher doses of the drug will increase not only the rate of reduction of bacteria but also the length of time of drug exposure to bactericidal concentrations. This dependence on the magnitude and the duration of exposure of bactericidal concentrations implies that concentration-dependent drugs are influenced by the Cmax and the area under the serum concentration curve (AUC), whereas for drugs with time-dependent activity, the extent of bactericidal activity will depend mainly on the duration of drug exposure at concentrations great than the MIC.

After drug levels at the site of infection decrease to concentrations that are less than the MIC, there may be persistent suppression of growth that is due to a PAE, the duration of which is also concentration-dependent for aminoglycosides and fluoroquinolones; the higher the drug concentration, the longer the duration of the PAE for these drugs, and the smaller the residual bacterial population at the time of the next dose.

Indeed, effective dosing regimens for concentration-dependent antibiotics require that either the 24-hour protein-free drug AUC/MIC value be at least 100 to 125 for aminoglycosides or fluoroquinolones against gram-negative bacilli[3,49,50] and from 25 to 30 for fluoroquinolones against S pneumoniae,[51,52] or that the Cmax/MIC value of the causative pathogen be more than 10.[53,54] For concentration-dependent drugs, dosing strategies that maximize the intensity of drug exposure, such as giving the total daily dose as a single dose every 24 hours rather than giving smaller divided doses, would maximize the Cmax and possibly allow for comparable efficacy at greater convenience and lower cost.[55]

The AUC/MIC or the Cmax/MIC ratios also can be used to compare the effectiveness of different concentration-dependent antibiotics. Drugs within a class having the greater potency (ie, lower MICs) will have higher AUC/MIC or Cmax/MIC ratios and therefore can be anticipated to have greater effectiveness. It is clear that an infection caused by susceptible pathogens that have relatively high MICs may not be adequately treated using the standard dosage of a concentration-dependent antimicrobial agent. For example, gentamicin-susceptible strains of P aeruginosa that have MICs close to the breakpoint for gentamicin of 4 µg/mL may respond suboptimally to standard dosing regimens that provide peak serum levels of gentamicin of

6 μg/mL. Similarly, ciprofloxacin-susceptible strains of *P aeruginosa* that have MICs close to the breakpoint of 2 μg/mL may respond suboptimally to standard dosing regimens that provide peak plasma levels of ciprofloxacin of about 3 to 4 μg/mL, and levofloxacin-susceptible strains of *S pneumoniae* with MICs close to the breakpoint of 2 μg/mL may respond suboptimally to 500-mg dosing regimens that provide peak plasma levels of levofloxacin of about 5 to 6 μg/mL and an AUC of 55. A 750-mg dose of levofloxacin doubles the peak level and the AUC.[56] The higher Cmax and AUC achieved using the higher dosage allow greater confidence in treating patients who may be infected with organisms for which levofloxacin MICs are high.

Higher rates of bactericidal action result in lower residual bacterial counts and longer intervals before significant regrowth occurs (see **Fig. 8**). Maximizing serum concentrations of drugs that exhibit concentration-dependent bactericidal activity by increasing the dose will maximize the rate and extent of bactericidal activity, if adverse effects are not also concentration-dependent. Dose-dependent toxicity was once believed to limit the ability to administer the total daily dose of an aminoglycoside as a single dose every 24 hours, but data from animal models of infection and human clinical trials suggest that dosing regimens that provide very high peak aminoglycoside concentrations relative to the MIC and prolonged periods of subinhibitory aminoglycoside concentrations have not resulted in greater nephrotoxicity than regimens that provide lower peaks but more persistent inhibitory concentrations,[57] although the relationship between the pharmacodynamic parameters and auditory and vestibular toxicity is unclear. Giving the total 24-hour dose as a single dose, rather than in smaller divided doses, and using extended dosing intervals has now become the standard in most clinical settings.[3] This strategy may be especially appropriate for treatment of many susceptible pathogens, (eg, *P aeruginosa*) that have MICs that are close to the breakpoint.[58] However, this same strategy may not be appropriate for fluoroquinolones that likely have concentration-dependent toxicity.

All aminoglycosides have similar pharmacokinetics, but there is significant variation in pharmacokinetics in normal individuals and certain patient populations. For example, volume of distribution tends to be elevated in critically ill patients, and clearance is elevated in children, in patients who have cystic fibrosis, and during pregnancy and the early postpartum period, and it is depressed in cases of renal insufficiency. The Cmax is primarily affected by the volume of distribution, and the AUC by the volume of distribution and clearance. Consequently, measurement of aminoglycoside levels is especially important early in the course of treatment, and doses should be adjusted to achieve therapeutic levels.[59]

Colistin, which is available as CMS, has been increasingly used intravenously for otherwise pan-resistant, nosocomial, gram-negative bacillary infections, especially those caused by *P aeruginosa*, *Klebsiella pneumoniae*, and *Acinetobacter* spp. Colistin demonstrates very rapid concentration-dependent killing action.[60–63] Although the concentration-dependent killing action of colistin suggests that single daily dosing rather than divided dosing may be necessary, its lack of a significant PAE at clinical achievable concentrations indicates that infrequent dosing regimens may be problematic.[62] Furthermore, the frequent emergence of colistin resistance after initial rapid killing of susceptible *P aeruginosa* and the emergence of colistin-heteroresistant strains of *K pneumoniae* and *Acinetobacter* spp suggest that colistin monotherapy may be inadequate.[61,63–67]

Bacteriostatic Activity

Erythromycin has exhibited time-dependent efficacy in various models; in contrast, it has been stated that the efficacy of azithromycin and the ketolide antibiotic telithromycin is correlated best with the AUC/MIC ratio.[68] It has been theorized that the prolonged PAE observed with azithromycin reduces the drug's dependency on the extent of time for which it should remain at concentrations greater than the MIC. However, the persistence of resistant subpopulations of S pneumoniae and their subsequent emergence may be encouraged by the presence of prolonged periods of sub-MIC concentrations of azithromycin in epithelial lining fluid.

A variety of in vitro and in vivo studies have demonstrated that the streptogramins exhibit concentration-independent killing action and produce prolonged PAEs in gram-positive organisms.[69] The efficacy of the streptogramins, which are characterized by this pattern of activity, is best correlated with the 24-hour AUC/MIC ratio. The 24-hour AUC/MIC ratio is also the pharmacodynamic parameter that can best be used to predict the in-vivo activity of clindamycin in a pneumococcal, neutropenic, murine thigh-infection model[70] The 24-hour AUC/MIC ratio is also the pharmacodynamic parameter that can best be used to predict the in-vivo activity of tigecycline.[1,71,72]

A review of the pharmacodynamics of linezolid was published.[31] In animal models, the 24-hour AUC/MIC ratio correlated best with the efficacy of a drug,[73] although the percentage of time that concentrations were greater than the MIC and the 24-hour AUC/MIC ratio was found to correlate with efficacy in clinical trials.[74] The chance of success in treating bacteremia, lower respiratory tract infection, and skin and skin structure infections was greater when linezolid plasma concentrations remained in excess of the MIC for the entire dosing interval. Although linezolid shows bactericidal action against S pneumoniae,[75] it is mainly bacteriostatic against S aureus. In a rabbit S aureus endocarditis model, linezolid was bactericidal if the levels were maintained constantly at concentrations that were greater than the MIC by using continuous infusion, and it was only bacteriostatic when administered by using intermittent infusion.[76] Linezolid penetrates epithelial lining fluid better than vancomycin, at levels threefold greater than simultaneous serum levels.[77]

PREVENTION OF RESISTANCE

Subpopulations that have reduced susceptibility to antibiotics are a normal feature of dense populations of some bacterial species, especially P aeruginosa, A baumanii, K pneumoniae, and S aureus. The likelihood that resistant subpopulations will emerge when using antimicrobial therapy will depend on the propensity for resistance within the population, that is, on the spontaneous mutation rate for antibiotic resistance, the ability of host defenses to control the growth of the resistant subpopulation, and the magnitude of the antimicrobial drug levels at the site of infection.[78] It is believed that drug levels should exceed at least 8 to 10 times the MIC to prevent emergence of resistant subpopulations, which could be accomplished by using a single daily dosing of an aminoglycoside, using the most potent fluoroquinolone, or using high doses of a beta-lactam. In vitro and animal models of infection have identified the peak MIC ratios and free-drug 24-hour AUC/MIC ratios for fluoroquinolones that are required to prevent the emergence of resistant subpopulations. The minimal prevention dose, which has been shown to vary among bacterial species, is higher for denser bacterial populations and is often higher than the ratios required for efficacy.[34,79] The clinical utility of high-dose antimicrobial therapy to prevent the emergence of resistance remains to be proved.[80]

USE OF PHARMACODYNAMIC BREAKPOINTS FOR ANTIMICROBIAL SUSCEPTIBILITY TESTING

For time-dependent drugs, the minimal serum concentration of free drug that is present for 40% to 50% of the dosing interval is the important parameter for predicting efficacy and can be determined if the peak serum level of free drug after a particular dose regimen and the serum T1/2 of the drug are known. This concentration is the pharmacodynamic breakpoint for time-dependent drugs. If the MIC of the drug that is effective against a particular pathogen or the MIC_{90} strains of the drug that is effective against a group of clinical isolates of a particular pathogen are at concentrations that are less than this breakpoint, the drug is likely to be clinically useful, and if concentrations are greater than this breakpoint, the drug may not be useful. For example, a 500-mg dose of amoxicillin given every 8 hours or an 875-mg dose given every 12 hours yields a concentration of at least 2 μg/mL for 40% to 50% of the dosing interval, and the MIC_{90} for amoxicillin against S pneumoniae in the United States is currently less than this breakpoint, allowing for the prediction of clinical success when using these dosing regimens of amoxicillin. The same calculations for defined dosing regimens can be done for other time-dependent drugs to determine their pharmacodynamic breakpoints.[81]

For concentration-dependent drugs, successful treatment of pneumococcal infections using the fluoroquinolones or azithromycin requires a 24-hour protein-free drug AUC/MIC ratio that is greater than 25 to 35, and successful treatment of gram-negative bacillary infections requires a 24-hour protein-free drug AUC/MIC ratio that is greater than 100–125 or a peak serum level that has a free-drug/MIC ratio that is greater than 8 to 10.[82] The pharmacodynamic clinical breakpoint MIC can be calculated by using the following formula: for S pneumoniae, AUC/25, and for gram-negative bacilli, AUC/100, when the average AUC from the dosing regimen is known.[81] Similarly, the pharmacodynamic clinical breakpoint MIC can be calculated by using the following formula: peak serum level of free drug/10. For ciprofloxacin, the peak serum level after a 400-mg IV dose is about 4 μg/mL of the total drug and 2.8 μg/mL of the free drug; the respective pharmacodynamic breakpoint MIC would be 0.4 and 0.28 μg/mL for the total drug and free drug; strains of S pneumoniae that have an MIC that is greater than 0.28 μg/mL would be considered to be resistant, those with an MIC of 0.28 μg/mL or less would be considered to be sensitive.

SUMMARY

The importance of pharmacodynamic factors in developing optimal treatment strategies has been confirmed in many studies of in vitro models, in models of infection in animals that attempt to simulate human infections, and in clinical studies. The requirements for bactericidal therapy for endocarditis and meningitis, for synergistic combinations to treat enterococcal endocarditis or to shorten the course of antimicrobial therapy, for obtaining Cmax/MIC ratios that are greater than 10 or 24 hour protein-free drug AUC/MIC ratios that are greater than 100–125 for concentration-dependent agents against gram-negative bacilli and 25 to 35 against S pneumoniae, and for the percentage of time that concentrations are greater than an MIC that is at least 40% to 50% of the dosing interval for time-dependent agents are a few important pharmacodynamic concepts that have been demonstrated in animal models and that that have successfully guided therapy of human infections. Pharmacodynamic concepts can also be used to optimize dosing to prevent the emergence of resistance and to rationalize the determination of antimicrobial susceptibility.

REFERENCES

1. Meagher AK, Ambrose PG, Grasela TH, et al. Pharmacokinetic/pharmacodynamic profile for tigecycline—a new glycylcycline antimicrobial agent. Diagn Microbiol Infect Dis 2005;52(3):165–71.

2. Turnidge J. Pharmacodynamics and dosing of aminoglycosides. Infect Dis Clin North Am 2003;17(3):503–28.

3. Buijk SE, Mouton JW, Gyssens IC, et al. Experience with a once-daily dosing program of aminoglycosides in critically ill patients. Intensive Care Med 2002; 28(7):936–42.

4. Tod M, Lortholary O, Seytre D, et al. Population pharmacokinetic study of amikacin administered once or twice daily to febrile, severely neutropenic adults. Antimicrob Agents Chemother 1998;42(4):849–56.

5. Leeming JP. Treatment of ocular infections with topical antibacterials. Clin Pharmacokinet 1999;37(5):351–60.

6. Smith A, Pennefather PM, Kaye SB, et al. Fluoroquinolones: place in ocular therapy. Drugs 2001;61(6):747–61.

7. Tamai I, Yamashita J, Kido Y, et al. Limited distribution of new quinolone antibacterial agents into brain caused by multiple efflux transporters at the blood–brain barrier. J Pharmacol Exp Ther 2000;295(1):146–52.

8. Barza M. Pharmacologic principles. In: Gorbach S, Bartlett JG, Blacklow NR, editors, Infectious diseases, vol. 3. Philadelphia: Lippincott Williams & Wilkins; 2004. p. 172–9.

9. Tan JS, Salstrom SJ. Levels of carbenicillin, ticrcillin, cephalothin, cefazolin, cefamandole, gentamicin, tobramycin, and amikacin in human serum and interstitial fluid. Antimicrob Agents Chemother 1977;11:698–700.

10. Lamer C, de Beco V, Soler P, et al. Analysis of vancomycin entry into pulmonary lining fluid by bronchoalveolar lavage in critically ill patients. Antimicrob Agents Chemother 1993;37:281–6.

11. Garrison MW, Vance-Bryan K, Larson TA, et al. Assessment of effects of protein binding on daptomycin and vancomycin killing of Staphylococcus aureus by using an in vitro pharmacodynamic model. Antimicrob Agents Chemother 1990;34:1925–31.

12. Chambers HF, Mills J, Drake TA, et al. Failure of a once-daily regimen of cefonicid for treatment of endocarditis due to Staphylococcus aureus. Rev Infect Dis 1984; 6(Suppl 4):s870–4.

13. Bryan LE, Van den Elzen HM. Streptomycin accumulation in susceptible and resistant strains of Escherichia coli and Pseudomonas aeruginosa. Antimicrob Agents Chemother 1976;9(6):928–38.

14. Bamberger DM, Herndon BL, Suvarna PR. The effect of zinc on microbial growth and bacterial killing by cefazolin in a Staphylococcus aureus abscess milieu. J Infect Dis 1993;168(4):893–6.

15. Neu HC. General concepts on the chemotherapy of infectious diseases. Med Clin North Am 1987;71(6):1051–64.

16. Plorde JJ, Hovland D, Garcia M, et al. Studies on the pathogenesis of meningitis. V. Action of penicillin in experimental pneumococcal meningitis. J Lab Clin Med 1965;65:71–80.

17. Quie PG, Belani KK. Coagulase-negative staphylococcal adherence and persistence. J Infect Dis 1987;156(4):543–7.

18. Stewart PS, Costerton JW. Antibiotic resistance of bacteria in biofilms. Lancet 2001;358(9276):135–8.

19. Carryn S, Van Bambeke F, Mingeot-Leclercq MP, et al. Comparative intracellular (THP-1 macrophage) and extracellular activities of beta-lactams, azithromycin, gentamicin, and fluoroquinolones against Listeria monocytogenes at clinically relevant concentrations. Antimicrob Agents Chemother 2002;46(7): 2095–103.

20. Pascual A, Ballesta S, Garcia I, et al. Uptake and intracellular activity of linezolid in human phagocytes and nonphagocytic cells. Antimicrob Agents Chemother 2002;46(12):4013–5.

21. Carryn S, Chanteux H, Seral C, et al. Intracellular pharmacodynamics of antibiotics. Infect Dis Clin North Am 2003;17(3):615–34.

22. Van Bambeke F, Michot JM, Tulkens PM. Antibiotic efflux pumps in eukaryotic cells: occurrence and impact on antibiotic cellular pharmacokinetics, pharmacodynamics and toxicodynamics. J Antimicrob Chemother 2003;51(5):1067–77.

23. Matzke GR, Zhanel GG, Guay DR. Clinical pharmacokinetics of vancomycin. Clin Pharmacokinet 1986;11:257–82.

24. Milne RW, Nation RL, Turnidge JD, et al. Pharmacokinetics of colistin methanesulphonate and colistin in rats following an intravenous dose of colistin methanesulphonate. J Antimicrob Chemother 2004;53:837–40.

25. Bush LM, Levison ME. Antibiotic selection and pharmacokinetics in the critically ill. Crit Care Clin 1988;4(2):299–324.

26. Beringer PM, Vinks AA, Jelliffe RW, et al. Pharmacokinetics of tobramycin in adults with cystic fibrosis: implications for once-daily administration. Antimicrob Agents Chemother 2000;44(4):809–13.

27. Verbeeck RK, Horsmans Y. Effect of hepatic insufficiency on pharmacokinetics and drug dosing. Pharm World Sci 1998;20(5):183–92.

28. Westphal JF, Brogard JM. Drug administration in chronic liver disease. Drug Saf 1997;17(1):47–73.

29. Ingerman MJ, Pitsakis PG, Rosenberg AF, et al. The importance of pharmacodynamics in determining the dosing interval in therapy for experimental *Pseudomonas endocarditis* in the rat. J Infect Dis 1986;153:707–14.

30. Stevens DL, Yan S, Bryant AE. Penicillin-binding protein expression at different growth stages determines penicillin efficacy in vitro and in vivo: an explanation for the inoculum effect. J Infect Dis 1993;167:1401–5.

31. Craig WA. Basic pharmacodynamics of antimicrobials with clinical applications to the use of beta-lactams, glycopeptides, and linezolid. Infect Dis Clin North Am 2003;17:479–502.

32. Barza M, Cuchural G. General principles of antibiotic tissue penetration. J Antimicrob Chemother 1985;15(Suppl A):59–75.

33. Lutsar I, McCracken GH, Friedland IA. Antibiotic pharmacodynamics in cerebrospinal fluid. Clin Infect Dis 1998;42:2650–9.

34. Ambrose PG, Bhavnani SM, Owens RC. Clinical pharmacodynamics of quinolones. Infect Dis Clin North Am 2003;17:529–43.

35. Brook I. Inoculum effect. Rev Infect Dis 1989;11:361–8.

36. Kasiakou SK, Lawrence KR, Choulis N, et al. Continuous versus intermittent administration of antibacterials with time-dependent action: a systematic review of pharmacokinetic and pharmacodynamic parameters. Drugs 2005;65(17): 2499–511.

37. Drusano GL, Preston SL, Fowler C, et al. Relationship between fluoroquinolone area under the curve: minimum inhibitory concentration ratio and the probability of eradication of the infecting pathogen, in patients with nosocomial pneumonia. J Infect Dis 2004;189(9):1590–7.

38. Roberts JA, Paratz J, Paratz E, et al. Continuous infusion of beta-lactam antibiotics in severe infections: a review of its role. Int J Antimicrob Agents 2007; 30(1):11–8.

39. Paterson DL, Ko WC, Von Gottberg A, et al. Outcome of cephalosporin treatment for serious infections due to apparently susceptible organisms producing

extended-spectrum beta-lactamases: implications for the clinical microbiology laboratory. J Clin Microbiol 2001;39:2206–12.

40. Chambers HF, Kennedy S. Effects of dosage peak and trough concentrations in serum, protein binding, and bactericidal rate on efficacy of teicoplanin in a rabbit model of endocarditis. Antimicrob Agents Chemother 1990;34:510–4.

41. Harding I, MacGowan AP, White LO, et al. Teicoplanin therapy for *Staphylococcus aureus* septicaemia: relationship between pre-dose serum concentrations and outcome. J Antimicrob Chemother 2000;45:835–41.

42. Wilson APR, Gruneberg RN, Neu H. A critical review of the dosage teicoplanin in Europe and the USA. Int J Antimicrob Agents 1991;4(Suppl 1):s1–30.

43. Moise-Broder PA, Forrest A, Birmingham MC, et al. Pharmacodynamics of vancomycin and other antimicrobials in patients with *Staphylococcus aureus* lower respiratory tract infections. Clin Pharmacokinet 2004;43(13):925–42.

44. Drew RH, Lu I, Joyce M, et al. Lack of relationship between predicted area under the time-concentration curve/minimum inhibitory concentration and outcome in vancomycin-treated patients with Staphylococcus aureus bacteremia, [abstract A-1493]. In: Program and abstracts of the 44th Interscience Conference on Antimicrobial Agents and Chemotherapy (Oct 30–Nov 2, 2004; Washington, DC). Washington, DC: American Society for Microbiology.

45. Rybak MJ, Lomaestro BM, Rotscahfer JC, et al. Vancomycin therapeutic guidelines: a summary of consensus recommendations from the Infectious Diseases Society of America, the American Society of Health-System Pharmacists, and the Society of Infectious Diseases Pharmacists. Clin Infect Dis 2009;49:325–7.

46. Lepper M, Dowling H. Treatment of pneumococcal meningitis with penicillin compared with penicillin plus aureomycin. Arch Intern Med 1951;88:489–94.

47. Drusano GL. Human pharmacodynamics of beta-lactams, aminoglycosides and their combination. Scand J Infect Dis Suppl 1991;74:235–48.

48. Lacy MK, Nicolau DP, Nightingale CH, et al. The pharmacodynamics of aminoglycosides. Clin Infect Dis 1998;27:23–7.

49. Lode H, Borner K, Koeppe P. Pharmacodynamics of fluoroquinolones. Clin Infect Dis 1998;27:33–9.

50. Forrest A, Nix DE, Ballow CH, et al. Pharmacodynamics of intravenous ciprofloxacin in seriously ill patients. Antimicrob Agents Chemother 1993;37:1073–81.

51. Woodnut G. Pharmacodynamics to combat resistance. J Antimicrob Chemother 2000;46:25–31.

52. Lister PD, Sanders CC. Pharmacodynamics of moxifloxacin, levofloxacin, and sparfloxacin against *Streptococcus pneumoniae* in an in vitro pharmacodynamic model. J Antimicrob Chemother 2001;47:811–8.

53. Preston SL, Dursano GL, Berman AL, et al. Pharmacodynamics of levofloxacin. A new paradigm for early clinical trials. JAMA 1998;279:125–9.

54. Moore RD, Leitman PS, Smith CR. Clinical response to aminoglycoside therapy: importance of the ration of peak concentration to minimum inhibitory concentration. J Infect Dis 1987;155:93–9.

55. Drusano GL, Ambrose PG, Bhavnani SM, et al. Back to the future: using aminoglycosides again and how to dose them optimally. Clin Infect Dis 2007;45(6):753–60.

56. Chow AT, Fowler C, Williams RR, et al. Safety and pharmacokinetics of multiple 750-milligram doses of intravenous levofloxacin in healthy volunteers. Antimicrob Agents Chemother 2001;45(7):2122–5.

57. Rybak MJ, Abate BJ, Kang SL, et al. Prospective evaluation of the effect of an aminoglycoside dosing regimen on rates of observed nephrotoxicity and ototoxicity. Antimicrob Agents Chemother 1999;43:1549–65.

58. Nicolau DP, Freeman CD, Belliveau, et al. Experience with once-daily aminogly-coside program administered to 2,184 adult patients. Antimicrob Agents Chemo-ther 1995;39:650–5.
59. Watling SM, Dasta JF. Aminoglycoside dosing considerations in intensive care unit patients. Ann Pharmacother 1993;27:351–6.
60. Li J, Turnidge J, Milne R, et al. In vitro pharmacodynamic properties of colistin and colistin methanesulfonate against *Pseudomonas aeruginosa* isolates from patients with cystic fibrosis. Antimicrob Agents Chemother 2001;45(3):781–5.
61. Owen RJ, Li J, Nation RL, et al. In vitro pharmacodynamics of colistin against *Acinetobacter baumanii* clinical isolates. J Antimicrob Chemother 2007;59:473–7.
62. Bergen PJ, Li J, Nation RL, et al. Comparison of once-, twice- and thrice-daily dosing of colistin on antibacterial effect and emergence of resistance: studies with *Pseudomonas aeruginosa* in an in vitro pharmacodynamic model. J Antimi-crob Chemother 2008;61(3):636–42.
63. Poudyal A, Howden BP, Bell JM, et al. In vitro pharmacodynamics of colistin against multidrug-resistant *Klebsiella pneumoniae*. J Antimicrob Chemother 2008;62(6):1311–8.
64. Rahal JJ. Novel antibiotic combinations against infections with almost completely resistant *Pseudomonas aeruginosa* and *Acinetobacter* species. Clin Infect Dis 2006;43(Suppl 2):S95–9.
65. Chitnis S, Chitnis V, Chitnis DS. In vitro synergistic activity of colistin with amino-glycosides, beta-lactams and rifampin against multidrug-resistant gram-negative bacteria. J Chemother 2007;19(2):226–9.
66. Petrosillo N, Ioannidou E, Falagas ME. Colistin monotherapy vs. combination therapy: evidence from microbiological, animal and clinical studies. Clin Micro-biol Infect 2008;14(9):816–27.
67. Song JY, Lee J, Heo JY, et al. Colistin and rifampicin combination in the treatment of ventilator-associated pneumonia caused by carbapenem-resistant *Acineto-bacter baumanii*. Int J Antimicrob Agents 2008;32(3):281–4.
68. Maglio D, Nicolau DP, Nightingale CH. Impact of pharmacodynamics on dosing of macrolides, azalides and ketolides. Infect Dis Clin North Am 2003;17:563–77.
69. Carbon C. Pharmacodynamics of macrolides, azalides, and streptogramins: effect on extracellular pathogens. Clin Infect Dis 1998;27:28–32.
70. Christianson J, Andes DR, Craig WA. Pharmacodynamic characteristics of clin-damycin against Streptococcus pneumoniae in a murine thigh-infection model. In: Program and abstracts of the 41st Interscience Conference on Antimicrobial Agents and Chemotherapy (2001: Chicago, IL). Abstr Intersci Conf Antimicrob Agents Chemother. 2001, Dec 16–19; 41: abstract no. A-1100. Washington, DC: American Society for Microbiology.
71. Passarell JA, Meagher AK, Liolios K, et al. Exposure-response analyses of tige-cycline efficacy in patients with complicated intra-abdominal infections. Antimi-crob Agents Chemother 2008;52(1):204–10 [Epub 2007 Oct 22].
72. Meagher AK, Passarell JA, Cirincione BB, et al. Exposure-response analyses of tigecycline efficacy in patients with complicated skin and skin-structure infections. Antimicrob Agents Chemother 2007;51(6):1939–45 [Epub 2007 Mar 12].
73. Andes D, van Ogtrop ML, Peng J, et al. In vivo pharmacodynamics of a new oxazolidinone (linezolid). Antimicrob Agents Chemother 2002;46:3484–9.
74. Rayner CR, Forrest A, Meagher AK, et al. Clinical pharmacodynamics of linezolid in seriously ill patients treated in a compassionate use programme. Clin Pharma-cokinet 2003;42:1411–23.

75. Cha R, Akins RL, Ryback MJ. Linezolid, levofloxacin and vancomycin against vancomycin-tolerant and fluoroquinolone-resistant *Streptococcus pneumoniae* in an in vitro pharmacodynamic model. Pharmacotherapy 2003;23:1531–7.
76. Jacqueline C, Batard E, Perez L, et al. In vivo efficacy of continuous infusion versus intermittent dosing of linezolid compared to vancomycin in a methicillin-resistant *Staphylococcus aureus* rabbit endocarditis model. Antimicrob Agents Chemother 2002;46:3706–11.
77. Conte JE, Golden JA, Kipps J, et al. Intrapulmonary pharmacokinetics of linezolid. Antimicrob Agents Chemother 2002;26:1475–80.
78. Rybak MJ. Pharmacodynamics: relation to antimicrobial resistance. Am J Infect Control 2006;34(5 Suppl 1):s38–45 [discussion: s64–73].
79. Wispelwey B. Clinical implications of pharmacokinetics and pharmacodynamics of fluoroquinolones. Clin Infect Dis 2005;41(Suppl 2):s127–35.
80. Falagas ME, Bliziotis IA, Rafailidis PI. Do high doses of quinolones decrease the emergence of antibacterial resistance? A systematic review of data from comparative clinical trials. J Infect 2007;55(2):97–105.
81. Jacobs MR. Optimization of antimicrobial therapy using pharmacokinetic and pharmacodynamic parameters. Clin Microbiol Infect 2001;7:589–96.
82. Craig WA. Does the dose matter? Clin Infect Dis 2001;33:s233–7.

Pathogens Resistant to Antibacterial Agents

Luke F. Chen, MBBS (Hons), CIC, FRACP[a],*, Teena Chopra, MD[b],
Keith S. Kaye, MD, MPH[c]

KEYWORDS

- Drug resistance • Methicillin-resistant *Staphylococcus aureus*
- Vancomycin-resistant *Enterococcus*
- Vancomycin intermediate-susceptible *Staphylococcus aureus*
- Extended-spectrum β-lactamase
- Penicillin-resistant *Streptococcus pneumoniae*
- *Klebsiella pneumoniae* carbapenemase
- *Acinetobacter baumanii*

Multidrug-resistant pathogens historically were limited to the hospital setting. In the 1990s, multidrug-resistant pathogens were described to be affecting outpatients in health care–associated settings (nursing homes, dialysis centers, infusion centers, among patients recently hospitalized). More recently, multidrug-resistant pathogens have become major issues in the community, affecting persons with limited or in many cases no contact with health care. This article reviews the molecular mechanisms by which resistance traits are conferred and disseminated and the epidemiology of such bacterial resistance.

MECHANISMS OF RESISTANCE

It is important to distinguish the many ways by which an organism may demonstrate resistance. Intrinsic resistance to an antimicrobial agent characterizes resistance that is an inherent attribute of a particular species; all organisms of the species may lack the appropriate drug-susceptible target or possess natural barriers that prevent an antimicrobial agent from reaching its target. Some examples are the natural resistance of gram-negative bacteria to vancomycin because the drug cannot penetrate the

---

[a] Department of Medicine, Division of Infectious Diseases and International Health, Duke University Medical Center, Box 102359, Hanes House, Durham, NC 27710, USA
[b] Department of Medicine, Division of Infectious Diseases, Harper Hospital, Detroit Medical Center and Wayne State University, 3990 John R. Street, 5 Hudson, Detroit, MI 48201, USA
[c] Department of Medicine, Division of Infectious Diseases, Detroit Medical Center and Wayne State University, 4201 Saint Antoine, Suite 2B, Box 331, Detroit, MI 48201, USA
* Corresponding author.
E-mail address: luke.chen@duke.edu (L.F. Chen).

Infect Dis Clin N Am 23 (2009) 817–845
doi:10.1016/j.idc.2009.06.002
0891-5520/09/$ – see front matter © 2009 Elsevier Inc. All rights reserved.

id.theclinics.com

gram-negative outer membrane, or the intrinsic resistance of the penicillin-binding proteins (PBPs) of enterococci to the effects of the cephalosporins.

Acquired resistance, the primary focus of this article, reflects a change in the genetic composition of a bacterium so that a drug that once was effective is no longer active, resulting in clinical resistance. Sometimes genetic change results in diminished antimicrobial activity, but not complete loss of drug effectiveness.

The major strategies used by bacteria to avoid the actions of antimicrobial agents are outlined in **Table 1**. These include limiting the intracellular concentration of an antimicrobial agent by decreased influx or increased efflux, neutralization of the antimicrobial agent by enzymes, alteration of the target so that the agent no longer interferes with it, and elimination of the target altogether by the creation of new metabolic pathways.[1] Bacteria may use one or multiple mechanisms against a single agent or class of agents or a single change may result in resistance to several different agents or even multiple unrelated drug classes.

Gram-positive and gram-negative bacteria possess different structural characteristics and these differences determine the mechanisms for primary resistance. The targets of most antimicrobial agents are located either in the cell wall, cytoplasmic membrane, or within the cytoplasm. In gram-negative bacteria, the outer membrane may provide an additional intrinsic barrier that prevents drugs from reaching these targets. Additionally, modifications in outer membrane permeability by both alterations in porin channels and by upregulation of multidrug efflux pumps may contribute to resistance in many gram-negative organisms. Moreover, inactivating enzymes released across the cytoplasmic membrane can function more efficiently within the confines of the periplasmic space.

The mechanisms by which intracellular concentrations of drugs are limited include decreased outer membrane permeability, decreased uptake through the cytoplasmic

Table 1
General mechanisms of resistance to antimicrobial agents

Resistance Mechanism	Specific Examples	References
Diminished intracellular drug concentration		
Decreased outer membrane permeability	β-Lactams (eg, OmpF, OprD)	2
Decreased cytoplasmic membrane transport	Quinolones (eg, OmpF)	1
	Aminoglycosides (decreased energy)	3
Increased efflux	Tetracyclines (eg, tetA)	195
	Quinolones (eg, norA)	196
	Macrolides (eg, mefA)	196
	Multiple drugs (eg, mexAB-OprF)	2
Drug inactivation (reversible or irreversible)	β-Lactams (β-lactamases)	95
	Carbapenemases (carbapenems)	105,96
	Aminoglycosides (modifying enzymes)	3
	Chloramphenicol (inactivating enzymes)	1
Target modification	Quinolones (gyrase modifications)	6
	Rifampin (DNA polymerase binding)	6
	β-Lactams (PBP changes)	6
	Macrolides (rRNA methylation)	5
	Linezolid (23srRNA modifications)	58
Target bypass	Glycopeptides (vanA, vanB)	7
	Trimethoprim (thymidine-deficient strains)	—

membrane, and active efflux out of both the cytoplasmic membrane and the outer membrane. Acquired outer membrane permeability changes in gram-negative organisms previously attributed solely to alterations in outer membrane porin proteins are now also understood to be related to the upregulation of complex multidrug efflux pumps whose expression is linked to that of outer membrane proteins, such as the MexAB-OprM system of Pseudomonas aeruginosa.[2] These efflux systems are widely distributed among gram-negative pathogens, such as P aeruginosa and Enterobacteriaceae, and may be an important component of resistance to β-lactams, but usually result in high-level resistance only when associated with β-lactamase production.[2] Imipenem resistance in P aeruginosa can be mediated by alteration of a specific porin OprD that is used preferentially by this agent.[2] Decreased outer membrane permeability through porin changes and efflux may also play a role in resistance to fluoroquinolones and aminoglycosides. Resistance mediated by decreased uptake across the metabolically active cytoplasmic membrane is best demonstrated by small-colony aminoglycoside-resistant mutants of staphylococci, but this mechanism is less important than other mechanisms of aminoglycoside resistance.[3] Active antimicrobial efflux systems play a role in resistance to many different agents, including macrolides, tetracyclines, quinolones, chloramphenicol, and β-lactams.

Inactivating enzymes remain the predominant mechanism of resistance to several major classes of antimicrobial agents. Resistance to β-lactams is mediated by a wide variety of β-lactamases that hydrolytically inactivate these drugs. β-lactamases can be either plasmid or chromosomally mediated, and their expression can be constitutive or induced. Unlike those of gram-positive organisms, β-lactamases of gram-negative organisms are confined to the periplasmic space, which may explain some of the differences in their phenotypic expression and ease of laboratory detection. Of particular importance in the hospital setting are the class I chromosomal β-lactamases in organisms, such as Enterobacter cloacae, which are produced in high levels after exposure to an inducing β-lactam agent (particularly to third-generation cephalosporins), and the extended-spectrum β-lactamases (ESBLs), mediating resistance to third-generation cephalosporins and aztreonam.[4] Carbapenemases are an emerging, and important class of inactivating enzymes that mediate resistance to carbapenem antibiotics in gram-negative organisms. Another major class of inactivating enzymes is the family of aminoglycoside-modifying enzymes. These enzymes are widely distributed in gram-positive and gram-negative bacteria, and usually are plasmid-mediated.[3] Resistance to chloramphenicol and macrolides also can be mediated by modifying or inactivating enzymes.[5]

Target modifications are widely used by bacteria to mediate resistance to a wide variety of antimicrobial agents.[6] Some of these alterations may require as little as a single mutational event at a critical gene sequence in the primary target to create a new, functional target with reduced affinity for the antimicrobial agent. Such changes account for the relative ease of selection of rifampin-resistant mutants of staphylococci and streptococci by changes in DNA polymerase or the selection of high-level streptomycin-resistant mutants with altered ribosomes. Although some resistance secondary to target modifications can be directly selected, others, such as development of resistance to semisynthetic penicillins in staphylococci, require acquisition of novel exogenous DNA. Modification of PBPs is the primary mode of penicillin resistance in Streptococcus pneumoniae, Neisseria meningitidis, and Enterococcus faecium. Modification of genes encoding DNA gyrases and topoisomerases is the main mechanism of resistance to quinolones, while target modification is important in resistance to macrolides, tetracyclines, rifampin, and mupirocin.[6]

Some bacteria have gone beyond simple target modification and have acquired novel systems in which the antimicrobial target is no longer necessary for survival of the organism. This is achieved by creation of new metabolic pathways to bypass the primary target. Perhaps the most elaborate examples of this are the *vanA* and *vanB* clusters that mediate resistance to glycopeptides in enterococci.[7] Target bypass also is the major mechanism of acquired resistance to folate antagonists.

MECHANISMS OF DISSEMINATION OF RESISTANCE GENES

In addition to the complex strategies used to express resistance to antimicrobial agents, bacteria also can avail themselves of a variety of efficient mechanisms for the transfer of resistance genes to other organisms and to other species.[8] The bacterial genome consists of chromosomal DNA, and encodes the following cellular characteristics: metabolic and repair pathways, smaller circular DNA elements or plasmids that encode for supplemental bacterial activities, such as virulence factors and resistance genes, and genes essential to the independent mobilization and transmission of the plasmid elements. Most resistance genes are plasmid-mediated, but plasmid-mediated traits can interchange with chromosomal elements. Transfer of genetic material from a plasmid to the chromosome can occur by simple recombination events, but the process is greatly facilitated by transposons. Transposons are small, mobile DNA elements capable of mediating transfer of DNA by removing and inserting themselves into host chromosomal and plasmid DNA. Many resistance genes, such as plasmid-mediated β-lactamases, tetracycline-resistance genes, and aminoglycoside-modifying enzymes, are organized on transposons, which may have a broader host range than their parent plasmids. Multiple resistance transposons can then be clustered together on even larger composite transposable elements capable of simultaneously transferring multiple unrelated resistance genes.[8]

Resistance determinants carried on the chromosome are vertically transmitted by clonal dissemination. Resistance determinants on plasmids can also be vertically transferred, although plasmids may be lost from the bacterial population if they no longer confer a particular selective advantage. Plasmids also are capable of horizontal transfer by conjugation, although the efficiency of plasmid transfer both within and between species can vary tremendously. Plasmid transfer between gram-positive and gram-negative bacteria, once thought to be an unlikely event, can occur both in the laboratory and in the gastrointestinal tract of gnotobiotic mice, suggesting that such transfer events between even remotely related organisms may be important in nature.[9]

Conjugative transposons of gram-positive bacteria are capable of directly mediating gene transfer without plasmids. Transformation, direct incorporation of free DNA by bacterial cells, may also be important for the evolution of resistance in *Neisseria* and streptococcal species.[6,8]

Resistant Gram-Positive Cocci

Multidrug-resistant enterococci
Epidemiology and characteristics of resistance Enterococci are naturally tolerant of penicillins, and are resistant to cephalosporins, clindamycin, and achievable serum levels of aminoglycosides. Cephalosporin resistance is caused by poor affinity of cephalosporins for enterococcal PBPs. Natural low-level aminoglycoside resistance is attributed to the inability of aminoglycosides to penetrate the enterococcal cell wall, but activity is enhanced in the presence of cell wall–active drugs, such as ampicillin or vancomycin.[10] Enterococci are usually intrinsically tolerant, or lysis resistant, to the

effects of penicillins and glycopeptides alone. Until the emergence of drug-resistant isolates, bactericidal therapy was reliably achieved with synergistic combinations of cell wall–active drugs plus aminoglycosides.

Enterococci demonstrate several types of penicillin resistance Penicillin resistance in *E faecalis* is mediated by β-lactamase production and has been reported from a few nosocomial outbreaks both within and outside of the United States,[11] but infections with such strains are still very uncommon. Chromosomal high-level penicillin resistance is a species-specific characteristic of *E faecium*, but is occasionally found in other species.[12] *E faecium* with low-level penicillin-resistance are found in normal fecal flora, but high-level resistant strains are likely to be nosocomially acquired.[13] Ampicillin resistance to an intermediate level (minimum inhibitory concentrations [MICs] of 16–64 μg/mL) is attributable to alterations in PBPs and in most cases, is associated with the overexpression of PBP5, a PBP with low affinity for penicillins.[14] High-level penicillin-resistant *E faecium* are also resistant to imipenem and β-lactam–β-lactamase inhibitors and are often also glycopeptide-resistant.[15]

High-level gentamicin resistance, mediated by a bifunctional inactivating enzyme, first appeared in 1978 and rapidly spread worldwide. As many as 60% of enterococci from some hospitals are high-level gentamicin resistant, but resistance remains strongly associated with nosocomial acquisition.[16] High-level gentamicin resistant enterococci are highly resistant to all other aminoglycosides in clinical use in the United States, with the possible exception of streptomycin. Importantly, highly resistant strains do not demonstrate synergistic killing of enterococci when aminoglycosides are combined with penicillin or vancomycin.[17] Most high-level gentamicin resistance is carried on transposons and is plasmid mediated.[17] Detection of high-level gentamicin resistance requires either special susceptibility wells or screening plates with high concentrations of gentamicin or streptomycin (eg, ≥500 μg/mL for gentamicin and ≥1,000 μg/mL for streptomycin) (see the article on antibacterial susceptibility testing in the clinical laboratory elsewhere in this issue).

Vancomycin-resistant enterococci (VRE) were first isolated in Europe in 1988 and in the United States in 1989. Since then, VRE have spread rapidly throughout the United States and the world and have become a significant infection control problem for many hospitals.[18] VRE are established throughout the United States and Europe, but are less frequently isolated in Asia and Latin America.[19] The prevalence of VRE remains low in true community-acquired isolates in the United States.

The increase in glycopeptide resistance in the United States followed the marked increase in vancomycin usage in many hospitals, just as methicillin-resistant *Staphylococcus aureus* (MRSA) strains became established in the 1980s. Most VRE seem to have been acquired nosocomially or institutionally, and spread of epidemic strains both within and between institutions is well documented.[20] From 1989 to 2002, the proportion of enterococcal isolates from ICUs that were resistant to vancomycin increased from 0.3% in 1989 to 23.9% in 1998, and further increased to 33.3% in 2008.[18] As of October 2008, the National Nosocomial Infections Surveillance system reported that more than one third of healthcare–associated enterococcal infections were associated with organisms resistant to vancomycin.[18] Some risk factors for VRE colonization or infection include the exposure to antibiotics, such as broad-spectrum cephalosporins, fluoroquinolones, vancomycin, and antianaerobic drugs, prolonged hospital and ICU stays, intrahospital transfer between patient floors, use of enteral tube feedings, or sucralfate and liver transplant requiring surgical re-exploration.[21]

Glycopeptides are large, complex molecules that do not enter the bacterial cell. They interfere with cell wall synthesis by tightly binding to the D-alanine-D-alanine terminal dipeptide on the peptidoglycan precursor, sterically blocking the subsequent transglycosylation and transpeptidation reactions. The vancomycin-resistance mechanism involves a complex series of reactions that ultimately result in the building of the cell wall by bypassing the D-alanine-D-alanine–containing pentapeptide intermediate structure, thereby eliminating the glycopeptide target.[22]

VRE initially were characterized phenotypically as *vanA*, *vanB*, and *vanC* strains based on levels of resistance to vancomycin, cross-resistance to teicoplanin, and the inducible or constitutive nature of resistance.[23] The genotype and molecular basis for each resistance type have now been characterized (**Table 2**). The *vanA* cluster has been identified predominantly in *E faecium* and *E faecalis* but has also been found in other enterococci, streptococci, *Oerskovia*, and *Bacillus*, and most recently has been found in *S aureus*.[24–28] Furthermore, there is evidence for in vivo transfer of *vanA* resistance on plasmids.[29]

vanB is found almost exclusively in *E faecium* and *E faecalis*. *vanC1, C2, C3, D, E,* and *G* are rarely found in enterococci causing human infections.[30–32]

Resistance to linezolid in enterococci is mediated by the G2576U mutation or similar mutations of the 23S ribosome.[33] Recent data document high rates of linezolid resistance among enterococcal isolates. In recent studies, 11% to 20% of VRE colonizing or infecting isolates were resistant to linezolid.[34,35] Risk factors found to be specifically associated with isolation of linezolid-resistant VRE were receipt of a solid organ transplant; receipt of parenteral nutrition; peripheral vascular disease; and prior receipt of linezolid, piperacillin-tazobactam, or cefepime.[35]

Enterococcal resistance to daptomycin rarely occurs and is associated with previous treatment with daptomycin. The mechanism of resistance is not well understood.[36]

Multidrug-Resistant *Staphylococcus Aureus*

The first strain of penicillinase-producing *S aureus* was reported in 1941[37] and 90% of *S aureus* isolates in the world are now penicillin-resistant as a result of β-lactamase production. Over the ensuing decades, *S aureus* continued to predominate as a major

Table 2
Glycopeptide-resistant enterococci

Genotype	Vancomycin MIC (µg/mL)	Teicoplanin MIC (µg/mL)	Expression	Typical Location
vanA	64–1024	≥16	Inducible	Plasmid[a]
vanB	4–1024	≤1[b]	Inducible[c]	Chromosome[d]
vanC[f]	2–32	≤1	Constitutive and inducible	Chromosome
vanD	64–256	4–32	Constitutive and inducible[e]	Chromosome
vanE	16	0.5	Inducible	Chromosome
vanG	16	0.5	Inducible	Chromosome

[a] Strains with *vanA* on the chromosome have been described.
[b] Teicoplanin-resistant strains have emerged with MIC ≥16.
[c] Constitutively expressing strains have been described.
[d] Plasmids containing *vanB* have been described.
[e] Both have been described.
[f] Species-specific variants *vanC-1, vanC-2,* and *vanC-3* have been described.

human pathogen and it became increasingly resistant to drugs in the face of antimicrobial selection pressure. For example, since 1996, there have been several reports of infections caused by MRSA with intermediate susceptibility to vancomycin (vancomycin-intermediate *S aureus* [VISA]; MIC 4–8 μg/mL).[38] Furthermore, there are now several strains of *S aureus* in the United States that are fully resistant to vancomycin (vancomycin-resistant *S aureus* [VRSA]; MIC ≥16 μg/mL)[39] and to other recently approved antibiotics specifically developed to treat MRSA, such as linezolid[40] and daptomycin.[41]

Mechanism of resistance in MRSA

Resistance to methicillin and other β-lactam antibiotics is mediated by the *mecA* gene, which encodes for an additional PBP (PBP2a), which has low affinity for β-lactams. Strains with *mecA*-mediated methicillin resistance are classically referred to as MRSA. These *mecA* genes are situated on a mobile genetic element, known as the Staphylococcal Cassette Chromosome mec (SCCmec). To date, eight types of SCCmec (I–VIII) have been reported, and these are widely distributed in both coagulase-positive and coagulase-negative staphylococci.[42–44] The SCCmec element also includes two regulatory loci, the repressor MecI and the trans-membrane β-lactam–sensing signal-transducer MecRI.[45] Some SCCmec components may contain additional genes encoding for resistance against non–β-lactam antibiotics.

The expression of *mecA* can be either constitutive or inducible. Additionally, expression of the resistance phenotype also depends, in part, on other chromosomal genes, which are part of cellular peptidoglycan metabolism and can regulate the degree of resistance without altering levels of PBP2a.

Community-acquired MRSA Community-acquired MRSA is both phenotypically and genotypically distinct from healthcare–associated MRSA. Frequently, community-acquired MRSA isolates produce toxins including Panton-Valentine leukocidin, which is an exotoxin encoded by two cotranscribed genes: lukF-PV and lukS-PV. Although the actual virulence of the Panton-Valentine leukocidin gene has not been determined, presence of the Panton-Valentine leukocidin protein has been associated with skin and soft tissue infections and severe necrotizing pneumonia.[46] Furthermore, community-acquired MRSA strains are susceptible to non–β-lactam antibiotics[47] and this is explained by the fact that resistance genes to non–β-lactam antibiotics are not usually included in the smaller type IV SCCmec elements that are common in community-acquired MRSA isolates. In contrast to nosocomial MRSA isolates, most community-acquired MRSA strains are susceptible to multiple classes of antibiotics other than β-lactams, including trimethoprim-sulfamethoxazole (TMP-SMX), clindamycin, aminoglycosides, tetracyclines, and fluoroquinolones.

Reduced susceptibility to vancomycin Vancomycin is the mainstay of treatment of MRSA infections. Failure of vancomycin therapy, however, is not uncommon and is increasing. Reduced susceptibility of MRSA to vancomycin, which occurs predominantly among strains of healthcare–associated MRSA, is being studied in the following three contexts: (1) VRSA; (2) VISA; and (3) the trend of MRSA isolates with increased vancomycin MICs (MIC creep).

VRSA, fortunately, continues to be rare. There have only been seven reports of clinical isolates of VRSA in the United States as of this writing; five of the seven occurred within the greater Michigan area.[39] MICs of VRSA isolates to vancomycin are generally greater than 128 μg/mL. In these isolates, vancomycin resistance has been conferred by the *vanA* resistance cluster, which also mediates glycopeptide resistance in some enterococcal species. In these patients from whom VRSA was isolated, prior dual infection with MRSA and VRE was documented in five patients, suggesting that the *vanA* gene was transferred from VRE to MRSA isolate. The transfer of the *vanA* gene has been demonstrated in vitro from enterococcus to *S aureus*.[48] Vancomycin acts by binding the D-Ala-D-Ala terminus of peptidoglycan precursors and the resistance to vancomycin in VRSA is mediated by the presence of enzymes that produce low-affinity precursors, such as D-Ala-D-lactate or D-Ala-D-Ser, or the presence of enzymes that eliminate the high-affinity peptidoglycan precursors that are normally produced in susceptible *S aureus*.[49]

Among VISA isolates, the MIC to vancomycin is 4 to 8 µg/mL. The mechanism conferring glycopeptide resistance in VISA is not well understood at the genetic level but seems to involve cell wall thickening with reduced levels of peptidoglycan cross-linking and does not seem to require the acquisition of new DNA. It is postulated that reduced levels of peptidoglycan cross-linking leads to more D-alanyl-D-alanine side chains. These side chains can bind vancomycin outside the cell membrane and prevent vancomycin from reaching its cell membrane targets.

Independent risk factors for infections caused by VISA include prior infection caused by MRSA and antecedent vancomycin use within 3 months before VISA infection. Most patients in the United States with VISA infections received repeated, prolonged exposures to vancomycin and received dialysis at the time of infection.

Several investigators have observed increased rates of vancomycin treatment failure in patients with MRSA infections where the isolates have increased vancomycin MICs but are still classified as susceptible by Clinical and Laboratory Standards Institute (CLSI) definitions.[50] One study showed less than 10% treatment success when vancomycin was used to treat bacteremia caused by MRSA strains with vancomycin MICs of 1 to 2 µg/mL, compared with 56% success when the vancomycin MIC was less than or equal to 0.5 µg/mL.[51] Partly in response to this study and others, in 2007 the susceptibility breakpoints for *S aureus* to vancomycin were lowered from 8 to 16 µg/mL to 4 to 8 µg/mL for intermediate and from less than or equal to 4 µg/mL to less than or equal to 2 µg/mL for susceptible.

Several investigators from different geographic locales have reported that the MICs of *S aureus* isolates to vancomycin have increased over time. This phenomenon has been described as "MIC creep."[52] Debate is ongoing with respect to the significance of the MIC creep and the degree to which it is actually occurring.[53] For example, a study of more than 35,000 *S aureus* isolates from the SENTRY database collected from sites around the world between 1997 and 2003 showed no evidence of increasing vancomycin MICs over time.[54] Another study of more than 6000 *S aureus* isolates collected over 5 years in southern California found a clear and statistically significant drift of vancomycin MICs toward reduced susceptibility, with an increase in the proportion of isolates with a MIC equal to 1 µg/mL from 19.9% in 2000 to 70.4% in 2004.[55] Despite these conflicting results, reports of vancomycin treatment failures for susceptible MRSA strains and reports of MIC creep from some geographic locales raise concerns about the future of vancomycin as an effective agent for treatment of invasive MRSA infections. Recently, guidelines were published regarding optimal dosing of vancomycin for the treatment of infections caused by *S aureus*.[56]

Resistance to other alternative agents for treatment of MRSA

Linezolid is bacteriostatic against *S aureus* and binds to the 50S subunit of the bacterial ribosome, resulting in the inhibition of bacterial protein synthesis.[57] In vitro resistance to linezolid have been reported in *S aureus*.[58] Fortunately, such resistant isolates remain a rare phenomenon. Linezolid may fail to bind its bacterial target site in the presence of single point mutations in the bacterial 23S rRNA of the 50S subunit.[59] Notably, 23S rRNA mutations that confer resistance to linezolid can produce cross-resistance to chloramphenicol and quinupristin-dalfopristin, which also bind to the same 23S rRNA domain.[59] Prior therapy with linezolid seems to be an important risk factor for subsequent isolation of linezolid-resistant S aureus.

Daptomycin is rapidly bactericidal against S aureus and its primary mechanism of action is a calcium-dependent depolarization of bacterial cell wall.[60] Daptomycin is inactivated by alveolar surfactants, and should not be used for pulmonary infections.[61] Clinical failures caused by emergence of resistance have been reported during daptomycin for chronic infections.[62] The exact mechanisms of resistance to daptomycin have not been completely elucidated. Studies have shown that daptomycin resistance gradually emerges by a multistep process[63] and generally results in a heteroresistant bacterial subpopulation with higher MICs to daptomycin. Current evidence suggests that resistance is caused by impairment of daptomycin binding by a change in cell membrane potential leading to (1) reduced daptomycin binding to the cell membrane, (2) changes in cell membrane surface charge, and (3) reduced susceptibility to daptomycin-induced depolarization.[64] Furthermore, there is a correlation between daptomycin-resistance and vancomycin nonsusceptibility in isolates of VISA.[65] The cross-resistance between vancomycin and daptomycin in VISA is thought to be caused by the thickened cell wall, which acts as a common obstacle to daptomycin and vancomycin cellular penetration.

Quinupristin-dalfopristin is a concentration-dependent antibiotic that is bactericidal against staphylococci. Staphylococcal isolates constitutively expressing macrolide-lincosamide-streptogramin B resistance (eg, erm A or erm C) may be resistant to the quinupristin component of quinupristin-dalfopristin. In such cases, the activity of quinupristin-dalfopristin may be significantly altered.[66]

Clinical failures associated with resistance to quinupristin-dalfopristin have already been described in some isolates of MRSA even in the relatively short timeframe that the drug has been available.[67] Isolates of staphylococci that are resistant to quinupristin-dalfopristin are more likely to have resistances to the dalfopristin component, which is caused by genes encoding acetyltransferases (vatA, vatB, and vatC) or efflux pumps (vgaA and vgaB).[68] Resistance to quinupristin-dalfopristin can also be mediated by resistance to the quinupristin component, caused by production of ribosomal methylases encoded by erm genes; and the macrolide-lincosamide-streptogramin B phenotype, which also confers cross-resistance to macrolides and lincosamides.

Resistance of MRSA to other classes of antibiotics

MRSA isolates containing mecA are resistant to all β-lactam antibiotics. Most nosocomial and health care–associated isolates frequently carry multiple other resistance determinants. Many of these resistance determinants can be found on transferable genetic elements or plasmids, whereas others are chromosomal in origin. The plasmid-mediated determinants include aminoglycoside-modifying enzymes, tetracycline efflux genes, and macrolide-methylating enzymes, and resistance determinants for TMP-SMX. Quinolone resistance is mediated primarily by alterations in DNA topoisomerases, but also by the staphylococcal norA gene by active efflux. Resistance to macrolide, lincosamide, and streptogramin antibiotics may be conferred by modifications of target sites, active efflux, and by inactivating enzymes. Gentamicin resistance also can occur by selection of small-colony, membrane energy-deficient mutants.

Penicillin and Multidrug-Resistant Pneumococci

Mechanisms of resistance

Penicillin-resistance in S pneumoniae is caused by reduced affinity between the PBPs and β-lactam antibiotics. Such resistance is mediated through changes in genes that encode one of the six high-molecular-weight PBPs of the organism.[69] There are two notable features of PBP-mediated resistance in pneumococci. First, highly resistant strains generally show more PBP alterations than do those of low-level resistant strains.[70] Second, pneumococcal resistance can occur by homologous recombination of PBP genes of different strains, in addition to direct clonal dissemination of resistant strains.[71] Such events can occur both between different pneumococcal species and between pneumococci and the closely related viridans streptococcal species. Oral streptococci have been postulated to be the major reservoir for the novel DNA required to create the genetic sequences demonstrated by some of the altered pneumococcal PBP genes.[6]

Tolerance to penicillins in pneumococci can also be mediated by altered peptidoglycan structures. Additionally, penicillin tolerance has been found in strains with reduced penicillin susceptibility that fails to lyse at penicillin concentrations far above the MIC; however, the clinical significance of this observation remains unclear.

Changes in PBP of penicillin-resistant strains also result in diminished susceptibility to other β-lactam agents.[72] The levels of resistance to different agents vary greatly. Penicillin-resistant strains are uniformly resistant to penicillin derivatives, such as ampicillin and the ureidopenicillins, and generally are resistant to first- and second-generation cephalosporins. Certain third-generation agents, particularly cefotaxime and ceftriaxone, are often effective, in part because of their high level of activity and in part because the tissue levels attained by these agents are high. Many strains of pneumococci also harbor high-level resistance to cefotaxime and ceftriaxone (MIC ≥2 µg/mL) (3.3% of all strains reported in a recent United States study were ceftriaxone-resistant and 5% of all isolates in a recent Taiwanese study were ceftriaxone-resistant).[73,74] Interestingly, several studies also show that isolates of penicillin-resistant pneumococci may be disproportionately more susceptible to ceftriaxone than to cefotaxime.[75] Regardless of the pattern of β-lactam nonsusceptibility, debate is still ongoing as to infections caused by these resistant strains are associated with poorer outcomes than infections caused by susceptible strains.[76]

Resistance of pneumococci to non–β-lactam antimicrobial agents

Penicillin-resistant strains are frequently resistant to non–β-lactam antimicrobial agents and are often multidrug resistant. Resistance to erythromycin, tetracycline, TMP-SMX, and chloramphenicol are the most common.

A recent surveillance study in the United States shows that prevalence of macrolide resistance in S pneumoniae is approximately 26.2%.[77] The most common mechanism of macrolide resistance in S pneumoniae is caused by target-site modification encoded by erythromycin ribosome methylation (erm) genes that provide inducible cross-resistance to all macrolides, lincosamides, and streptogramin B. Two other mechanisms of resistance to macrolides include active efflux pump encoded by macrolide efflux genes (mefA, mefE) that result in resistance to macrolides alone (M phenotype); and ribosomal mutations in the 23S rRNA gene for ribosomal protein L4 or L22.

Although vancomycin-tolerant pneumococcal isolates have recently been isolated, no strains fully resistant to vancomycin have been reported.[78]

Fluoroquinolone resistance has developed during therapy, especially in patients with prior fluoroquinolone exposures, leading to clinical failure.[79] The older fluoroquinolones (eg, ciprofloxacin) lack reliable activity against pneumococci (18.6% of pneumococcal isolates in a 2008 study were nonsusceptible to ciprofloxacin).[77] Newer fluoroquinolones, such as levofloxacin, moxifloxacin, and gemifloxacin, inhibit most strains at achievable levels (only 1.3% of the isolates were nonsusceptible to levofloxacin in a study by Sahm and colleagues[77]). The mechanism of decreased susceptibility to the newer fluoroquinolones is primarily caused by mutations in the *parC* gene of topoisomerase IV and the *gyrA* gene of DNA gyrase.

RESISTANT GRAM-NEGATIVE MICROORGANISMS
Escherichia Coli and *Klebsiella spp* Resistant to Broad-Spectrum Cephalosporins

Resistance of *Escherichia coli* and *Klebsiella* spp to broad-spectrum cephalosporins is largely mediated by ESBLs, designated as Bush-Jacoby-Medeiros Group 2be. These enzymes confer resistance to oxyimino-β-lactam antibiotics. Most ESBLs are derivatives of TEM and SHV, which have undergone amino acid substitutions at the active site of the enzyme. Such ESBL enzymes are often plasmid-borne. Depending on the location of the substitution, the resultant β-lactamase can cause variably diminished susceptibility to cefotaxime, ceftazidime, and aztreonam. ESBLs are most commonly expressed in *Klebsiella pneumoniae*, *Klebsiella oxytoca*, and *E coli*, although they have been detected in other organisms including *Salmonella* spp, *Pseudomonas aeruginosa*, *Proteus mirabilis*, and other Enterobacteriaceae. Plasmids that encode ESBLs often carry resistance to other antibiotics. The effective control and treatment of ESBLs are a growing challenge because of the role of ESBLs in outbreaks in hospitals and nursing homes, and because of the ability of ESBLs to be transferred to other bacterial species by plasmids.

Epidemiology and mechanisms of resistance

ESBLs were first discovered in Europe in 1983 and soon after in the United States. Since then their prevalence has increased. By 1990, 14% of all *K pneumoniae* isolated from French hospitals were ESBL producers, with rates approaching 50% in some hospitals.[80] In some United States hospitals, the prevalence of ESBLs in *K pneumoniae* has been reported to be as high as 40%.[81] The Centers for Disease Control and Prevention reported, in 2006 to 2007, the rate of ceftazidime-resistant *K pneumoniae* strains associated with device-related infection exceeded 20%, and the rate of ceftazidime-resistant *E coli* ranged between 5% and 11%.[82] Teaching hospitals have a higher prevalence of ESBL resistance.[83]

ESBL-producing organisms are generally found in hospitals, although nursing home outbreaks have been reported.[84] Outbreaks can occur through either clonal spread of a specific plasmid-carrying strain or through transfer of a particular plasmid to other bacterial strains, or even to different bacterial genera.[84] Resistant organisms can pass from patient to patient on the hands of healthcare providers.[85] Risk factors for acquisition of ESBLs are similar to those reported for other hospital-acquired organisms and include emergency abdominal surgery, mechanical ventilation, presence of percutaneous devices, tracheostomy, prolonged hospital stay, and increased patient morbidity.[83,84,86] Risk factors associated with antibiotics are of increasing interest to researchers. Exposure to antibiotics, particularly to ceftazidime and aztreonam, has been associated with an increased prevalence of ESBL-producing organisms.[87,88] Other studies, however, have found no association between use of third-generation cephalosporins and emergence of ESBL resistance.[84,89] Exposure to TMP-SMX has also been associated with acquisition of ESBLs.[84] Restriction of cephalosporin use has been associated with control of hospital outbreaks.[90,91]

Recently, a study showed use of piperacillin-tazobactam and vancomycin was an independent risk factor for colonization with ESBL organisms.[92]

Many different types of ESBLS have been described, including greater than 160 in the TEM class, over 100 in the SHV family, over 80 in the CTX-M class, and more than 140 in the OXA family. A Web site maintains an up-to-date, complete listing of all identified ESBLs: http://www.lahey.org/studies/.[93]

Each ESBL has unique amino acid substitutions at active sites of the enzyme, affecting its isoelectric point and affecting the enzyme's affinity for and hydrolytic activity of oxyimino-β-lactams.[83] Most ESBLs have higher hydrolytic activity against ceftazidime and aztreonam and less activity against cefotaxime, although the opposite may be true in some cases. For example, in SHV and TEM β-lactamases a serine substitution for glycine at amino acid 238 causes decreased hydrolytic activity against ceftazidime but increases activity against cefotaxime.[83] CTX-M–type ESBLs, however, generally have higher hydrolytic activity against cefotaxime than ceftazidime.[94] Multiple β-lactamases conferring resistance to different classes of β-lactam antibiotics can be found within a single bacterial strain. The diversity of cephalosporin susceptibility profiles manifested by different ESBL enzymes makes detection of some ESBL-producing strains a major challenge for the clinical laboratory. These enzymes are not capable of hydrolyzing cephamycins and carbapenems.[95]

Carbapenemase-producing gram-negative organisms can hydrolyze all penicillins, cephalosporins, and carbapenems and they have been reported in several large outbreaks in hospitalized patients since 2001.[96] KPC,[97] a class A plasmid-mediated β-lactamase, has been associated with outbreaks in hospitals in the northeastern regions of the United States,[98–100] and in other countries, such as China, Brazil, and Israel. KPCs are classically associated with *K pneumoniae*; however, outbreaks of KPCs have been reported with *E coli*, *K oxytoca*, *Enterobacter* spp, *Salmonella*,[101] and *Pseudomonas*.[102] Some preliminary evidence demonstrates propagation of KPC-producing organisms in diverse geographic regions in the United States; inside and outside of hospitals; and in community-based health care services, such as nursing homes.

Metallo-β-lactamases are class B β-lactam hydrolyzing enzymes that contain a zinc moiety and have caused several extended outbreaks of nosocomial infections in patients in ICUs and burns units in Europe and Australia.[103] VIM and IMP metallo-β-lactamases are more commonly found in *Pseudomonas* and *Acinetobacter* species. These metallo-β-lactamases can also rapidly hydrolyze cephalosporins and penicillins (but not aztreonam), and can be encoded by integrins, raising concerns regarding horizontal spread of this resistance mechanism. OXA-type carbapenemases are class D β-lactamases that have caused limited outbreaks in the United States.[104] Metallo-β-lactamases are a diverse group of β-lactamases that are active not only against the oxyimino-cephalosporins and cephamycins but also against carbapenems.[105] There are two major groups of metalloid-β-lactamases: the IMP-type carbapenemases and the Verona integron-encoded metallo-β-lactamase (VIM) carbapenemases.[106]

Another mechanism facilitating β-lactamase activity involves loss of porin channels in the outer cellular membrane and upregulation of efflux pumps, decreasing antibiotic concentrations in the periplasmic space and facilitating hydrolysis by β-lactamases. This mechanism often results in increased resistance to cephalosporins, cephamycins, and β-lactamase inhibitors.[83,107,108] Plasmids producing ESBLs often carry resistance to other antibiotics, including aminoglycosides, tetracyclines, chloramphenicol, TMP, and sulfonamides.[83]

Escherichia coli and *Klebsiella* possess other mechanisms of β-lactam antibiotic resistance unrelated to ESBL production. Resistance to extended-spectrum cephalosporins, cephamycins, oxyimino-β-lactams, and β-lactamase inhibitors in *E coli* and *K pneumoniae* can be mediated by plasmid-mediated β-lactamases similar to those chromosomal AmpC enzymes produced in species such as *E cloacae* and *Serratia marcescens*.[109,110] Additional porin mutations can result in carbapenem resistance.[83] Resistance to β-lactam–β-lactamase inhibitor combinations can occur by alterations in porin channels, TEM and SHV hyperproduction, by the production of inhibitor-resistant TEM enzymes (Bush-Jacoby-Medeiros Group 2br) and in *E coli*, by chromosomal cephalosporinase AmpC production.[83,95,109]

β-lactam–resistant *Klebsiella* and *E coli* strains are often resistant to quinolones and aminoglycosides, leaving few alternatives for treatment.[111] Alterations in DNA gyrase (topoisomerase II and to a lesser extent topoisomerase IV), porin channel mutations, and efflux mechanisms can confer quinolone resistance.[112] Enzymatic modifications can lead to aminoglycoside resistance.[113]

Tigecycline has potent in vitro activity against multidrug-resistant gram-negative bacilli including ESBL-producing organisms.[25] Unfortunately, there are few data from the clinical setting to support the use of tigecycline as a single agent for the treatment of invasive infections caused by multidrug-resistant gram-negative bacilli. A recent study reported failure of tigecycline among patients with serious infections caused by gram-negative bacilli. Of note, these treatment failures occurred among isolates considered to be susceptible to tigecycline.[114]

Pseudomonas and Other Gram-Negative Rods Producing AmpC

AmpC β-lactamase production is another important mechanism of antimicrobial resistance in gram-negative organisms.[115] These hydrolyzing enzymes were discovered in the 1980s and were extensively studied. AmpC enzymes were initially identified only as inducible, chromosome-encoded β-lactamases found in certain species of *Enterobacter*, *Serratia*, *Pseudomonas*, *Providencia*, *Citrobacter*, and indole-positive *Proteus*.[116] Further research into gram-negative resistance also detected AmpC genes on transferrable plasmids in gram-negative bacilli, which do not chromosomally express these types of β-lactamases, including *Klebsiella* spp, *E coli*, or *Salmonella* spp.[117] Plasmid-mediated AmpC hyperproduction and antimicrobial resistance caused by chromosome-encoded AmpC enzymes can substantially complicate the management of gram-negative infections and adversely impact the clinical outcomes of patients.[118]

β-Lactam resistance among gram-negative organisms can also be mediated by two other classes of plasmid-mediated β-lactamases: hydrolyzing carbapenemases and ESBL. The former is briefly discussed in this section, whereas ESBL resistance was covered previously in the section on multidrug-resistant Enterobacteriaceae.

Epidemiology and mechanisms of resistance

The production of AmpC is regulated through a series of complex interactions among chromosomal bacterial genes. Such interactions are influenced by changes in the cytoplasmic concentrations of intermediates of murein peptidoglycan synthesis and degradation.[119] AmpC is usually not produced at high levels initially, but exposure to particular β-lactam antibiotics, including cephalosporins, cephamycins, monobactams, and extended-spectrum penicillins, can "induce" or "derepress" the production of AmpC enzymes.[120] Additionally, certain genetic mutations lead to constitutive cephalosporinase production.[121] In both of these cases, the increase in AmpC production is regulated by changes in the homeostatic levels of intermediate products of murein synthesis.[119] There is a 20% to 30% risk of clinical failure when a third-generation cephalosporin is used to treat bacteremia secondary to AmpC-producing

Enterobacter. The risk of such failure is much lower in urinary tract infections because of the high local cephalosporin concentrations.[122] AmpC-mediated resistance can be partially overcome by fourth-generation cephalosporins cefepime and cefpirome, which are more stable against AmpC-derepressed strains.[123]

Although AmpC production mediates much of the antibiotic resistance in certain gram-negative organisms, the impermeability of the outer cellular membrane and alterations in the outer membrane often also contribute to β-lactam resistance.[124] Cefepime, a fourth-generation cephalosporin, has neutral charge and a lower affinity for β-lactamases than third-generation cephalosporins, penetrates the outer membrane more effectively, and exhibits increased affinity for some essential PBP.[125] Cefepime often exhibits greater activity against AmpC-producing organisms than other cephalosporins.[126]

Acinetobacter spp

Resistance mechanisms to β-lactam antibiotics in *Acinetobacter* are not clearly understood, but resistance is common. Resistance frequently seems to be related to β-lactamase production, but other mechanisms have been identified. TEM-I and CARB enzymes seem to confer resistance to penicillins and some narrow-spectrum cephalosporins, whereas chromosomally produced cephalosporinases and plasmid-mediated ESBLs are thought to modulate resistance to broader-spectrum cephalosporins.[95,127] Carbapenem resistance is conferred by multiple different mechanisms including carbapenemase production of the IMP- and VIM-type, production of OXA-type β-lactamases, reduced cellular uptake, target mutations, and alterations in the PBP.[128–131] IMP metallo-β-lactamases were first described in a strain of *P aeruginosa* in Japan in 1988. In *Acinetobacter baumannii* IMP metallo-β-lactamases are usually present as part of a class 1 integron. Although metallo-β-lactamases are not the predominant carbapenemases in *A baumannii*, several have been described including IMP-1, IMP-2, IMP-4, IMP-5, IMP-6, and IMP-11.[132] Aminoglycoside resistance is mediated by aminoglycoside-modifying enzymes, and quinolone resistance by mutational changes of topoisomerase IV.[133,134]

Carbapenems are the most reliable therapeutic agents for infections caused by *Acinetobacter*, but resistance has begun to emerge in multiple geographic areas. Recent studies have reported rates of carbapenem resistance in *A baumannii*, the more resistant *Acinetobacter* species, as high as 11%.[135] A recent Centers for Disease Control and Prevention report noted that greater than 25% of *Acinetobacter* strains associated with device-related infections were carbapenem-resistant. A 1999 study reported meropenem resistance at greater than 50% in all isolates of *A baumannii* recovered from 15 hospitals in Brooklyn, New York.[136] A more recent study from the same area reported that rates of carbapenem resistance have exceeded 60% in some hospitals.[137] β-lactam–β-lactamase inhibitor combination antibiotics have good in vitro activity against *Acinetobacter lwoffi* (approximately 15% are resistant) but are less effective against *A baumannii* (20%–30% are resistant to piperacillin-tazobactam).[135] Ampicillin-sulbactam may be active against strains of *Acinetobacter* resistant to all other β-lactam agents, perhaps because of the unique antimicrobial activity of the sulbactam component against some acinetobacters. Ceftazidime and cefepime have modest activity, but approximately 35% of *A lwoffi* and *A baumannii* strains are resistant.[135] Aminoglycoside resistance occurs in approximately 20% to 30% of *A baumannii* isolates.[138] Resistance to quinolones is variable–precluding use of these drugs empirically before the results of susceptibility tests are known. In one study, approximately 80% of isolates tested were found to be ciprofloxacin-resistant.[139] Tigecycline, a relatively new glycylcycline agent, has bacteriostatic activity against multidrug-resistant *Acinetobacter* species. High-level resistance to tigecycline has been detected among some multidrug-resistant *Acinetobacter* isolates, and there is concern that the organism can rapidly evade this antimicrobial agent by upregulating chromosomally mediated efflux pumps. Given these findings and concern about whether adequate peak serum concentrations can be achieved, currently tigecycline is best reserved for salvage therapy.[140]

Stenotrophomonas Maltophilia

Stenotrophomonas maltophilia (formerly *Xanthomonas maltophilia*) is an aerobic gram-negative rod that causes bacteremia, respiratory tract infection, skin and soft tissue infection, and endocarditis. The virulence factors associated with *S maltophilia* include the production of proteases and elastases and the ability to adhere to synthetic materials. Nosocomial *S maltophilia* pneumonia is associated with adverse outcomes, particularly when the pneumonia is postobstructive or associated with bacteremia. In uncontrolled clinical trials, mortality rates associated with *S maltophilia* bacteremia range from 21% to 69%.[141]

The inducible, chromosomal enzymes *L1* and *L2* in *S maltophilia* confer resistance to β-lactam antibiotics. *L1* is a Bush-Jacoby-Medeiros class 3 enzyme (or metallo-β-lactamase) with broad activity against penicillins, carbapenems, cephalosporins, and β-lactamase inhibitors.[106,142] *L2* is a cephalosporinase (Bush-Jacoby-Medeiros class 2e) active against cephalosporins and monobactams. A TEM-2 β-lactamase encoded on a Tn-1 like transposon was also recently cloned from an *S maltophilia* isolate.[143] Decreased membrane permeability secondary to porin mutations often leads to quinolone resistance.[144] Aminoglycosides generally are not active against *S maltophilia*, probably caused by inactivating enzymes and alterations in the cell surface.[142] Overexpression of the multidrug efflux pump *SmeDEF* in *S maltophilia* may contribute to decreased susceptibility to tetracyclines, erythromycin, quinolones, and chloramphenicol.[145] Recent studies have reported that TMP-SMX resistance is mediated by the sul2 gene, which is associated with production by plasmids and class 1 integrons.[146,147]

TMP-SMX, a bacteriostatic agent, is the treatment of choice for infections caused by *S maltophilia*. Ticarcillin-clavulanate is the only β-lactam–β-lactamase inhibitor combination antibiotic that is reliably effective and may be used in patients who are intolerant of or infected with an isolate resistant to TMP-SMX.[142] Resistance to both of these agents is increasing; studies have reported that 5% of *S maltophilia* in the United States and 10% of isolates in Europe were resistant to TMP-SMX.[148] Ceftazidime does not possess reliable activity and should not be used empirically.[148] Cefepime has greater activity than ceftazidime (susceptibility was 88.7% versus 35.3% of United States bloodstream isolates in one study).[149] Resistance to imipenem approaches 100%.[149] Among the available fluoroquinolones, levofloxacin and moxifloxacin have better in vitro activity than ciprofloxacin. Minocycline has good in vitro activity,[150] but clinical experience is limited.

Tigecycline, a glycylcycline derived from minocycline, is a compound that has demonstrated good in vitro activity against *S maltophilia* strains including TMP-SMX–resistant *S maltophilia*, so it may be considered as a promising therapeutic option for the treatment of nosocomial infections caused by *S maltophilia*.[151] Use of antibiotic combinations, including TMP-SMX plus ticarcillin-clavulanate or a third-generation cephalosporin, and TMP-SMX plus minocycline plus ticarcillin-clavulanate, is being explored for the treatment of serious *S maltophilia* infections.[152] Although aztreonam is usually inactive against *S maltophilia*, one study demonstrated synergistic activity in vitro when combined with ticarcillin-clavulanate.[152] Although data are limited, resistance to TMP-SMX seems to be emerging, and recent in vitro modeling studies suggest that combination therapies of TMP-SMX plus ciprofloxacin and TMP-SMX plus tobramycin exhibit a greater killing capacity than TMP-SMX alone.[153]

The choice of monotherapy or combination therapy remains controversial. Use of multidrug therapy should be considered in cases of severe infection, particularly if local rates of resistance to TMP-SMX are high.[141]

Salmonella spp

Nontyphoidal species of Salmonella, such as S enteritidis and S enterica, are foodborne pathogens that can asymptomatically colonize the human intestine or cause clinical illnesses, such as gastroenteritis and bacteremia. Resistance to antimicrobial agents used to treat typhoidal and nontyphoidal species has rapidly emerged and disseminated around the world.[154]

Resistance to chloramphenicol in Salmonella typhi emerged in the 1970s, and several major outbreaks have been caused by chloramphenicol-resistant strains.[155] Resistance to chloramphenicol is often mediated by a self-transferable plasmid (IncHl) that also mediates resistance to sulfonamides, tetracycline, amoxicillin, TMP-SMX, and streptomycin.[154,156,157]

Resistance to the fluoroquinolones is an emerging problem, particularly in Asia,[158,159] and is usually mediated by chromosomal point mutations in the gyrA gene.[160] These quinolone-resistant strains are usually sensitive to ceftriaxone, cefixime, and azithromycin but the clinical response to treatment is usually slower and, with clearance of fever, sometimes exceeding taking 7 days or more. Failure rates are higher (>20%) when infection is caused by quinolone-resistant strains.[161] Resistance to nalidixic acid may predict clinical failure of quinolone therapy, even among isolates with in vitro quinolone susceptibility.[162] Such resistance to nalidixic acid was detected among 23% of S typhi isolates identified through the National Antimicrobial Resistance Monitoring System in 2000.[163] Resistance to third-generation cephalosporins (eg, ceftriaxone and cefotaxime) has occurred sporadically.[164]

The quinolones, such as ciprofloxacin, are considered the drugs of choice for empiric treatment of typhoid fever, except in areas of the world where quinolone resistance is common (eg, Asia).[165] So far, resistance to ciprofloxacin is infrequent in the United States, but was found in up to 23% of S typhi isolates in the United Kingdom in 1999.[166] In that study, multidrug resistance to chloramphenicol, ampicillin, and TMP was reported in 26% of all S typhi isolates.[166] Other potential oral alternatives for treatment of S typhi infections include amoxicillin, TMP-SMX, cefixime, azithromycin, and chloramphenicol, as long as these agents possess in vitro activity against a given strain.[154] Third-generation cephalosporins, such as ceftriaxone and cefotaxime, remain active but require intravenous administration.[167]

Resistance among nontyphoidal strains of salmonellae emerged in the 1990s and spread rapidly.[154] Emergence of multiresistance to ampicillin, chloramphenicol, and TMP-SMX is caused in part by the widespread dissemination of Salmonella typhimurium definitive phage type 104 (DT 104).[168] This strain contains chromosomal determinants that mediate resistance to ampicillin, chloramphenicol, TMP-SMX, streptomycin, and tetracycline.[169] Resistance to fluoroquinolones has also emerged among nontyphoidal salmonellae in the United Kingdom (including DT104) and in the United States. Resistance to the fluoroquinolones is often mediated by gyrA mutations and fortunately this remains uncommon in isolates in the United States.[170] Resistance to broad-spectrum cephalosporins is conferred by plasmid-mediated AmpC-type cephalosporinase production[171] and sometimes by ESBL production.[172] Resistance to the carbapenems has been reported and is mediated by porin loss; cephalosporinase production; and carbapenemase production (including KPCs).[101,173]

Campylobacter Jejuni

Campylobacter spp are fastidious, curved, seagull-shaped, motile gram-negative bacilli and are the leading cause of foodborne diarrhea and a common cause of travelers' diarrhea.[174] Fluoroquinolone resistance in *Campylobacter* spp has been present since the early 1990s in Asia and Europe, which coincided with the addition of enrofloxacin to animal feed. In Spain, quinolone resistance is well above 50%. Elsewhere in Europe, resistance rates are approximately 10% to 20% and many of the resistant strains are acquired outside the reporting country.[175,176] Thailand experienced a similar increase in the rates of fluoroquinolone resistance in campylobacter during the 1990s (0% in 1990 to 84% in 1995).[177] Rates of fluoroquinolone resistance among *Campylobacter* are lower in the United States, but agricultural use of fluoroquinolones again coincided with increased resistance. In one United States study, resistance increased from 1.3% in 1992 to 10.2% in 1998.[178] Imported isolates can contribute significantly to local resistance patterns.

Resistance to the macrolides is low (<5% in most regions).[179] Most isolates are still susceptible to aminoglycosides, chloramphenicol, clindamycin, nitrofurantoin, and imipenem.[180] A point mutation at codon 86 in the *gyrA* DNA gyrase gene is the most common mutation conferring quinolone resistance.[179] Mutations in the *parC* gene occur less frequently,[181] but the presence of mutations in both regions confers high-level quinolone resistance.[181] Multidrug efflux pumps may also have a role in the development of quinolone resistance.[182] Erythromycin resistance in *Campylobacter* is caused by ribosomal alterations.[179]

Neisseria Gonorrhoeae

Antimicrobial resistance has been a concern with *Neisseria gonorrhoeae* since the 1940s when resistance to sulfonamides was first noted; this was followed by penicillin resistance in the 1950s, tetracycline resistance in the 1980s, and fluoroquinolone resistance in the 1990s.[183,184]

High-level penicillin resistance (MIC ≥ 16 µg/mL) in *N gonorrhoeae* is most often mediated by penicillinase production.[185] Penicillin resistance caused by production of a plasmid-encoded TEM-1 type β-lactamase was first detected in *N gonorrhoeae* in 1976 and has now disseminated worldwide.[186] In the United States, the percentage of penicillinase-producing *N gonorrhoeae* peaked in 1991 at 11% but declined to 0.4% in 2006.[187]

Multiple chromosomal mutations can mediate lower-level penicillin (MIC >2 µg/mL) resistance. Resistance genes typically accumulate in a stepwise fashion, leading to gradually increasing penicillin MICs.[185] These resistance genes include *penA*, which encodes an altered PBP 2; *mtr*, which increases expression of an efflux pump; and *penB*, which decreases antibiotic permeability across the cell membrane through a porin gene mutation.[185,188] Chromosomally mediated resistance to penicillin was present in 1.2% of isolates in a recent United States survey.[187]

Resistance to tetracycline occurs through chromosomally mediated changes in cell membrane porins or by ribosomal protection by the plasmid mediated tetM resistance gene. Additional chromosomal mutations led to resistance to spectinomycin.[189] Macrolide resistance can occur through efflux pumps, *erm* methylases, and changes in the 23S ribosome.[190]

Fluoroquinolone-resistant *N gonorrhoeae* (MIC ≥ 1 μg/mL) has disseminated to many countries,[191] and is widespread in certain parts of Asia. In a recent study, greater than 35% of *N gonorrhoeae* isolates in the Philippines and Vietnam were quinolone resistant.[192] There have also been alarming increases in quinolone resistance reported recently in England and Wales.[191] The overall prevalence of quinolone-resistant gonococci in the United States was 2.2% in 2002, but this increased to greater than 13% by 2005.[183] The rate of quinolone resistance is particularly high among men who have sex with men (29%). Decreased susceptibility to fluoroquinolones is caused by mutations in the *parC* gene of topoisomerase IV and *gyrA* of DNA gyrase.[193,194]

SUMMARY

The emergence of resistance to antimicrobial agents continues to evolve substantially, influencing the evaluation and treatment of infections in nosocomial and health care–associated settings and in the community. Bacteria use several strategies to avoid the effects of antimicrobial agents, and have evolved highly efficient means for clonal spread and for the dissemination of resistance traits. Control of antibiotic-resistant pathogens provides a major challenge for the medical and public health communities and for society. Control of the emergence of resistant pathogens requires adherence to infection control guidelines, such as those issued by the Centers for Disease Control and Prevention (http://www.cdc.gov/ncidod/dhqp/guidelines.html), and physicians, patients, and health care consumers must all understand the need for judicious use of antibiotics (http://www.cdc.gov/drugresistance/healthcare/default.htm).

REFERENCES

1. Neu HC. The crisis in antibiotic resistance [see comments]. Science 1992; 257(5073):1064–73.
2. Nikaido H. Preventing drug access to targets: cell surface permeability barriers and active efflux in bacteria. Semin Cell Dev Biol 2001;12(3):215–23.
3. Davies J, Wright GD. Bacterial resistance to aminoglycoside antibiotics. Trends Microbiol 1997;5(6):234–40.
4. Helfand MS, Bonomo RA. Beta-lactamases: a survey of protein diversity. Curr Drug Targets Infect Disord 2003;3(1):9–23.
5. Davies J. Inactivation of antibiotics and the dissemination of resistance genes. Science 1994;264(5157):375–82.
6. Spratt BG. Resistance to antibiotics mediated by target alterations. Science 1994;264(5157):388–93.
7. Fraimow H, Courvalin P. Resistance to glycopeptides in gram-positive pathogens. In: Novick R, Fischetti V, Feretti J, et al, editors. Gram positive pathogens. Washington, DC: ASM Press; 2000. p. 621–34.
8. Normark BH, Normark S. Evolution and spread of antibiotic resistance. J Intern Med 2002;252(2):91–106.
9. Courvalin P. Transfer of antibiotic resistance genes between gram-positive and gram- negative bacteria. Antimicrob Agents Chemother 1994;38(7):1447–51.
10. Moellering RC Jr. Therapeutic options for infections caused by multiply-resistant enterococci. Abstracts of the 34th Interscience Conference on Antimicrobial Agents and Chemotherapy. American Society for Microbiology. Orlando (FL); 4–7 October, 1994.
11. Murray BE, Singh KV, Markowitz SM, et al. Evidence for clonal spread of a single strain of beta-lactamase-producing *Enterococcus (Streptococcus) faecalis* to six hospitals in five states. J Infect Dis 1991;163(4):780–5.

12. Grayson ML, Eliopoulos GM, Wennersten CB, et al. Increasing resistance to beta-lactam antibiotics among clinical isolates of *Enterococcus faecium*: a 22-year review at one institution. Antimicrob Agents Chemother 1991;35(11): 2180–4.

13. Boyce JM, Opal SM, Potter-Bynoe G, et al. Emergence and nosocomial transmission of ampicillin-resistant enterococci. Antimicrob Agents Chemother 1992;36(5):1032–9.

14. Williamson R, le Bouguenec C, Gutmann L, et al. One or two low affinity penicillin-binding proteins may be responsible for the range of susceptibility of *Enterococcus faecium* to benzylpenicillin. J Gen Microbiol 1985;131(8):1933–40.

15. Rupp ME, Marion N, Fey PD, et al. Outbreak of vancomycin-resistant *Enterococcus faecium* in a neonatal intensive care unit. Infect Control Hosp Epidemiol 2001;22(5):301–3.

16. Patterson JE, Zervos MJ. High-level gentamicin resistance in *Enterococcus*: microbiology, genetic basis, and epidemiology. Rev Infect Dis 1990;12(4): 644–52.

17. Krogstad DJ, Korfhagen TR, Moellering RC Jr, et al. Aminoglycoside-inactivating enzymes in clinical isolates of *Streptococcus faecalis*: an explanation for resistance to antibiotic synergism. J Clin Invest 1978;62(2):480–6.

18. Hidron AI, Edwards JR, Patel J, et al. NHSN annual update: antimicrobial-resistant pathogens associated with healthcare-associated infections: annual summary of data reported to the National Healthcare Safety Network at the Centers for Disease Control and Prevention, 2006–2007. Infect Control Hosp Epidemiol 2008;29(11):996–1011.

19. Mutnick AH, Biedenbach DJ, Jones RN. Geographic variations and trends in antimicrobial resistance among *Enterococcus faecalis* and *Enterococcus faecium* in the SENTRY Antimicrobial Surveillance Program (1997–2000). Diagn Microbiol Infect Dis 2003;46(1):63–8.

20. Livornese LL Jr, Dias S, Samel C, et al. Hospital-acquired infection with vancomycin-resistant *Enterococcus faecium* transmitted by electronic thermometers. Ann Intern Med 1992;117(2):112–6.

21. Carmeli Y, Eliopoulos GM, Samore MH. Antecedent treatment with different antibiotic agents as a risk factor for vancomycin-resistant *Enterococcus*. Emerg Infect Dis 2002;8(8):802–7.

22. Arthur M, Courvalin P. Genetics and mechanisms of glycopeptide resistance in enterococci. Antimicrob Agents Chemother 1993;37(8):1563–71.

23. Shlaes DM, Etter L, Gutmann L. Synergistic killing of vancomycin-resistant enterococci of classes A, B, and C by combinations of vancomycin, penicillin, and gentamicin. Antimicrob Agents Chemother 1991;35(4):776–9.

24. Power EG, Abdulla YH, Talsania HG, et al. vanA genes in vancomycin-resistant clinical isolates of *Oerskovia turbata* and *Arcanobacterium (Corynebacterium) haemolyticum*. J Antimicrob Chemother 1995;36(4):595–606.

25. Ligozzi M, Lo Cascio G, Fontana R. vanA gene cluster in a vancomycin-resistant clinical isolate of *Bacillus circulans*. Antimicrob Agents Chemother 1998;42(8):2055–9.

26. Mevius D, Devriese L, Butaye P, et al. Isolation of glycopeptide resistant *Streptococcus gallolyticus* strains with vanA, vanB, and both vanA and vanB genotypes from faecal samples of veal calves in The Netherlands. J Antimicrob Chemother 1998;42(2):275–6.

27. Dutka-Malen S, Blaimont B, Wauters G, et al. Emergence of high-level resistance to glycopeptides in *Enterococcus gallinarum* and *Enterococcus casseliflavus*. Antimicrob Agents Chemother 1994;38(7):1675–7.

28. Centers for Disease Control and Prevention (CDC) *Staphylococcus aureus* resistant to vancomycin—United States, 2002. MMWR Morb Mortal Wkly Rep 2002; 51(26):565–7.

29. Noble WC, Virani Z, Cree RG. Co-transfer of vancomycin and other resistance genes from *Enterococcus faecalis* NCTC 12201 to *Staphylococcus aureus*. FEMS Microbiol Lett 1992;72(2):195–8.

30. Perichon B, Reynolds P, Courvalin P. VanD-type glycopeptide-resistant *Enterococcus faecium* BM4339. Antimicrob Agents Chemother 1997;41(9):2016–8.

31. McKessar SJ, Berry AM, Bell JM, et al. Genetic characterization of vanG, a novel vancomycin resistance locus of *Enterococcus faecalis*. Antimicrob Agents Chemother 2000;44(11):3224–8.

32. Fines M, Perichon B, Reynolds P, et al. VanE, a new type of acquired glycopeptide resistance in *Enterococcus faecalis* BM4405. Antimicrob Agents Chemother 1999;43(9):2161–4.

33. Prystowsky J, Siddiqui F, Chosay J, et al. Resistance to linezolid: characterization of mutations in rRNA and comparison of their occurrences in vancomycin-resistant enterococci. Antimicrob Agents Chemother 2001;45:2154–6.

34. Bonora MG, Solbiati M, Stepan E, et al. Emergence of linezolid resistance in the vancomycin-resistant *Enterococcus faecium* multilocus sequence typing C1 epidemic lineage. J Clin Microbiol 2006;44(3):1153–5.

35. Pogue JM, Paterson DL, Pasculle AW, et al. Determination of risk factors associated with isolation of linezolid-resistant strains of vancomycin-resistant *Enterococcus*. Infect Control Hosp Epidemiol 2007;28(12):1382–8.

36. Montero CI, Stock F, Murray PR. Mechanisms of resistance to daptomycin in *Enterococcus faecium*. Antimicrob Agents Chemother 2008;52(3):1167–70.

37. Kirby WM. Extraction of a highly potent penicillin inactivator from penicillin resistant staphylococci. Science 1944;99(2579):452–3.

38. Clinical and Laboratory Standards Institute (CLSI) Performance standards for antimicrobial susceptibility testing. Wayne (PA): Clinical and Laboratory Standards Institute (CLSI); 2008.

39. Sievert DM, Rudrik JT, Patel JB, et al. Vancomycin-resistant *Staphylococcus aureus* in the United States, 2002–2006. Clin Infect Dis 2008;46(5):668–74.

40. Cunha BA, Mikail N, Eisenstein L. Persistent methicillin-resistant *Staphylococcus aureus* (MRSA) bacteremia due to a linezolid tolerant strain. Heart Lung 2008; 37(5):398–400.

41. Murthy MH, Olson ME, Wickert RW, et al. Daptomycin non-susceptible methicillin-resistant *Staphylococcus aureus* USA 300 isolate. J Med Microbiol 2008; 57(Pt 8):1036–8.

42. Higuchi W, Takano T, Teng LJ, et al. Structure and specific detection of staphylococcal cassette chromosome mec type VII. Biochem Biophys Res Commun 2008;377(3):752–6.

43. Oliveira DC, Milheirico C, de Lencastre H. Redefining a structural variant of staphylococcal cassette chromosome mec, SCCmec type VI. Antimicrob Agents Chemother 2006;50(10):3457–9.

44. Zhang K, McClure JA, Elsayed S, et al. Novel staphylococcal cassette chromosome mec type carrying class A mec and type 4 ccr gene complexes in a Canadian epidemic strain of methicillin-resistant *Staphylococcus aureus*. 2009;53(2): 531–40.

45. Katayama Y, Ito T, Hiramatsu K. Genetic organization of the chromosome region surrounding mecA in clinical staphylococcal strains: role of IS431-mediated mecI deletion in expression of resistance in mecA-carrying, low-level

methicillin-resistant *Staphylococcus haemolyticus*. Antimicrob Agents Chemother 2001;45(7):1955–63.

46. Boyle-Vavra S, Daum RS. Community-acquired methicillin-resistant *Staphylococcus aureus*: the role of Panton-Valentine leukocidin. Lab Invest 2007;87(1):3–9.

47. Martinez-Aguilar G, Hammerman WA, Mason EO Jr, et al. Clindamycin treatment of invasive infections caused by community-acquired, methicillin-resistant and methicillin-susceptible *Staphylococcus aureus* in children. Pediatr Infect Dis J 2003;22(7):593–8.

48. Weigel LM, Clewell DB, Gill SR, et al. Genetic analysis of a high-level vancomycin-resistant isolate of *Staphylococcus aureus*. Science 2003;302(5650):1569–71.

49. Reynolds PE, Courvalin P. Vancomycin resistance in enterococci due to synthesis of precursors terminating in D-alanyl-D-serine. Antimicrob Agents Chemother 2005;49(1):21–5.

50. Soriano A, Marco F, Martinez JA, et al. Influence of vancomycin minimum inhibitory concentration on the treatment of methicillin-resistant *Staphylococcus aureus* bacteremia. Clin Infect Dis 2008;46(2):193–200.

51. Sakoulas G, Moise-Broder PA, Schentag J, et al. Relationship of MIC and bactericidal activity to efficacy of vancomycin for treatment of methicillin-resistant *Staphylococcus aureus* bacteremia. J Clin Microbiol 2004;42(6):2398–402.

52. Steinkraus G, White R, Friedrich L. Vancomycin MIC creep in non-vancomycin-intermediate *Staphylococcus aureus* (VISA), vancomycin-susceptible clinical methicillin-resistant *S. aureus* (MRSA) blood isolates from 2001–05. J Antimicrob Chemother 2007;60(4):788–94.

53. Alos JI, Garcia-Canas A, Garcia-Hierro P, et al. Vancomycin MICs did not creep in *Staphylococcus aureus* isolates from 2002 to 2006 in a setting with low vancomycin usage. J Antimicrob Chemother 2008;62(4):773–5.

54. Jones RN. Microbiological features of vancomycin in the 21st century: minimum inhibitory concentration creep, bactericidal/static activity, and applied breakpoints to predict clinical outcomes or detect resistant strains. Clin Infect Dis 2006;42(Suppl 1):S13–24.

55. Wang G, Hindler JF, Ward KW, et al. Increased vancomycin MICs for *Staphylococcus aureus* clinical isolates from a university hospital during a 5-year period. J Clin Microbiol 2006;44(11):3883–6.

56. Rybak M, Lomaestro B, Rotschafer JC, et al. Therapeutic monitoring of vancomycin in adult patients: a consensus review of the American Society of Health-System Pharmacists, the Infectious Diseases Society of America, and the Society of Infectious Diseases Pharmacists. Am J Health Syst Pharm 2009;66(1):82–98.

57. Champney WS, Miller M. Linezolid is a specific inhibitor of 50S ribosomal subunit formation in *Staphylococcus aureus* cells. Curr Microbiol 2002;44(5):350–6.

58. Tsiodras S, Gold HS, Sakoulas G, et al. Linezolid resistance in a clinical isolate of *Staphylococcus aureus*. Lancet 2001;358(9277):207–8.

59. Besier S, Ludwig A, Zander J, et al. Linezolid resistance in *Staphylococcus aureus*: gene dosage effect, stability, fitness costs, and cross-resistances. Antimicrob Agents Chemother 2008;52(4):1570–2.

60. Silverman JA, Perlmutter NG, Shapiro HM. Correlation of daptomycin bactericidal activity and membrane depolarization in *Staphylococcus aureus*. Antimicrob Agents Chemother 2003;47(8):2538–44.

61. Silverman JA, Mortin LI, Vanpraagh AD, et al. Inhibition of daptomycin by pulmonary surfactant: in vitro modeling and clinical impact. J Infect Dis 2005;191(12):2149–52.

62. Skiest DJ. Treatment failure resulting from resistance of *Staphylococcus aureus* to daptomycin. J Clin Microbiol 2006;44(2):655–6.
63. Sakoulas G, Alder J, Thauvin-Eliopoulos C, et al. Induction of daptomycin heterogeneous susceptibility in *Staphylococcus aureus* by exposure to vancomycin. Antimicrob Agents Chemother 2006;50(4):1581–5.
64. Jones T, Yeaman MR, Sakoulas G, et al. Failures in clinical treatment of *Staphylococcus aureus* infection with daptomycin are associated with alterations in surface charge, membrane phospholipid asymmetry, and drug binding. Antimicrob Agents Chemother 2008;52(1):269–78.
65. Cui L, Tominaga E, Neoh HM, et al. Correlation between reduced daptomycin susceptibility and vancomycin resistance in vancomycin-intermediate *Staphylococcus aureus*. Antimicrob Agents Chemother 2006;50(3):1079–82.
66. Schmitz FJ, Witte W, Werner G, et al. Characterization of the translational attenuator of 20 methicillin-resistant, quinupristin/dalfopristin-resistant *Staphylococcus aureus* isolates with reduced susceptibility to glycopeptides. J Antimicrob Chemother 2001;48(6):939–41.
67. Drago L, Nicola L, De Vecchi E. A comparative in-vitro evaluation of resistance selection after exposure to teicoplanin, vancomycin, linezolid and quinupristin-dalfopristin in *Staphylococcus aureus* and *Enterococcus* spp. Clin Microbiol Infect 2008;14(6):608–11.
68. Allignet J, el Solh N. Diversity among the gram-positive acetyltransferases inactivating streptogramin A and structurally related compounds and characterization of a new staphylococcal determinant, vatB. Antimicrob Agents Chemother 1995;39(9):2027–36.
69. Markiewicz Z, Tomasz A. Variation in penicillin-binding protein patterns of penicillin-resistant clinical isolates of pneumococci. J Clin Microbiol 1989;27(3):405–10.
70. Nagai K, Davies TA, Jacobs MR, et al. Effects of amino acid alterations in penicillin-binding proteins (PBPs) 1a, 2b, and 2x on PBP affinities of penicillin, ampicillin, amoxicillin, cefditoren, cefuroxime, cefprozil, and cefaclor in 18 clinical isolates of penicillin-susceptible, -intermediate, and -resistant pneumococci. Antimicrob Agents Chemother 2002;46(5):1273–80.
71. Zapun A, Contreras-Martel C, Vernet T. Penicillin-binding proteins and beta-lactam resistance. FEMS Microbiol Rev 2008;32(2):361–85.
72. Pernot L, Chesnel L, Le Gouellec A, et al. A PBP2x from a clinical isolate of *Streptococcus pneumoniae* exhibits an alternative mechanism for reduction of susceptibility to beta-lactam antibiotics. J Biol Chem 2004;279(16):16463–70.
73. Sahm DF, Brown NP, Draghi DC, et al. Tracking resistance among bacterial respiratory tract pathogens: summary of findings of the TRUST Surveillance Initiative, 2001–2005. Postgrad Med 2008;120(3 Suppl 1):8–15.
74. Chiu CH, Su LH, Huang YC, et al. Increasing ceftriaxone resistance and multiple alterations of penicillin-binding proteins among penicillin-resistant *Streptococcus pneumoniae* isolates in Taiwan. Antimicrob Agents Chemother 2007; 51(9):3404–6.
75. Gums JG, Boatwright DW, Camblin M, et al. Differences between ceftriaxone and cefotaxime: microbiological inconsistencies. Ann Pharmacother 2008;42(1):71–9.
76. Cardoso MR, Nascimento-Carvalho CM, Ferrero F, et al. Penicillin-resistant pneumococcus and risk of treatment failure in pneumonia. Arch Dis Child 2008;93(3):221–5.
77. Sahm DF, Brown NP, Thornsberry C, et al. Antimicrobial susceptibility profiles among common respiratory tract pathogens: a GLOBAL perspective. Postgrad Med 2008;120(3 Suppl 1):16–24.

78. Rodriguez CA, Atkinson R, Bitar W, et al. Tolerance to vancomycin in pneumococci: detection with a molecular marker and assessment of clinical impact. J Infect Dis 2004;190(8):1481–7.

79. Low DE. Quinolone resistance among pneumococci: therapeutic and diagnostic implications. Clin Infect Dis 2004;38(Suppl 4):S357–62.

80. Sirot DL, Goldstein FW, Soussy CJ, et al. Resistance to cefotaxime and seven other beta-lactams in members of the family Enterobacteriaceae: a 3-year survey in France. Antimicrob Agents Chemother 1992;36(8):1677–81.

81. Burwen DR, Banerjee SN, Gaynes RP. Ceftazidime resistance among selected nosocomial gram-negative bacilli in the United States. National Nosocomial Infections Surveillance System. J Infect Dis 1994;170(6):1622–5.

82. Edwards JR, Peterson KD, Andrus ML, et al. National Healthcare Safety Network (NHSN) Report, data summary for 2006 through 2007, issued November 2008. Am J Infect Control 2008;36(9):609–26.

83. Jacoby GA. Extended-spectrum beta-lactamases and other enzymes providing resistance to oxyimino-beta-lactams. Infect Dis Clin North Am 1997;11(4): 875–87.

84. Wiener J, Quinn JP, Bradford PA, et al. Multiple antibiotic-resistant Klebsiella and Escherichia coli in nursing homes [see comments]. JAMA 1999;281(6):517–23.

85. Montgomerie JZ. Epidemiology of Klebsiella and hospital-associated infections. Rev Infect Dis 1979;1(5):736–53.

86. Lin MF, Huang ML, Lai SH. Risk factors in the acquisition of extended-spectrum beta-lactamase Klebsiella pneumoniae: a case-control study in a district teaching hospital in Taiwan. J Hosp Infect 2003;53(1):39–45.

87. Lautenbach E, Patel JB, Bilker WB, et al. Extended-spectrum beta-lactamase-producing Escherichia coli and Klebsiella pneumoniae: risk factors for infection and impact of resistance on outcomes. Clin Infect Dis 2001;32(8):1162–71.

88. Du B, Long Y, Liu H, et al. Extended-spectrum beta-lactamase-producing Escherichia coli and Klebsiella pneumoniae bloodstream infection: risk factors and clinical outcome. Intensive Care Med 2002;28(12):1718–23.

89. D'Agata E, Venkataraman L, DeGirolami P, et al. The molecular and clinical epidemiology of enterobacteriaceae-producing extended-spectrum beta-lactamase in a tertiary care hospital. J Infect 1998;36(3):279–85.

90. Rahal JJ, Urban C, Horn D, et al. Class restriction of cephalosporin use to control total cephalosporin resistance in nosocomial Klebsiella [see comments]. JAMA 1998;280(14):1233–7.

91. Pena C, Pujol M, Ardanuy C, et al. Epidemiology and successful control of a large outbreak due to Klebsiella pneumoniae producing extended-spectrum beta-lactamases. Antimicrob Agents Chemother 1998;42(1):53–8.

92. Harris AD, McGregor JC, Johnson JA, et al. Risk factors for colonization with extended-spectrum beta-lactamase-producing bacteria and intensive care unit admission. Emerg Infect Dis 2007;13(8):1144–9.

93. Amino acid sequences for TEM, SHV and OXA extended-spectrum beta-lactamases. Available at: http://www.lahey.org/studies/inc_webt.asp. Accessed July, 2009.

94. Bonnet R. Growing group of extended-spectrum beta-lactamases: the CTX-M enzymes. Antimicrob Agents Chemother 2004;48(1):1–14.

95. Livermore DM. beta-Lactamases in laboratory and clinical resistance. Clin Microbiol Rev 1995;8(4):557–84.

96. Nordmann P, Poirel L. Emerging carbapenemases in gram-negative aerobes. Clin Microbiol Infect 2002;8(6):321–31.

97. Patel G, Huprikar S, Factor SH, et al. Outcomes of carbapenem-resistant *Klebsiella pneumoniae* infection and the impact of antimicrobial and adjunctive therapies. Infect Control Hosp Epidemiol 2008;29(12):1099–106.
98. Martinez-Martinez L, Hernandez-Alles S, Alberti S, et al. In vivo selection of porin-deficient mutants of *Klebsiella pneumoniae* with increased resistance to cefoxitin and expanded-spectrum-cephalosporins. Antimicrob Agents Chemother 1996;40(2):342–8.
99. Pangon B, Bizet C, Bure A, et al. In vivo selection of a cephamycin-resistant, porin-deficient mutant of *Klebsiella pneumoniae* producing a TEM-3 beta-lactamase. J Infect Dis 1989;159(5):1005–6.
100. Kaye KS, Gold HS, Schwaber MJ, et al. Variety of beta-lactamases produced by amoxicillin-clavulanate-resistant *Escherichia coli* isolated in the northeastern United States. Antimicrob Agents Chemother 2004;48(5):1520–5.
101. Coudron PE, Moland ES, Thomson KS. Occurrence and detection of AmpC beta-lactamases among *Escherichia coli*, *Klebsiella pneumoniae*, and *Proteus mirabilis* isolates at a veterans medical center. J Clin Microbiol 2000;38(5):1791–6.
102. Bell JM, Turnidge JD, Gales AC, et al. Prevalence of extended spectrum beta-lactamase (ESBL)-producing clinical isolates in the Asia-Pacific region and South Africa: regional results from SENTRY Antimicrobial Surveillance Program (1998–99). Diagn Microbiol Infect Dis 2002;42(3):193–8.
103. Andriole VT. The quinolones. 2nd edition. New York: Academic Press; 1998.
104. Mandell GL, Bennett JE, Mandell Dolin R. Douglas and Bennett's principles and practice of infectious diseases. 6th edition. New York: Churchill Livingstone; 2004.
105. Anthony KB, Fishman NO, Linkin DR, et al. Clinical and microbiological outcomes of serious infections with multidrug-resistant gram-negative organisms treated with tigecycline. Clin Infect Dis 2008;46(4):567–70.
106. Yang K, Guglielmo BJ. Diagnosis and treatment of extended-spectrum and AmpC beta-lactamase-producing organisms. Ann Pharmacother 2007;41(9):1427–35.
107. Sanders WE Jr, Sanders CC. Inducible beta-lactamases: clinical and epidemiologic implications for use of newer cephalosporins. Rev Infect Dis 1988;10(4):830–8.
108. Tenover FC, Emery SL, Spiegel CA, et al. Identification of plasmid-mediated AmpC {beta}-lactamases in *Escherichia coli*, *Klebsiella pneumoniae*, and *Proteus* species can potentially improve reporting of cephalosporin susceptibility testing results. J Clin Microbiol 2009;47(2):294–9.
109. Fakioglu E, Queenan AM, Bush K, et al. Amp C beta-lactamase-producing *Escherichia coli* in neonatal meningitis: diagnostic and therapeutic challenge. J Perinatol 2006;26(8):515–7.
110. Jacobs C, Frere JM, Normark S. Cytosolic intermediates for cell wall biosynthesis and degradation control inducible beta-lactam resistance in gram-negative bacteria. Cell 1997;88(6):823–32.
111. Korsak D, Liebscher S, Vollmer W. Susceptibility to antibiotics and beta-lactamase induction in murein hydrolase mutants of *Escherichia coli*. Antimicrob Agents Chemother 2005;49(4):1404–9.
112. Medeiros AA. Evolution and dissemination of beta-lactamases accelerated by generations of beta-lactam antibiotics. Clin Infect Dis 1997;24(Suppl 1):S19–45.
113. Kaye KS, Cosgrove S, Harris A, et al. Risk factors for emergence of resistance to broad-spectrum cephalosporins among *Enterobacter* spp. Antimicrob Agents Chemother 2001;45(9):2628–30.

114. Mammeri H, Poirel L, Bemer P, et al. Resistance to cefepime and cefpirome due to a 4-amino-acid deletion in the chromosome-encoded AmpC beta-lactamase of a *Serratia marcescens* clinical isolate. Antimicrob Agents Chemother 2004;48(3):716–20.

115. Ceccarelli M, Ruggerone P. Physical insights into permeation of and resistance to antibiotics in bacteria. Curr Drug Targets 2008;9(9):779–88.

116. Kessler RE. Cefepime microbiologic profile and update. Pediatr Infect Dis J 2001;20(3):331–6.

117. Ishii Y, Tateda K, Yamaguchi K. Evaluation of antimicrobial susceptibility for beta-lactams using the Etest method against clinical isolates from 100 medical centers in Japan (2006). Diagn Microbiol Infect Dis 2008;60(2):177–83.

118. Poirel L, Pitout JD, Nordmann P. Carbapenemases: molecular diversity and clinical consequences. Future Microbiol 2007;2(5):501–12.

119. Yigit H, Queenan AM, Anderson GJ, et al. Novel carbapenem-hydrolyzing beta-lactamase, KPC-1, from a carbapenem-resistant strain of *Klebsiella pneumoniae*. Antimicrob Agents Chemother 2001;45(4):1151–61.

120. Bratu S, Brooks S, Burney S, et al. Detection and spread of *Escherichia coli* possessing the plasmid-borne carbapenemase KPC-2 in Brooklyn, New York. Clin Infect Dis 2007;44(7):972–5.

121. Lomaestro BM, Tobin EH, Shang W, et al. The spread of *Klebsiella pneumoniae* carbapenemase-producing *K. pneumoniae* to upstate New York. Clin Infect Dis 2006;43(3):e26–8.

122. Bratu S, Mooty M, Nichani S, et al. Emergence of KPC-possessing *Klebsiella pneumoniae* in Brooklyn, New York: epidemiology and recommendations for detection. Antimicrob Agents Chemother 2005;49(7):3018–20.

123. Miriagou V, Tzouvelekis LS, Rossiter S, et al. Imipenem resistance in a *Salmonella* clinical strain due to plasmid-mediated class A carbapenemase KPC-2. Antimicrob Agents Chemother 2003;47(4):1297–300.

124. Villegas MV, Lolans K, Correa A, et al. First identification of *Pseudomonas aeruginosa* isolates producing a KPC-type carbapenem-hydrolyzing beta-lactamase. Antimicrob Agents Chemother 2007;51(4):1553–5.

125. Peleg AY, Franklin C, Bell JM, et al. Dissemination of the metallo-beta-lactamase gene blaIMP-4 among gram-negative pathogens in a clinical setting in Australia. Clin Infect Dis 2005;41(11):1549–56.

126. Lolans K, Rice TW, Munoz-Price LS, et al. Multicity outbreak of carbapenem-resistant *Acinetobacter baumannii* isolates producing the carbapenemase OXA-40. Antimicrob Agents Chemother 2006;50(9):2941–5.

127. Danes C, Navia MM, Ruiz J, et al. Distribution of beta-lactamases in *Acinetobacter baumannii* clinical isolates and the effect of Syn 2190 (AmpC inhibitor) on the MICs of different beta-lactam antibiotics. J Antimicrob Chemother 2002;50(2):261–4.

128. Livermore DM. Acquired carbapenemases. J Antimicrob Chemother 1997;39(6):673–6.

129. Afzal-Shah M, Woodford N, Livermore DM. Characterization of OXA-25, OXA-26, and OXA-27, molecular class D beta-lactamases associated with carbapenem resistance in clinical isolates of *Acinetobacter baumannii*. Antimicrob Agents Chemother 2001;45(2):583–8.

130. Bou G, Cervero G, Dominguez MA, et al. Characterization of a nosocomial outbreak caused by a multiresistant *Acinetobacter baumannii* strain with a carbapenem-hydrolyzing enzyme: high-level carbapenem resistance in *A. baumannii* is not due solely to the presence of beta-lactamases. J Clin Microbiol 2000;38(9):3299–305.

131. Quale J, Bratu S, Landman D, et al. Molecular epidemiology and mechanisms of carbapenem resistance in *Acinetobacter baumannii* endemic in New York City. Clin Infect Dis 2003;37(2):214–20.

132. Perez F, Hujer AM, Hujer KM, et al. Global challenge of multidrug-resistant *Acinetobacter baumannii*. Antimicrob Agents Chemother 2007;51(10): 3471–84.

133. Miller GH, Sabatelli FJ, Hare RS, et al. The most frequent aminoglycoside resistance mechanisms–changes with time and geographic area: a reflection of aminoglycoside usage patterns? Aminoglycoside Resistance Study Groups. Clin Infect Dis 1997;24(Suppl 1):S46–62.

134. Vila J, Ruiz J, Goni P, et al. Quinolone-resistance mutations in the topoisomerase IV parC gene of *Acinetobacter baumannii*. J Antimicrob Chemother 1997;39(6): 757–62.

135. Turner PJ, Greenhalgh JM. The activity of meropenem and comparators against *Acinetobacter* strains isolated from European hospitals, 1997–2000. Clin Microbiol Infect 2003;9(6):563–7.

136. Landman D, Quale JM, Mayorga D, et al. Citywide clonal outbreak of multiresistant *Acinetobacter baumannii* and *Pseudomonas aeruginosa* in Brooklyn, NY: the preantibiotic era has returned. Arch Intern Med 2002;162(13):1515–20.

137. Landman D, Bratu S, Kochar S, et al. Evolution of antimicrobial resistance among Pseudomonas aeruginosa, Acinetobacter baumannii and Klebsiella pneumoniae in Brooklyn, NY. J Antimicrob Chemother 2007;60(1):78–82.

138. Seifert H, Strate A, Pulverer G. Nosocomial bacteremia due to *Acinetobacter baumannii*: clinical features, epidemiology, and predictors of mortality. Medicine (Baltimore) 1995;74(6):340–9.

139. Vila J, Ribera A, Marco F, et al. Activity of clinafloxacin, compared with six other quinolones, against *Acinetobacter baumannii* clinical isolates. J Antimicrob Chemother 2002;49(3):471–7.

140. Maragakis LL, Perl TM. *Acinetobacter baumannii*: epidemiology, antimicrobial resistance, and treatment options. Clin Infect Dis 2008;46(8):1254–63.

141. Nicodemo AC, Paez JI. Antimicrobial therapy for *Stenotrophomonas maltophilia* infections. Eur J Clin Microbiol Infect Dis 2007;26(4):229–37.

142. Denton M, Kerr KG. Microbiological and clinical aspects of infection associated with *Stenotrophomonas maltophilia*. Clin Microbiol Rev 1998;11(1):57–80.

143. Avison MB, von Heldreich CJ, Higgins CS, et al. A TEM-2beta-lactamase encoded on an active Tn1-like transposon in the genome of a clinical isolate of *Stenotrophomonas maltophilia*. J Antimicrob Chemother 2000;46(6):879–84.

144. Cullmann W. Antibiotic susceptibility and outer membrane proteins of clinical *Xanthomonas maltophilia* isolates. Chemotherapy 1991;37(4):246–50.

145. Alonso A, Martinez JL. Expression of multidrug efflux pump SmeDEF by clinical isolates of *Stenotrophomonas maltophilia*. Antimicrob Agents Chemother 2001; 45(6):1879–81.

146. Barbolla R, Catalano M, Orman BE, et al. Class 1 integrons increase trimethoprim-sulfamethoxazole MICs against epidemiologically unrelated *Stenotrophomonas maltophilia* isolates. Antimicrob Agents Chemother 2004;48(2): 666–9.

147. Toleman MA, Bennett PM, Bennett DM, et al. Global emergence of trimethoprim/sulfamethoxazole resistance in *Stenotrophomonas maltophilia* mediated by acquisition of sul genes. Emerg Infect Dis 2007;13(4):559–65.

148. Gales AC, Jones RN, Forward KR, et al. Emerging importance of multidrug-resistant *Acinetobacter* species and *Stenotrophomonas maltophilia* as

pathogens in seriously ill patients: geographic patterns, epidemiological features, and trends in the SENTRY Antimicrobial Surveillance Program (1997–1999). Clin Infect Dis 2001;32(Suppl 2):S104–13.

149. Jones RN, Pfaller MA, Marshall SA, et al. Antimicrobial activity of 12 broad-spectrum agents tested against 270 nosocomial blood stream infection isolates caused by non-enteric gram-negative bacilli: occurrence of resistance, molecular epidemiology, and screening for metallo-enzymes. Diagn Microbiol Infect Dis 1997;29(3):187–92.

150. Canton R, Valdezate S, Vindel A, et al. Antimicrobial susceptibility profile of molecular typed cystic fibrosis *Stenotrophomonas maltophilia* isolates and differences with noncystic fibrosis isolates. Pediatr Pulmonol 2003;35(2):99–107.

151. Insa R, Cercenado E, Goyanes MJ, et al. In vitro activity of tigecycline against clinical isolates of *Acinetobacter baumannii* and *Stenotrophomonas maltophilia*. J Antimicrob Chemother 2007;59(3):583–5.

152. Krueger TS, Clark EA, Nix DE. In vitro susceptibility of *Stenotrophomonas maltophilia* to various antimicrobial combinations. Diagn Microbiol Infect Dis 2001;41(1–2):71–8.

153. Al-Jasser AM. *Stenotrophomonas maltophilia* resistant to trimethoprim-sulfamethoxazole: an increasing problem. Ann Clin Microbiol Antimicrob 2006;5:23.

154. Parry CM, Threlfall EJ. Antimicrobial resistance in typhoidal and nontyphoidal salmonellae. Curr Opin Infect Dis 2008;21(5):531–8.

155. Parry CM, Hien TT, Dougan G, et al. Typhoid fever. N Engl J Med 2002;347(22):1770–82.

156. Taylor DE, Chumpitaz JC, Goldstein F. Variability of IncHI1 plasmids from *Salmonella typhi* with special reference to Peruvian plasmids encoding resistance to trimethoprim and other antibiotics. Antimicrob Agents Chemother 1985;28(3):452–5.

157. Gilmour MW, Thomson NR, Sanders M, et al. The complete nucleotide sequence of the resistance plasmid R478: defining the backbone components of incompatibility group H conjugative plasmids through comparative genomics. Plasmid 2004;52(3):182–202.

158. Capoor MR, Nair D, Deb M, et al. Enteric fever perspective in India: emergence of high-level ciprofloxacin resistance and rising MIC to cephalosporins. J Med Microbiol 2007;56(Pt 8):1131–2.

159. Ko WC, Yan JJ, Yu WL, et al. A new therapeutic challenge for old pathogens: community-acquired invasive infections caused by ceftriaxone- and ciprofloxacin-resistant *Salmonella enterica* serotype choleraesuis. Clin Infect Dis 2005;40(2):315–8.

160. Shirakawa T, Acharya B, Kinoshita S, et al. Decreased susceptibility to fluoroquinolones and gyrA gene mutation in the *Salmonella enterica* serovar typhi and paratyphi A isolated in Katmandu, Nepal, in 2003. Diagn Microbiol Infect Dis 2006;54(4):299–303.

161. Crump JA, Kretsinger K, Gay K, et al. Clinical response and outcome of infection with *Salmonella enterica* serotype typhi with decreased susceptibility to fluoroquinolones: a United States foodnet multicenter retrospective cohort study. Antimicrob Agents Chemother 2008;52(4):1278–84.

162. Kownhar H, Shankar EM, Rajan R, et al. Emergence of nalidixic acid-resistant *Salmonella enterica* serovar typhi resistant to ciprofloxacin in India. J Med Microbiol 2007;56(Pt 1):136–7.

163. Crump JA, Barrett TJ, Nelson JT, et al. Reevaluating fluoroquinolone breakpoints for *Salmonella enterica* serotype typhi and for non-typhi salmonellae. Clin Infect Dis 2003;37(1):75–81.

164. Su LH, Wu TL, Chia JH, et al. Increasing ceftriaxone resistance in *Salmonella* isolates from a university hospital in Taiwan. J Antimicrob Chemother 2005; 55(6):846–52.
165. Thaver D, Zaidi AK, Critchley JA, et al. Fluoroquinolones for treating typhoid and paratyphoid fever (enteric fever). Cochrane Database Syst Rev 2008;(4): CD004530.
166. Threlfall EJ, Ward LR. Decreased susceptibility to ciprofloxacin in *Salmonella enterica* serotype typhi, United Kingdom. Emerg Infect Dis 2001;7(3):448–50.
167. Connor BA, Schwartz E. Typhoid and paratyphoid fever in travellers. Lancet Infect Dis 2005;5(10):623–8.
168. Skov MN, Andersen JS, Baggesen DL. Occurrence and spread of multiresistant *Salmonella typhimurium* DT104 in Danish animal herds investigated by the use of DNA typing and spatio-temporal analysis. Epidemiol Infect 2008;136(8):1124–30.
169. Meakins S, Fisher IS, Berghold C, et al. Antimicrobial drug resistance in human nontyphoidal *Salmonella* isolates in Europe 2000–2004: a report from the Enter-net International Surveillance Network. Microb Drug Resist 2008;14(1):31–5.
170. Gay K, Robicsek A, Strahilevitz J, et al. Plasmid-mediated quinolone resistance in non-typhi serotypes of *Salmonella enterica*. Clin Infect Dis 2006;43(3):297–304.
171. Li WC, Huang FY, Liu CP, et al. Ceftriaxone resistance of nontyphoidal *Salmonella enterica* isolates in Northern Taiwan attributable to production of CTX-M-14 and CMY-2 beta-lactamases. J Clin Microbiol 2005;43(7):3237–43.
172. Gupta A, Fontana J, Crowe C, et al. Emergence of multidrug-resistant *Salmonella enterica* serotype Newport infections resistant to expanded-spectrum cephalosporins in the United States. J Infect Dis 2003;188(11):1707–16.
173. Armand-Lefevre L, Leflon-Guibout V, Bredin J, et al. Imipenem resistance in *Salmonella enterica* serovar Wien related to porin loss and CMY-4 beta-lactamase production. Antimicrob Agents Chemother 2003;47(3):1165–8.
174. Shlim DR. Update in traveler's diarrhea. Infect Dis Clin North Am 2005;19(1): 137–49.
175. Little CL, Richardson JF, Owen RJ, et al. *Campylobacter* and *Salmonella* in raw red meats in the United Kingdom: prevalence, characterization and antimicrobial resistance pattern, 2003–2005. Food Microbiol 2008;25(3):538–43.
176. Ruiz J, Marco F, Oliveira I, et al. Trends in antimicrobial resistance in *Campylobacter* spp. causing traveler's diarrhea. APMIS 2007;115(3):218–24.
177. Serichantalergs O, Dalsgaard A, Bodhidatta L, et al. Emerging fluoroquinolone and macrolide resistance of *Campylobacter jejuni* and *Campylobacter coli* isolates and their serotypes in Thai children from 1991 to 2000. Epidemiol Infect 2007;135(8):1299–306.
178. Smith KE, Besser JM, Hedberg CW, et al. Quinolone-resistant *Campylobacter jejuni* infections in Minnesota, 1992–1998. Investigation team. N Engl J Med 1999;340(20):1525–32.
179. Gibreel A, Taylor DE. Macrolide resistance in *Campylobacter jejuni* and *Campylobacter coli*. J Antimicrob Chemother 2006;58(2):243–55.
180. Allos BM. *Campylobacter jejuni* infections: update on emerging issues and trends. Clin Infect Dis 2001;32(8):1201–6.
181. Engberg J, Aarestrup FM, Taylor DE, et al. Quinolone and macrolide resistance in *Campylobacter jejuni* and *C. coli*: resistance mechanisms and trends in human isolates. Emerg Infect Dis 2001;7(1):24–34.
182. Yan M, Sahin O, Lin J, et al. Role of the CmeABC efflux pump in the emergence of fluoroquinolone-resistant *Campylobacter* under selection pressure. J Antimicrob Chemother 2006;58(6):1154–9.

183. Centers for Disease Control and Prevention (CDC). Increases in fluoroquino-lone-resistant *Neisseria gonorrhoeae*—Hawaii and California, 2001 [see comment]. MMWR Morb Mortal Wkly Rep 2002;51(46):1041–4.

184. Erbelding E, Quinn TC. The impact of antimicrobial resistance on the treatment of sexually transmitted diseases. Infect Dis Clin North Am 1997;11(4): 889–903.

185. Ropp PA, Hu M, Olesky M, et al. Mutations in ponA, the gene encoding penicillin-binding protein 1, and a novel locus, penC, are required for high-level chromosomally mediated penicillin resistance in *Neisseria gonorrhoeae*. Antimicrob Agents Chemother 2002;46(3):769–77.

186. Ison CA, Dillon JA, Tapsall JW. The epidemiology of global antibiotic resistance among *Neisseria gonorrhoeae* and *Haemophilus ducreyi*. Lancet 1998; 351(Suppl 3):8–11 [erratum appears in Lancet 1998 Oct 17;352(9136):1316].

187. Gonococcal Isolate Surveillance Project (GISP) Annual Report. Centers for Disease Control and Prevention. 2006. Available at: http://www.cdc.gov/std/GISP2006/GISPSurvSupp2006Short.pdf. Accessed August 1, 2009.

188. Gill MJ, Simjee S, Al-Hattawi K, et al. Gonococcal resistance to beta-lactams and tetracycline involves mutation in loop 3 of the porin encoded at the penB locus. Antimicrob Agents Chemother 1998;42(11):2799–803.

189. Galimand M, Gerbaud G, Courvalin P. Spectinomycin resistance in *Neisseria* spp. due to mutations in 16S rRNA. Antimicrob Agents Chemother 2000; 44(5):1365–6.

190. Cousin SL Jr, Whittington WL, Roberts MC. Acquired macrolide resistance genes and the 1 bp deletion in the mtrR promoter in *Neisseria gonorrhoeae*. J Antimicrob Chemother 2003;51(1):131–3.

191. Fenton KA, Ison C, Johnson AP, et al. Ciprofloxacin resistance in *Neisseria gonorrhoeae* in England and Wales in 2002 [see comment]. Lancet 2003;361(9372): 1867–9.

192. Anonymous. Surveillance of antibiotic resistance in *Neisseria gonorrhoeae* in the WHO Western Pacific Region, 2000. Commun Dis Intell 2001;25(4):274–6.

193. Kam KM, Kam SS, Cheung DT, et al. Molecular characterization of quinolone-resistant *Neisseria gonorrhoeae* in Hong Kong. Antimicrob Agents Chemother 2003;47(1):436–9.

194. Trees DL, Sandul AL, Neal SW, et al. Molecular epidemiology of *Neisseria gonorrhoeae* exhibiting decreased susceptibility and resistance to ciprofloxacin in Hawaii, 1991–1999. Sex Transm Dis 2001;28(6):309–14.

195. McMurry L, Petrucci RE Jr, Levy SB. Active efflux of tetracycline encoded by four genetically different tetracycline resistance determinants in *Escherichia coli*. Proc Natl Acad Sci U S A 1980;77(7):3974–7.

196. Li XZ, Nikaido H. Efflux-mediated drug resistance in bacteria. Drugs 2004;64(2): 159–204.

Controlling Antimicrobial Resistance in the Hospital

Deverick J. Anderson, MD, MPH[a], Keith S. Kaye, MD, MPH[b],*

KEYWORDS

- Infection control • Antimicrobial resistance
- Hospital-acquired infection • Surveillance
- Prevention • Antibiotic stewardship

The hospital has historically been regarded as the epicenter for antimicrobial resistance. In many ways, it represents the "perfect storm" for emergence and spread of antimicrobial resistance: acutely and chronically ill patients with indwelling devices are exposed to high levels of antibiotic use and busy hospital staff that come into contact with multiple patients during a single day. Although antimicrobial resistance has moved to health care settings outside of the hospital (eg, nursing homes and dialysis centers) and to the community at large, the hospital remains the predominant environment where antimicrobial resistance emerges and spreads.

This article discusses methods used in hospitals to control antimicrobial resistance. The various methods can be categorized into two broad categories: infection control and antibiotic stewardship.

INFECTION CONTROL

Infection control and health care epidemiology is the discipline focused on preventing the spread of infections within the health care setting. Monitoring the emergence and spread of antimicrobial resistance within the hospital (ie, nosocomial spread) is a key component to infection control practices. To optimize efforts to control the spread of multidrug-resistant organisms (MDROs) in a hospital, the program must be adequately staffed, have adequate microbiology information provided on a routine basis, have database support, and have knowledgeable leadership.[1] This section discusses surveillance for and feedback of data pertaining to antimicrobial resistance and

[a] Department of Medicine, Duke University Medical Center, Durham, NC, USA
[b] Department of Medicine, Wayne State University, Detroit Medical Center, Detroit, MI, USA
* Corresponding author.
E-mail address: kkaye@med.wayne.edu (K.S. Kaye).

Infect Dis Clin N Am 23 (2009) 847–864
doi:10.1016/j.idc.2009.06.005   id.theclinics.com
0891-5520/09/$ – see front matter © 2009 Elsevier Inc. All rights reserved.

specific methods to control the emergence and spread of antimicrobial resistance in the hospital.

Surveillance for and Feedback of Antimicrobial Resistance Data

Surveillance is the hallmark of infection control. Surveillance of antimicrobial resistance in the hospital involves tracking the incidence and frequency of certain antimicrobial-resistant pathogens, such as methicillin-resistant *Staphylococcus aureus* (MRSA); vancomycin-resistant enterococcus (VRE); *Clostridium difficile*; extended-spectrum β-lactamase (ESBL)–producing gram-negative bacilli; and other multidrug-resistant gram-negative bacilli, such as *Acinetobacter* spp and *Pseudomonas aeruginosa*. Surveillance is conducted through two major methods: passive (or routine) surveillance, which includes review of clinical test and culture results; and active surveillance.[1] Routine surveillance is the most common method of surveillance and is practiced to some degree in almost all United States hospitals. Active surveillance is a method used to detect MDROs in patients who are asymptomatically colonized with these organisms. In contrast to routine surveillance, active surveillance uses specimens that are collected for epidemiologic and infection control purposes as opposed to clinical purposes. Methods used to identify resistant organisms from specimens obtained through active surveillance include standard culture; modified culture methods to decrease the time needed to obtain results (eg, chromogenic agar for MRSA detection); and rapid detection methods, such as polymerase chain reaction, which can provide active surveillance results within hours after specimen collection.[1]

Surveillance data should be regularly evaluated by infection preventionists and fed back to providers to raise awareness regarding rates and trends of MDROs in the hospital. Surveillance data can be rapidly reported to providers so that interventions can be immediately implemented to prevent spread of MDROs (eg, implementation of barrier precautions) and to identify and control clusters or an outbreak of MDROs. Surveillance data can also be collated over time and presented to providers to demonstrate trends in MDRO spread and to identify problem areas where interventions are needed to control high endemic rates of MDROs.

MDRO surveillance data are typically presented as number of unique patients infected or colonized with nosocomially acquired MDROs and as a rate, the number of nosocomially acquired cases of MDROs per 1000 patient days. Rates can be benchmarked among different units to stimulate improvement among poorly performing units and to promote pride and satisfaction among health care workers within highly performing units. Benchmarked surveillance data and rates of MDRO spread should be routinely fed back to leadership of clinical units (often monthly or quarterly). Incentives, such as raffles and prizes for highest performing or most improved units, can help to improve behavior, morale, and hygiene of health care workers and decrease rate of MDRO acquisition.

Methods to Control Antimicrobial Resistance in the Hospital

Hand hygiene

Hand hygiene is the single most important method to control nosocomial spread of pathogens in the hospital, including MDROs. Hand hygiene should be performed by health care workers before and after every patient encounter (ie, every time a health care worker enters a patient's room or comes into contact with a patient) to prevent the spread of pathogens from patient to patient by the contaminated hands of health care workers.[2] Hand hygiene can be performed with soap and water (for a minimum of 15 seconds). Regular soap is as effective as antimicrobial soap (soap containing an antiseptic agent) when hands are visibly soiled with proteinaceous material, blood, or other body fluids. Otherwise, antimicrobial soap is recommended for most clinical scenarios in the hospital.[2] Hand hygiene can also be performed with waterless rubs that are alcohol-based. Waterless agents have been demonstrated to be more effective than soap and water for most hospital pathogens. Notable exceptions include spore-forming organisms, such as *C difficile*, and certain nonenveloped viruses, such as norovirus. As a result, soap and water are recommended for hand hygiene after caring for a patient with *C difficile* or norovirus infection. Finally, soap and water should be used if hands are visibly soiled.[2]

Although hand hygiene is critically important for patient safety and the prevention of spread of MDROs, compliance with hand hygiene by health care workers is extremely poor. National studies quote rates of hand hygiene compliance among health care workers to be consistently under 40%. Numerous methods to improve hand hygiene compliance have been implemented, including the following: improving the number and quality of hand hygiene stations to facilitate hand hygiene opportunities, education, observation of compliance and feedback, hand hygiene reminders, sanctions and rewards, patient education and patient reminders, promoting and facilitating skin care, and instituting a culture of safety and excellence in the hospital.[2] Many of these methods result in temporary improvement in hand hygiene compliance, but more often than not, compliance returns to low, preintervention levels over time.

Artificial nails should not be worn by health care workers providing direct patient care, and natural nails should be no longer than 0.25 in long. Health care workers with artificial nails or long natural nails are more likely to harbor pathogens on their hands before and after handwashing and have been tied to outbreaks of infections.[3,4]

Contact precautions

Barrier precautions typically involve wearing a gown and gloves when coming into contact with patients. Traditionally, barrier precautions have been reserved for patients who have draining wounds or are soiled with urine, feces, or blood to prevent contamination and infection of the provider. Barrier precautions have also been used to help control the spread of MDROs of epidemiologic importance, however, such as MRSA and VRE. MDROs of epidemiologic significance are generally pathogens that are susceptible to only a few antimicrobial agents.[1] The rationale for using barrier precautions to prevent spread of MDROs is to prevent contamination of the clothes and body of the health care worker. Gowns and gloves should be put on after hand hygiene has been performed and on entering the patient room. Gowns and gloves should be discarded before exiting the room. Hand hygiene should be performed after gowns and gloves are discarded.[1] Ideally, patients placed on contact isolation should reside in a private room. Dedicated patient equipment, such as stethoscopes and blood pressure cuffs that remain in the patient room, should be used whenever possible. Alternatively, if dedicated equipment is not available, stethoscopes and blood pressure cuffs should be cleaned (eg, with alcohol) before coming into contact with another patient.

Recommendations for when it is appropriate to discontinue contact precautions are not available. Patients can remain colonized with MDROs for a long duration after their infection has resolved (particularly long periods of colonization have been described for gram-positive MDROs, such as MRSA and VRE); many experts advocate continuing contact precautions for the duration of hospitalization and, in many cases, on readmission to the hospital. For VRE and MRSA, some experts remove a patient from isolation if they are off antibiotics and have three negative surveillance cultures over a 1- to 2-week period (anatomic source of culture is usually nares for MRSA and perirectal swab for VRE).[1,5]

Contact precautions have primarily been studied in outbreak settings. Although it is widely accepted that contact precautions are an important component of controlling the spread of *C difficile*, data demonstrating the effect of contact precautions in controlling the spread of other MDROs in endemic settings are few and conflicting.[1,6,7] Current guidelines recommend implementing contact precautions routinely for all patients colonized or infected with a target MDRO.[1] A target MDRO is not clearly defined, however, in the guidelines. Many hospitals consider one or more of the following to be target MDROs: MRSA, VRE, ESBL-producing organisms, *Acinetobacter*, and *Pseudomonas*.

Contact precautions have been shown adversely to affect patient well-being. Specifically, patients on contact precautions are visited and examined less often than patients not on contact precautions and have higher levels of anxiety.[8–10] Contact precautions are only effective if health care workers are compliant. Compliance with contact precautions is often a problem, because these measures increase the time required for health care workers to complete routine patient care. It is important to understand the local patterns of antimicrobial resistance and nosocomial spread of MDROs before deciding which MDROs to target for control by using contact precautions.

Screening of high-risk patients with active surveillance

Active surveillance is a method used to increase the detection of MDROs and, by doing so, decrease the silent transmission of MDROs. This type of surveillance typically is performed in hospitalized patients by culturing the nares of patients for MRSA or the rectum for VRE and other MDR gram-negative pathogens (eg, ESBL and *Klebsiella pneumoniae* carbapenemase (KPC)-producing Enterobacteriaceae). Rapid detection methods, including polymerase chain reaction, have been used to increase the rapidity with which screening results are obtained. The rationale behind active surveillance is that MDROs can be spread by asymptomatic patients who are simply colonized rather than infected (ie, a silent reservoir).

Over 100 studies have evaluated the efficacy of such active surveillance programs in hospitalized patients. The conclusions from these studies have been conflicting and, in some cases, contradictory. Many studies of active surveillance of high-risk hospitalized patients (eg, patients in ICUs, burn units, or patients involved in an outbreak) have concluded that this strategy is a cost-effective way to prevent infection with and nosocomial transmission of MDRO.[11,12] For example, Huang and colleagues[13] performed a study in eight ICUs in an 800-bed tertiary care hospital and demonstrated that routine surveillance cultures followed by contact isolation precautions for all MRSA culture-positive patients led to a 67% decrease in the incidence of nosocomial MRSA bloodstream infection in both the ICUs and the general hospital wards. Other studies, however, have failed to demonstrate a clear benefit of performing active surveillance.[14–17] A recent systematic review of studies on active surveillance concluded that existing evidence favors the use of active surveillance (ie, more studies than not support active surveillance), but much of the evidence is of poor quality and definitive recommendations cannot be made.[18]

Universal active surveillance

The issue of universal active surveillance (eg, screening all patients admitted to the hospital, not just those admitted to high-risk units) is no less controversial. One recently published large, multicenter study evaluated the use of universal active surveillance for MRSA in conjunction with implementation of barrier precautions and decolonization regimens.[19] This study was a three-period quasiexperimental study comparing standard methods (period 1); ICU-based surveillance (period 2); and universal admission surveillance (period 3). The rate of MRSA infection decreased substantially during the universal screening period (period 3) compared with period 1 and period 2. Although this study was one of the first to examine active surveillance outside of high-risk units, it was limited by potential methodologic issues.[20] A recent large prospective study also evaluated the use of universal active surveillance but showed no effect of active surveillance, even in conjunction with implementation of barrier precautions and decolonization regimens.[21] The study was performed at a large, tertiary care hospital in Switzerland over approximately 2 years and included over 20,000 adult surgical patients. Overall, there was no decrease in the rate of nosocomial MRSA infection, no decrease in the rate of MRSA surgical infection, nor a decrease in rate of nosocomial acquisition of MRSA.

Despite the lack of consistent benefit in studies, several organizations have recommended performing active surveillance in settings other than high-risk units or an ongoing outbreak. For example, consumer interest groups, the Institute for Healthcare Improvement, and some state legislatures recommend or mandate active surveillance for MRSA in all hospitalized patients. In contrast, most scientific organizations, including the Centers for Disease Control and Prevention, the Association of Professionals in Infection Control, and the Society for Healthcare Epidemiology of America, recommend that active surveillance should be reserved for specific patient populations and specific scenarios. In November 2006, Healthcare Infection Control Practices Advisory Committee published its recommendations that introduced the concept of a two-tiered prevention system.[1] Healthcare Infection Control Practices Advisory Committee recommends that active surveillance for MDROs only be implemented if the incidence or prevalence is not decreasing despite the use of routine control measures; or after an epidemiologically important organism has been isolated for the first time at an institution or if an outbreak of an epidemiologically important organism is occurring within a health care facility.[1]

It is important to understand that active surveillance alone likely has no effect on the nosocomial spread of targeted pathogens. The processes used with the data generated by active surveillance ultimately dictate the use and effectiveness of active surveillance. For example, active surveillance cultures might be coupled with cohorting of colonized patients, immediate use of barrier precautions, attempts at decolonization, or combinations of some or all of these processes.

Decolonization

Colonization is an important precursor to infection; several studies have demonstrated that patients colonized with MDROs are at increased risk of infections caused by their colonizing MDRO.[22] Decolonization is eradication of colonizing bacteria to reduce the risk of subsequent infection or to decrease the risk of spread of the organism to other patients. This strategy has been primarily used in patients colonized with S aureus (and MRSA in particular) but has not been shown to be of any benefit in patients colonized with VRE.[23] Two approaches for decolonization of S aureus and MRSA are topical therapy and systemic therapy (given in combination with topical therapy).[24,25]

Decolonization may be beneficial in the setting of an MRSA outbreak, but it has not been consistently effective in other settings.[26] Notably, many "search and destroy" processes in hospitals involve active surveillance to identify patients colonized with MRSA followed by decolonization of identified patients. Decolonization regimens have potential adverse side effects and unintended consequences. Resistance to mupirocin and other antibiotics used for decolonization has been well documented.[25,27] Systemic therapy with antibiotics can and often does lead to side effects, such as nausea, vomiting, rash, and C difficile–associated diarrhea.

Although decolonization strategies may initially eradicate MRSA from the nose in 85% to 95% of cases, this effect is typically short-lived.[28] MRSA seems to recolonize many patients within 90 days of decolonization; as many as 50% to 75% of patients (including healthy health care workers) again have MRSA within 1 year. A systematic review of studies on decolonization of MRSA concluded that the available evidence is inadequate to recommend the use of topical or systemic agents to eliminate MRSA colonization.[26]

Source control

Source control is the process of reducing the bacterial bioburden on the skin by regularly applying chlorhexidine gluconate. Source control with chlorhexidine gluconate has primarily been studied in patients in ICUs. ICU patients who received daily bathing with chlorhexidine gluconate had lower rates of skin contamination with VRE than patients who were washed with soap and water alone.[29] Two additional benefits were also noted from this intervention. First, the number of health care workers with VRE on their hands was significantly reduced in units where source control was practiced. Furthermore, a reduction in the density of bacteria found in the environment was noted in these same units. Source control may also prevent health care–acquired infections. One multicenter study showed that daily bathing of ICU patients with chlorhexidine gluconate led to lower rates of MRSA colonization, VRE colonization, and all types of bloodstream infections.[30]

Cohorting of patients and staff

Cohorting is the practice of grouping patients either infected or colonized with a specific MDRO in the same physical location (eg, room, ward, or unit) or assigning dedicated health care workers to care exclusively for this group of patients. Several published reports include cohorting of patients and staff as one of several interventions to control an ongoing MDRO outbreak, including MRSA,[31,32] VRE,[33,34] ESBL-producing organisms,[35] and KPC-producing organisms.[36] Healthcare Infection Control Practices Advisory Committee includes cohorting as a potential intervention for controlling the spread of MDRO when standard interventions have not been effective.[1]

Antimicrobial prophylaxis and decontamination to prevent infections

Several prophylactic interventions have been used to prevent hospital-acquired infections, including perioperative antimicrobial prophylaxis and various types of decontamination. Perioperative antimicrobial prophylaxis is the standard of care for (1) clean-contaminated surgical procedures, (2) procedures involving insertion of vascular prostheses, and (3) procedures in which an incisional or organ-space surgical site infection would result in catastrophic risk.[37] Antimicrobial prophylaxis with a recommended agent should be administered within 1 hour before incision (2 hours are allowed for the administration of vancomycin and fluoroquinolones) and should be discontinued within 24 hours after surgery (discontinuation at 48 hours is allowable for cardiothoracic procedures).[38,39]

Different strategies have been used to decrease the burden of colonizing organisms on hospitalized patients and decrease the risk of infection. Source control and decolonization are described previously in this article. Chlorhexidine gluconate oropharyngeal and nasal washing before cardiothoracic surgery decreases the risk of hospital-acquired infection.[40] Chlorhexidine gluconate nasal rinses, however, are not yet available in the United States. Similarly, oral care with chlorhexidine gluconate reduces the risk of ventilator-associated pneumonia.[41,42]

Selective digestive decontamination, the prevention of secondary gastrointestinal colonization with gram-negative bacteria, S aureus, or yeast by administering antimicrobial therapy, has also been used to reduce the risk of ventilator-associated pneumonia, but remains controversial. Numerous regimens for selective digestive decontamination have been used; most include a nonabsorbable antimicrobial agent, such as polymyxin, in combination with other systemic antimicrobial agents including aminoglycosides and antifungal agents. Several studies have examined the effectiveness of selective digestive decontamination and shown that the practice may decrease the risk of ventilator-associated pneumonia.[43–46] Although a recent report suggests that selective digestive decontamination may improve mortality among ICU patients,[47] the usefulness of selective digestive decontamination remains "unresolved" because of methodologic concerns with the studies (ie, how to diagnose ventilator-associated pneumonia) and the concern for emergence of resistance with widespread use of antibiotics.[48]

Implementation of evidence-based best practices for invasive procedures and devices
Rates of hospital-acquired infections associated with invasive procedures and devices can be decreased by implementing best practices. The Institute for Healthcare Improvement has championed implementation of "bundles" of best practices to prevent surgical site infections, catheter-related bloodstream infections, and ventilator-associated pneumonia.[49]

In addition to antimicrobial prophylaxis before surgical procedures, rates of surgical site infections can be decreased by not shaving hair with a razor before surgery and controlling postoperative blood glucose levels.[39,50] Similarly, rates of central venous catheter-associated bloodstream infection can be greatly decreased by performing five evidence-based practices: (1) handwashing before line insertion, (2) use of full-barrier precautions during line insertion, (3) skin cleaning with chlorhexidine before line insertion, (4) avoidance of the femoral site for line insertions, and (5) prompt removal of unnecessary catheters.[51–53] Adding all of these components onto a checklist helps to ensure bundle compliance and improve outcomes.[53,54] Finally, rates of ventilator-associated pneumonia can be decreased by maintaining ventilated patients in a semirecumbent position, performing oral disinfection with chlorhexidine, and monitoring for the ability to wean from the ventilator.[48]

Disinfection and sterilization
Disinfection and sterilization are important interventions to prevent the cross-transmission of potentially infectious agents from patient to patient by medical devices. Approved chemical disinfectants include alcohols, glutaraldehyde, formaldehyde, hydrogen peroxide, iodophors, orthophthalaldehyde, peracetic acid, phenolics, quaternary ammonium compounds, and chlorine. The choice of disinfectant and exposure time of the disinfectant to medical equipment are based on the risk for infection associated with different types of medical devices, equipment, and the invasiveness of procedures. Sterilization can be achieved with steam, ethylene oxide, hydrogen peroxide gas plasma, and liquid peracetic acid. Equipment must be cleaned to remove proteinaceous material before disinfection and sterilization. Although rare, several outbreaks have occurred as a result of improper disinfection and sterilization.[55–58] Official guidelines for disinfection and sterilization have been recently updated.[59]

Cleaning the hospital environment

Patients can rarely acquire infections from environmental sources in the hospital. The relationship between the degree of environmental contamination and the risk of transmission of infection, however, is unknown. Several studies have demonstrated that potentially infectious agents can regularly be cultured from surfaces of hospital rooms, including MRSA,[60] VRE,[61] and C difficile.[62,63] Authors of some studies have concluded that some patient infections were acquired from environmental sources.[61] In contrast, other studies have failed to demonstrate that environmental contamination or changes in environmental cleaning practices impacted rates of hospital-acquired infections.[64,65]

Quaternary ammonium-containing cleaning agents are effective for killing almost all important pathogens.[66] Two notable exceptions, however, include C difficile and norovirus. Hypochlorite (bleach)-containing solutions are more effective for these pathogens.[67] The use of a hypochlorite-containing cleaning solution for terminal cleaning of patient rooms can lead to a decrease in rates of C difficile.[68] Despite effective cleaning agents and official recommendations regarding hospital room cleaning, many patients and personnel believe that rooms in many hospitals remain inadequately cleaned. Specific methods for monitoring compliance with room cleaning (eg, UV-visible markers[62]) may improve overall environmental cleaning in hospitals.

ANTIBIOTIC STEWARDSHIP
Introduction

Use and overuse of antibiotics have been the main driving factors for emergence of resistance. As a result, fewer agents are available for treatment of multidrug-resistant pathogens. Furthermore, patients infected with MDRO have worse outcomes than patients infected with susceptible organisms. Antibiotic stewardship, also known as "antimicrobial management plans," can help minimize the emergence of MDROs, improve patient outcomes, and save money for hospitals by promoting prudent usage of antibiotics.[69] Antibiotic stewardship involves optimizing antibiotic selection, dosing, route, and duration of therapy. One of the goals of hospital antibiotic stewardship programs is to minimize the emergence and spread of MDROs. This section discusses some of the basic concepts involved in the relationship between antibiotic stewardship and MDROs and different strategies of antimicrobials to minimize the emergence and spread of MDROs.

Effects of Antibiotics on MDROs

Antibiotics can facilitate the emergence and spread of MDROs through multiple mechanisms. First, antibiotics can give MDROs a selective advantage for colonizing a susceptible (uncolonized) host by inhibiting selective commensal flora of a patient. In addition, antimicrobials can also affect the structure and function of an MDRO giving it a selective structural advantage to colonize a susceptible host. An example of these two phenomena can be demonstrated by studying the relationship between fluoroquinolone exposure and MRSA. Fluoroquinolone exposure can suppress commensal bacteria that are fluoroquinolone susceptible but has little effect on most strains of MRSA (because most strains are resistant to fluoroquinolones). In addition, fluoroquinolones can induce changes in fibronectin binding of MRSA strains providing an additional selective advantage for MRSA to colonize a susceptible host. As a result, fluoroquinolone use is a risk factor for MRSA infection and colonization.[70,71]

Antibiotics can also promote the emergence of resistance in susceptible pathogens that are already colonizing or infecting a host. One example involves *Enterobacter* spp. This AmpC-producing organism is often susceptible to cephalosporins when it is initially isolated in culture. If third-generation cephalosporins are used for therapy of an *Enterobacter* infection, therapy fails and the *Enterobacter* strain emerges as an AmpC-hyperproducer in approximately 20% of cases, leading to high-level resistance to cephalosporins.[72] An important associated concept related to the emergence of resistance during therapy is "collateral damage." In this scenario, resistance emerges not in the primary pathogen being treated, but among other bacteria colonizing the patient (often in the intestine). An example of collateral damage is levofloxacin therapy for a nonpseudomonal infection leading to subsequent colonization or infection with a fluoroquinolone-resistant *Pseudomonas* strain.[73]

Specific relationships between MDROs and antibiotics

Although use (and overuse) of practically any antibiotic can promote or select for one or more MDROs, there are certain specific associations between use of antimicrobials or a class of antimicrobials and emergence and spread of a MDRO. In some cases, antimicrobial resistance in the hospital can be controlled, in part through formulary interventions or antibiotic stewardship interventions specifically targeted to decrease use of a specific antimicrobial agent or class of antimicrobial agents. These "bug-drug" associations often are considered when formulary decisions are being made or when interventions are considered to control an MDRO outbreak.

Some correlations between decreased use of an antimicrobial agent or class of agents at the level of hospital use and a decreased incidence of specific MDRO include fluoroquinolone use and MRSA;[74] vancomycin and VRE;[23] third-generation cephalosporins and VRE;[23] aztreonam and cephalosporin use (primarily third-generations) and ESBL-producing enterobacteriaciae;[75,76] third-generation cephalosporin use and cephalosporin-resistant *Enterobacter*;[77] and carbapenem use (antipseudomonal or type 2) and carbapenem-resistant *Acinetobacter*, *Pseudomonas*, and Enterobacteriaciae.[78,79] In almost all instances cited previously, decreases in MDROs occurred after antibiotic efforts were coupled with enhanced infection control practices. Antibiotic restriction alone is often not sufficient to control an MDRO outbreak or decrease high endemic levels of an MDRO.

Strategies to Prevent the Emergence of Resistance

If antibiotic usage leads to antibiotic resistance, then the key to decreasing emerging resistance is to minimize or eliminate unnecessary antimicrobial usage. Several methods are available to prevent the overuse of antimicrobial agents, including antibiotic restrictions, avoiding unnecessary antimicrobial therapy, de-escalation of broad-spectrum antimicrobial therapy, clinical decision support, and use of antibiograms.

Antibiotic restriction

The most effective method for controlling the use of antimicrobial agents is by restricting access to these drugs.[69] Restriction can be achieved by two main methods: restriction of antimicrobial agents at the level of the hospital formulary (ie, limiting the number of available antimicrobial agents); and requiring preauthorization before antibiotics are dispensed. These restrictive policies can lead to substantial decreases in the use of targeted antimicrobial agents.[80–82] Studies have provided conflicting results, however, regarding whether restrictive policies actually lead to a decrease in the emergence of antimicrobial resistance.[83,84] The caveat of these restrictive policies is that antibiotic usage may simply shift to other agents, leading to emergence of a different type of resistance.[85]

Decreasing unnecessary or inappropriate antimicrobial use

Restrictive policies may reduce antimicrobial use in hospitals, but they may not be effectively implemented in all hospital settings and are typically not effective in outpatient settings. Broader strategies are needed to improve antimicrobial usage in diverse settings. Two strategies to decrease unnecessary antimicrobial usage include education and adherence to guidelines and clinical pathways. Although education regarding appropriate antimicrobial therapy is a cornerstone of any antimicrobial stewardship program, it is a passive intervention and typically only leads to modest, short-term improvement in prescribing practices.[86,87]

Implementation of and adherence to published evidence-based guidelines from national organizations can improve antimicrobial use. It remains difficult, however, to ensure that providers are aware of and buy into national evidence-based guidelines.[88] In contrast, clinical pathways for specific diagnoses can be created using hospital-specific data (eg, microbiology and patient characteristics) to optimize antimicrobial use and eliminate unnecessary antibiotic prescription, particularly in ICUs.[89,90]

De-escalation of therapy

It is often difficult to convince physicians caring for sick, unstable patients that empiric broad-spectrum therapy might be unnecessary and that alternative regimens with narrower antimicrobial focus might be sufficient. Several studies have shown that early, effective therapy is key to improving survival in septic patients.[91–93] Nevertheless, an important intervention to improve antimicrobial use is narrowing coverage based on culture and susceptibility results (ie, 48–72 hours after antimicrobial therapy has been initiated and cultures have been obtained). This modification of "consolidative" antimicrobial therapy is sometimes known as "de-escalation" of therapy. Antimicrobial de-escalation decreases unnecessary antibiotic use and hospital costs, and improves patient outcomes.[91,94,95]

Clinical decision support

The age of the electronic medical record and computer physician order entry has allowed for the creation of sophisticated decision support and feedback systems for providers. Electronic systems can be developed to prompt providers with treatment recommendations based on local patient and microbiologic data and national guidelines.[96,97] These systems can be quite complex and difficult to implement and require clinical expertise to develop appropriate, effective, and safe algorithms. Such decision support systems must be validated before they are widely used. Rarely, decision support systems have led to adverse patient events and inappropriate discontinuation of therapy.[98] Validated decision support systems, however, have often led to improved compliance with practice guidelines, fewer adverse antimicrobial-related reactions, and improved antimicrobial dosing.[99–101]

Antibiograms

Antibiograms represent cumulative microbiologic data for specific institutions and, as such, provide information on the local bacteriologic ecology. Antibiograms can be used to guide empiric antibiotic choices[102] and monitor resistance patterns.[103] Unit-specific antibiograms provide more useful information for guidance of empiric antibiotic usage than hospital-wide antibiograms but are limited by including fewer isolates than the hospital-wide antibiogram.[104]

Unproved strategies

Insufficient data exist to support the routine use of double-coverage for treatment of gram-negative pathogens and antimicrobial cycling as methods to decrease antimicrobial resistance.[69] Double-coverage is the practice of administering two antimicrobial agents from different classes to improve the likelihood that an infected patient receives effective empiric therapy. Although use of double or multidrug therapy is well proved to limit the emergence or antimicrobial resistance in the treatment of HIV and tuberculosis, few data support the role of double coverage in preventing the emergence of resistance in bacteria, such as *Pseudomonas* or *Enterobacter*.[105–108] In one study, double coverage was actually associated with increased rates of superinfection compared with single-agent therapy.[109]

Similarly, there are few data to support the concept of antimicrobial cycling, the practice of rotating routine empiric or "workhorse" antibiotics in an individual unit or hospital. Substituting one empiric antimicrobial agent for another may temporarily decrease reduced resistance to the restricted agent, but reintroduction of the restricted agent has been associated with the re-emergence of resistance.[110,111] Rather than rotating agents, stewardship programs should focus on limiting unnecessary antibiotic use or de-escalation strategies.

SUMMARY

MDROs continue to proliferate and spread in both the hospital and community, but the hospital remains the primary source for emergence and spread of MDROs. Controlling the emergence and spread of MDROs presents many challenges to physicians, hospital epidemiologists, and infection preventionists. Several interventions and strategies are currently available and reasonably effective, but further studies are needed to determine the best methods for controlling antimicrobial resistance. Currently, hospitals must use a combination of infection control and antibiotic stewardship interventions to control and limit the emergence and spread of MDROs in their institutions.

REFERENCES

1. Siegel JD, Rhinehart E, Jackson M, et al. Management of multidrug-resistant organisms in health care settings, 2006. Am J Infect Control 2007;35(10 Suppl 2): S165–93.
2. Boyce JM, Pittet D. Guideline for hand hygiene in health-care settings. Recommendations of the Healthcare Infection Control Practices Advisory Committee and the HICPAC/SHEA/APIC/IDSA Hand Hygiene Task Force. Society for Healthcare Epidemiology of America/Association for Professionals in Infection Control/Infectious Diseases Society of America. MMWR Recomm Rep 2002;51(RR-16):1–45, quiz CE41–44.
3. Moolenaar RL, Crutcher JM, San Joaquin VH, et al. A prolonged outbreak of *Pseudomonas aeruginosa* in a neonatal intensive care unit: did staff fingernails play a role in disease transmission? Infect Control Hosp Epidemiol 2000;21(2): 80–5.
4. Pottinger J, Burns S, Manske C. Bacterial carriage by artificial versus natural nails. Am J Infect Control 1989;17(6):340–4.
5. Byers KE, Anglim AM, Anneski CJ, et al. Duration of colonization with vancomycin-resistant Enterococcus. Infect Control Hosp Epidemiol 2002;23(4):207–11.
6. Puzniak LA, Leet T, Mayfield J, et al. To gown or not to gown: the effect on acquisition of vancomycin-resistant enterococci. Clin Infect Dis 2002;35(1): 18–25.

7. Srinivasan A, Dick JD, Perl TM. Vancomycin resistance in staphylococci. Clin Microbiol Rev 2002;15(3):430–8.
8. Kirkland KB, Weinstein JM. Adverse effects of contact isolation. Lancet 1999; 354(9185):1177–8.
9. Saint S, Higgins LA, Nallamothu BK, et al. Do physicians examine patients in contact isolation less frequently? A brief report. Am J Infect Control 2003; 31(6):354–6.
10. Stelfox HT, Bates DW, Redelmeier DA. Safety of patients isolated for infection control. JAMA 2003;290(14):1899–905.
11. Karchmer TB, Durbin LJ, Simonton BM, et al. Cost-effectiveness of active surveillance cultures and contact/droplet precautions for control of methicillin-resistant Staphylococcus aureus. J Hosp Infect 2002;51(2):126–32.
12. West TE, Guerry C, Hiott M, et al. Effect of targeted surveillance for control of methicillin-resistant Staphylococcus aureus in a community hospital system. Infect Control Hosp Epidemiol 2006;27(3):233–8.
13. Huang SS, Yokoe DS, Hinrichsen VL, et al. Impact of routine intensive care unit surveillance cultures and resultant barrier precautions on hospital-wide methicillin-resistant Staphylococcus aureus bacteremia. Clin Infect Dis 2006;43(8): 971–8.
14. Troche G, Joly LM, Guibert M, et al. Detection and treatment of antibiotic-resistant bacterial carriage in a surgical intensive care unit: a 6-year prospective survey. Infect Control Hosp Epidemiol 2005;26(2):161–5.
15. Nijssen S, Bonten MJ, Weinstein RA. Are active microbiological surveillance and subsequent isolation needed to prevent the spread of methicillin-resistant Staphylococcus aureus? Clin Infect Dis 2005;40(3):405–9.
16. Huang SS, Rifas-Shiman SL, Warren DK, et al. Improving methicillin-resistant Staphylococcus aureus surveillance and reporting in intensive care units. J Infect Dis 2007;195(3):330–8.
17. Huang SS, Rifas-Shiman SL, Pottinger JM, et al. Improving the assessment of vancomycin-resistant enterococci by routine screening. J Infect Dis 2007; 195(3):339–46.
18. McGinigle KL, Gourlay ML, Buchanan IB. The use of active surveillance cultures in adult intensive care units to reduce methicillin-resistant Staphylococcus aureus-related morbidity, mortality, and costs: a systematic review. Clin Infect Dis 2008;46(11):1717–25.
19. Robicsek A, Beaumont JL, Paule SM, et al. Universal surveillance for methicillin-resistant Staphylococcus aureus in 3 affiliated hospitals. Ann Intern Med 2008; 148(6):409–18.
20. Lautenbach E. Expanding the universe of methicillin-resistant Staphylococcus aureus prevention. Ann Intern Med 2008;148(6):474–6.
21. Harbarth S, Fankhauser C, Schrenzel J, et al. Universal screening for methicillin-resistant Staphylococcus aureus at hospital admission and nosocomial infection in surgical patients. JAMA 2008;299(10):1149–57.
22. Huang SS, Platt R. Risk of methicillin-resistant Staphylococcus aureus infection after previous infection or colonization. Clin Infect Dis 2003;36(3):281–5.
23. Harbarth S, Cosgrove S, Carmeli Y. Effects of antibiotics on nosocomial epidemiology of vancomycin-resistant enterococci. Antimicrob Agents Chemother 2002;46(6):1619–28.
24. Kauffman CA, Terpenning MS, He X, et al. Attempts to eradicate methicillin-resistant Staphylococcus aureus from a long-term-care facility with the use of mupirocin ointment. Am J Med 1993;94(4):371–8.

25. Simor AE, Phillips E, McGeer A, et al. Randomized controlled trial of chlorhexidine gluconate for washing, intranasal mupirocin, and rifampin and doxycycline versus no treatment for the eradication of methicillin-resistant *Staphylococcus aureus* colonization. Clin Infect Dis 2007;44(2):178–85.

26. Loeb M, Main C, Walker-Dilks C, et al. Antimicrobial drugs for treating methicillin-resistant *Staphylococcus aureus* colonization. Cochrane Database Syst Rev 2003;(4):CD003340.

27. Miller MA, Dascal A, Portnoy J, et al. Development of mupirocin resistance among methicillin-resistant *Staphylococcus aureus* after widespread use of nasal mupirocin ointment. Infect Control Hosp Epidemiol 1996;17(12):811–3.

28. Mody L, Kauffman CA, McNeil SA, et al. Mupirocin-based decolonization of *Staphylococcus aureus* carriers in residents of 2 long-term care facilities: a randomized, double-blind, placebo-controlled trial. Clin Infect Dis 2003; 37(11):1467–74.

29. Vernon MO, Hayden MK, Trick WE, et al. Chlorhexidine gluconate to cleanse patients in a medical intensive care unit: the effectiveness of source control to reduce the bioburden of vancomycin-resistant enterococci. Arch Intern Med 2006;166(3):306–12.

30. Milstone AM, Passaretti CL, Perl TM. Chlorhexidine: expanding the armamentarium for infection control and prevention. Clin Infect Dis 2008;46(2):274–81.

31. Haley RW, Cushion NB, Tenover FC, et al. Eradication of endemic methicillin-resistant *Staphylococcus aureus* infections from a neonatal intensive care unit. J Infect Dis 1995;171(3):614–24.

32. Kotilainen P, Routamaa M, Peltonen R, et al. Eradication of methicillin-resistant *Staphylococcus aureus* from a health center ward and associated nursing home. Arch Intern Med 2001;161(6):859–63.

33. Jochimsen EM, Fish L, Manning K, et al. Control of vancomycin-resistant enterococci at a community hospital: efficacy of patient and staff cohorting. Infect Control Hosp Epidemiol 1999;20(2):106–9.

34. Rupp ME, Marion N, Fey PD, et al. Outbreak of vancomycin-resistant *Enterococcus faecium* in a neonatal intensive care unit. Infect Control Hosp Epidemiol 2001;22(5):301–3.

35. Lucet JC, Decre D, Fichelle A, et al. Control of a prolonged outbreak of extended-spectrum beta-lactamase-producing enterobacteriaceae in a university hospital. Clin Infect Dis 1999;29(6):1411–8.

36. Schwaber MJ, Israel pCRE Working Group. Infection control at the national level: containment of an outbreak of carbapenem-resistant Klebsiella pneumoniae (CRKP) in Israeli hospitals. Paper presented at: Proceedings of 48th Annual Interscience Conference on Anitmicrobial Agents and Chemotherapy/Infectious Disease Society of America 46th Annual Meeting; October 27, 2008; Washington, DC.

37. Mangram AJ, Horan TC, Pearson ML, et al. Guideline for prevention of surgical site infection, 1999. Centers for Disease Control and Prevention (CDC) Hospital Infection Control Practices Advisory Committee. Am J Infect Control 1999;27(2): 97–132, quiz 133–4 [discussion: 196].

38. Bratzler DW, Hunt DR. The surgical infection prevention and surgical care improvement projects: national initiatives to improve outcomes for patients having surgery. Clin Infect Dis 2006;43(3):322–30.

39. Bratzler DW, Houck PM. Antimicrobial prophylaxis for surgery: an advisory statement from the National Surgical Infection Prevention Project. Clin Infect Dis 2004;38(12):1706–15.

40. Klevens RM, Morrison MA, Nadle J, et al. Invasive methicillin-resistant *Staphylococcus aureus* infections in the United States. JAMA 2007;298(15): 1763–71.
41. Bergmans DC, Bonten MJ, Gaillard CA, et al. Prevention of ventilator-associated pneumonia by oral decontamination: a prospective, randomized, double-blind, placebo-controlled study. Am J Respir Crit Care Med 2001;164(3):382–8.
42. Chan EY, Ruest A, Meade MO, et al. Oral decontamination for prevention of pneumonia in mechanically ventilated adults: systematic review and meta-analysis. BMJ 2007;334(7599):889.
43. D'Amico R, Pifferi S, Leonetti C, et al. Effectiveness of antibiotic prophylaxis in critically ill adult patients: systematic review of randomised controlled trials. BMJ 1998;316(7140):1275–85.
44. de Jonge E, Schultz MJ, Spanjaard L, et al. Effects of selective decontamination of digestive tract on mortality and acquisition of resistant bacteria in intensive care: a randomised controlled trial. Lancet 2003;362(9389):1011–6.
45. Sanchez Garcia M, Cambronero Galache JA, Lopez Diaz J, et al. Effectiveness and cost of selective decontamination of the digestive tract in critically ill intubated patients: a randomized, double-blind, placebo-controlled, multicenter trial. Am J Respir Crit Care Med 1998;158(3):908–16.
46. Silvestri L, van Saene HK, Casarin A, et al. Impact of selective decontamination of the digestive tract on carriage and infection due to gram-negative and gram-positive bacteria: a systematic review of randomised controlled trials. Anaesth Intensive Care 2008;36(3):324–38.
47. de Smet AM, Kluytmans JA, Cooper BS, et al. Decontamination of the digestive tract and oropharynx in ICU patients. N Engl J Med 2009;360(1):20–31.
48. Coffin SE, Klompas M, Classen D, et al. Strategies to prevent ventilator-associated pneumonia in acute care hospitals. Infect Control Hosp Epidemiol 2008; 29(Suppl 1):S31–40.
49. Improvement IfH. A resource from the Institute of Healthcare Improvement. Available at: www.ihi.org. Accessed January 31, 2007.
50. Anderson DJ, Kaye KS, Classen D, et al. Strategies to prevent surgical site infections in acute care hospitals. Infect Control Hosp Epidemiol 2008;29 (Suppl 1):S51–61.
51. Berenholtz SM, Pronovost PJ, Lipsett PA, et al. Eliminating catheter-related bloodstream infections in the intensive care unit. Crit Care Med 2004;32(10): 2014–20.
52. Marschall J, Mermel LA, Classen D, et al. Strategies to prevent central line-associated bloodstream infections in acute care hospitals. Infect Control Hosp Epidemiol 2008;29(Suppl 1):S22–30.
53. Pronovost P, Needham D, Berenholtz S, et al. An intervention to decrease catheter-related bloodstream infections in the ICU. N Engl J Med 2006; 355(26):2725–32.
54. Tsuchida T, Makimoto K, Toki M, et al. The effectiveness of a nurse-initiated intervention to reduce catheter-associated bloodstream infections in an urban acute hospital: an intervention study with before and after comparison. Int J Nurs Stud 2007;44(8):1324–33.
55. Centers for Disease Control. *Pseudomonas aeruginosa* infections associated with transrectal ultrasound-guided prostate biopsies—Georgia, 2005. MMWR Morb Mortal Wkly Rep 2006;55(28):776–7.
56. Meyers H, Brown-Elliott BA, Moore D, et al. An outbreak of *Mycobacterium chelonae* infection following liposuction. Clin Infect Dis 2002;34(11):1500–7.

57. Spach DH, Silverstein FE, Stamm WE. Transmission of infection by gastrointestinal endoscopy and bronchoscopy. Ann Intern Med 1993;118(2):117–28.
58. Weber DJ, Rutala WA. Lessons from outbreaks associated with bronchoscopy. Infect Control Hosp Epidemiol 2001;22(7):403–8.
59. Rutala WA, Weber DJ, the Healthcare Infection Control Practices Advisory Committee (HICPAC). Guideline for disinfection and sterilization in healthcare facilities, 2008. Available at: http://www.cdc.gov/ncidod/dhqp/pdf/guidelines/Disinfection_Nov_2008.pdf. Accessed December 15, 2008.
60. Boyce JM, Potter-Bynoe G, Chenevert C, et al. Environmental contamination due to methicillin-resistant *Staphylococcus aureus*: possible infection control implications. Infect Control Hosp Epidemiol 1997;18(9):622–7.
61. Martinez JA, Ruthazer R, Hansjosten K, et al. Role of environmental contamination as a risk factor for acquisition of vancomycin-resistant enterococci in patients treated in a medical intensive care unit. Arch Intern Med 2003; 163(16):1905–12.
62. Alfa MJ, Dueck C, Olson N, et al. UV-visible marker confirms that environmental persistence of *Clostridium difficile* spores in toilets of patients with *C. difficile*-associated diarrhea is associated with lack of compliance with cleaning protocols. BMC Infect Dis 2008;8:1–7.
63. Samore MH, Venkataraman L, DeGirolami PC, et al. Clinical and molecular epidemiology of sporadic and clustered cases of nosocomial *Clostridium difficile* diarrhea. Am J Med 1996;100(1):32–40.
64. Bradley SF, Terpenning MS, Ramsey MA, et al. Methicillin-resistant *Staphylococcus aureus*: colonization and infection in a long-term care facility. Ann Intern Med 1991;115(6):417–22.
65. Maki DG, Alvarado CJ, Hassemer CA, et al. Relation of the inanimate hospital environment to endemic nosocomial infection. N Engl J Med 1982;307(25):1562–6.
66. Sehulster L, Chinn RY. Guidelines for environmental infection control in healthcare facilities. Recommendations of CDC and the Healthcare Infection Control Practices Advisory Committee (HICPAC). MMWR Recomm Rep 2003; 52(RR-10):1–42.
67. Hota B. Contamination, disinfection, and cross-colonization: are hospital surfaces reservoirs for nosocomial infection? Clin Infect Dis 2004;39(8):1182–9.
68. McMullen KM, Zack J, Coopersmith CM, et al. Use of hypochlorite solution to decrease rates of *Clostridium difficile*-associated diarrhea. Infect Control Hosp Epidemiol 2007;28(2):205–7.
69. Dellit TH, Owens RC, McGowan JE Jr, et al. Infectious Diseases Society of America and the Society for Healthcare Epidemiology of America guidelines for developing an institutional program to enhance antimicrobial stewardship. Clin Infect Dis 2007;44(2):159–77.
70. Charbonneau P, Parienti JJ, Thibon P, et al. Fluoroquinolone use and methicillin-resistant *Staphylococcus aureus* isolation rates in hospitalized patients: a quasi experimental study. Clin Infect Dis 2006;42(6):778–84.
71. Weber SG, Gold HS, Hooper DC, et al. Fluoroquinolones and the risk for methicillin-resistant *Staphylococcus aureus* in hospitalized patients. Emerg Infect Dis 2003;9(11):1415–22.
72. Kaye KS, Cosgrove S, Harris A, et al. Risk factors for emergence of resistance to broad-spectrum cephalosporins among *Enterobacter* spp. Antimicrob Agents Chemother 2001;45(9):2628–30.

73. Kaye KS, Kanafani ZA, Dodds AE, et al. Differential effects of levofloxacin and ciprofloxacin on the risk for isolation of quinolone-resistant *Pseudomonas aeruginosa*. Antimicrob Agents Chemother 2006;50(6):2192–6.

74. Madaras-Kelly KJ, Remington RE, Lewis PG, et al. Evaluation of an intervention designed to decrease the rate of nosocomial methicillin-resistant *Staphylococcus aureus* infection by encouraging decreased fluoroquinolone use. Infect Control Hosp Epidemiol 2006;27(2):155–69.

75. Meyer KS, Urban C, Eagan JA, et al. Nosocomial outbreak of *Klebsiella* infection resistant to late-generation cephalosporins. Ann Intern Med 1993;119(5):353–8.

76. Rahal JJ, Urban C, Horn D, et al. Class restriction of cephalosporin use to control total cephalosporin resistance in nosocomial *Klebsiella*. JAMA 1998;280(14): 1233–7.

77. Calil R, Marba ST, von Nowakonski A, et al. Reduction in colonization and nosocomial infection by multiresistant bacteria in a neonatal unit after institution of educational measures and restriction in the use of cephalosporins. Am J Infect Control 2001;29(3):133–8.

78. Go ES, Urban C, Burns J, et al. Clinical and molecular epidemiology of acinetobacter infections sensitive only to polymyxin B and sulbactam. Lancet 1994; 344(8933):1329–32.

79. Rahal JJ, Urban C, Segal-Maurer S. Nosocomial antibiotic resistance in multiple gram-negative species: experience at one hospital with squeezing the resistance balloon at multiple sites. Clin Infect Dis 2002;34(4):499–503.

80. Coleman RW, Rodondi LC, Kaubisch S, et al. Cost-effectiveness of prospective and continuous parenteral antibiotic control: experience at the Palo Alto Veterans Affairs Medical Center from 1987 to 1989. Am J Med 1991;90(4):439–44.

81. White AC Jr, Atmar RL, Wilson J, et al. Effects of requiring prior authorization for selected antimicrobials: expenditures, susceptibilities, and clinical outcomes. Clin Infect Dis 1997;25(2):230–9.

82. Woodward RS, Medoff G, Smith MD, et al. Antibiotic cost savings from formulary restrictions and physician monitoring in a medical-school-affiliated hospital. Am J Med 1987;83(5):817–23.

83. de Man P, Verhoeven BA, Verbrugh HA, et al. An antibiotic policy to prevent emergence of resistant bacilli. Lancet 2000;355(9208):973–8.

84. Quale J, Landman D, Saurina G, et al. Manipulation of a hospital antimicrobial formulary to control an outbreak of vancomycin-resistant enterococci. Clin Infect Dis 1996;23(5):1020–5.

85. Burke JP. Antibiotic resistance: squeezing the balloon? JAMA 1998;280(14): 1270–1.

86. Bantar C, Sartori B, Vesco E, et al. A hospitalwide intervention program to optimize the quality of antibiotic use: impact on prescribing practice, antibiotic consumption, cost savings, and bacterial resistance. Clin Infect Dis 2003; 37(2):180–6.

87. Belongia EA, Knobloch MJ, Kieke BA, et al. Impact of statewide program to promote appropriate antimicrobial drug use. Emerg Infect Dis 2005;11(6): 912–20.

88. Lomas J, Anderson GM, Domnick-Pierre K, et al. Do practice guidelines guide practice? The effect of a consensus statement on the practice of physicians. N Engl J Med 1989;321(19):1306–11.

89. Ibrahim EH, Ward S, Sherman G, et al. Experience with a clinical guideline for the treatment of ventilator-associated pneumonia. Crit Care Med 2001;29(6): 1109–15.

90. Price J, Ekleberry A, Grover A, et al. Evaluation of clinical practice guidelines on outcome of infection in patients in the surgical intensive care unit. Crit Care Med 1999;27(10):2118–24.

91. Centers for Disease Control. Guidelines for the management of adults with hospital-acquired, ventilator-associated, and healthcare-associated pneumonia. Am J Respir Crit Care Med 2005;171(4):388–416.

92. Harbarth S, Garbino J, Pugin J, et al. Inappropriate initial antimicrobial therapy and its effect on survival in a clinical trial of immunomodulating therapy for severe sepsis. Am J Med 2003;115(7):529–35.

93. Hyle EP, Lipworth AD, Zaoutis TE, et al. Impact of inadequate initial antimicrobial therapy on mortality in infections due to extended-spectrum beta-lactamase-producing enterobacteriaceae: variability by site of infection. Arch Intern Med 2005;165(12):1375–80.

94. Briceland LL, Nightingale CH, Quintiliani R, et al. Antibiotic streamlining from combination therapy to monotherapy utilizing an interdisciplinary approach. Arch Intern Med 1988;148(9):2019–22.

95. Kollef MH, Kollef KE. Antibiotic utilization and outcomes for patients with clinically suspected ventilator-associated pneumonia and negative quantitative BAL culture results. Chest 2005;128(4):2706–13.

96. Evans RS, Pestotnik SL, Classen DC, et al. A computer-assisted management program for antibiotics and other antiinfective agents. N Engl J Med 1998;338(4):232–8.

97. Pestotnik SL, Classen DC, Evans RS, et al. Implementing antibiotic practice guidelines through computer-assisted decision support: clinical and financial outcomes. Ann Intern Med 1996;124(10):884–90.

98. Koppel R, Metlay JP, Cohen A, et al. Role of computerized physician order entry systems in facilitating medication errors. JAMA 2005;293(10):1197–203.

99. Burke JP. Maximizing appropriate antibiotic prophylaxis for surgical patients: an update from LDS Hospital, Salt Lake City. Clin Infect Dis 2001;33(Suppl 2):S78–83.

100. Classen DC, Pestotnik SL, Evans RS, et al. Computerized surveillance of adverse drug events in hospital patients. JAMA 1991;266(20):2847–51.

101. Evans RS, Pestotnik SL, Classen DC, et al. Evaluation of a computer-assisted antibiotic-dose monitor. Ann Pharmacother 1999;33(10):1026–31.

102. Munson EL, Diekema DJ, Beekmann SE, et al. Detection and treatment of bloodstream infection: laboratory reporting and antimicrobial management. J Clin Microbiol 2003;41(1):495–7.

103. Peterson LR, Hamilton JD, Baron EJ, et al. Role of clinical microbiology laboratories in the management and control of infectious diseases and the delivery of health care. Clin Infect Dis 2001;32(4):605–11.

104. Binkley S, Fishman NO, LaRosa LA, et al. Comparison of unit-specific and hospital-wide antibiograms: potential implications for selection of empirical antimicrobial therapy. Infect Control Hosp Epidemiol 2006;27(7):682–7.

105. Leibovici L, Paul M, Poznanski O, et al. Monotherapy versus beta-lactam-aminoglycoside combination treatment for gram-negative bacteremia: a prospective, observational study. Antimicrob Agents Chemother 1997;41(5):1127–33.

106. Paul M, Benuri-Silbiger I, Soares-Weiser K, et al. Beta lactam monotherapy versus beta lactam-aminoglycoside combination therapy for sepsis in immunocompetent patients: systematic review and meta-analysis of randomised trials. BMJ 2004;328(7441):668.

107. Safdar N, Handelsman J, Maki DG. Does combination antimicrobial therapy reduce mortality in gram-negative bacteraemia? A meta-analysis. Lancet Infect Dis 2004;4(8):519–27.

108. Vidal F, Mensa J, Almela M, et al. Epidemiology and outcome of *Pseudomonas aeruginosa* bacteremia, with special emphasis on the influence of antibiotic treatment: analysis of 189 episodes. Arch Intern Med 1996;156(18):2121–6.

109. Bliziotis IA, Samonis G, Vardakas KZ, et al. Effect of aminoglycoside and beta-lactam combination therapy versus beta-lactam monotherapy on the emergence of antimicrobial resistance: a meta-analysis of randomized, controlled trials. Clin Infect Dis 2005;41(2):149–58.

110. Gerding DN, Larson TA, Hughes RA, et al. Aminoglycoside resistance and aminoglycoside usage: ten years of experience in one hospital. Antimicrob Agents Chemother 1991;35(7):1284–90.

111. Young EJ, Sewell CM, Koza MA, et al. Antibiotic resistance patterns during aminoglycoside restriction. Am J Med Sci 1985;290(6):223–7.

Antibacterial Agents in Pediatrics

Susana Chavez-Bueno, MD[a], Terrence L. Stull, MD[b],*

KEYWORDS

- Antibiotics • Antimicrobials • Antibacterials • Pediatrics
- Children • Pharmacokinetics

Antibiotics are the therapeutic agents most frequently used in pediatrics. The majority of prescriptions for antibacterial drugs are to treat common pediatric infections such as otitis media, pharyngitis, pneumonia, and other respiratory infections that are diagnosed primarily in the ambulatory setting.[1] In many of these cases, however, antimicrobials are inappropriately prescribed; thus, antibiotic overuse is a persistent problem, especially in outpatient pediatric practices.[2] Antibiotics are also widely used to treat infections of the skin and soft tissues, genitourinary tract, bones and joints, central nervous system (CNS), and other sites in patients who require hospitalization.

Despite their widespread use in pediatrics, few antibiotics have been studied adequately to be considered safe and effective for use in children. Unfortunately, data regarding antibiotic pharmacokinetics, efficacy, and side effects are often extrapolated from studies performed in adults or animals when selecting dosing regimens for children. The US Food and Drug Administration (FDA) addressed the issue with the Pediatric Rule, which became effective in 1999. Under this rule, any application for approval of a human drug or biologic agent is expected to contain data assessing the safety and effectiveness in pediatric patients. Two recent laws, which were reauthorized in 2007, the Best Pharmaceuticals for Children Act and the Pediatric Research Equity Act, further encourage the research and development of drugs in children.

When using antibiotics in children, many factors that are different from those for adults should be considered. A discussion of the general principles of pharmacokinetics and pharmacodynamics pertinent to the pediatric population is included in this article, followed by a discussion of selected antibiotics that are most commonly used in pediatrics.

[a] Department of Pediatrics, Section of Pediatric Infectious Diseases, University of Oklahoma Health Sciences Center, 940 NE 13th Street, Room 2B 2311, Oklahoma City, OK 73104, USA
[b] Department of Pediatrics, University of Oklahoma Health Sciences Center, 940 NE 13th Street, Room 2B 2308, Oklahoma City, OK 73104, USA
* Corresponding author.
E-mail address: terrence-stull@ouhsc.edu (T.L. Stull).

Infect Dis Clin N Am 23 (2009) 865–880
doi:10.1016/j.idc.2009.06.011
0891-5520/09/$ – see front matter © 2009 Elsevier Inc. All rights reserved.

id.theclinics.com

PHARMACOKINETICS

Antibiotic pharmacokinetics describe their absorption, metabolism, elimination, and distribution. Gestational and chronologic age are factors to consider when administering antibiotics to children because various organs mature at different rates as children grow, affecting the pharmacokinetics.[3] Other factors affecting pharmacokinetics include underlying diseases, drug interactions, and tissue distribution.

Parenteral antibiotic administration often results in higher and more predictable serum concentrations compared with the oral route. Oral bioavailability of most beta-lactam antibiotics, for example, is approximately 5% to 10% compared with the intravenous (IV) route. However, certain antibiotics, including clindamycin, trimethoprim/sulfamethoxazole, and linezolid, on the other hand, have excellent bioavailability after administration by the oral route, and the serum concentrations are similar to those found after an IV dose.

Hepatic function changes over time as the result of variations in blood flow and the maturation of enzyme systems. In neonates, both phase I (primarily oxidation) and phase II enzymes (conjugation) may be reduced, although they are more active by 2 months of age.[4] After the first year of life, the levels of most liver enzymes are similar to the levels in adults.[5,6] Besides the changes in hepatic metabolism, it is also important to consider the protein binding properties of different antibiotics at different stages of life. The bilirubin-albumin binding capacity in neonates is very low, and it does not reach adult levels until approximately 5 months of age. Excess unconjugated bilirubin can result in bilirubin encephalopathy (kernicterus). Certain antibacterial agents (eg, ceftriaxone and the sulfonamides) can increase toxic bilirubin levels as the result of displacement from albumin. Because the risk for kernicterus is directly related to the serum concentration of unbound, unconjugated bilirubin, these agents should be avoided in newborns and young infants. Cefotaxime and ceftazidime pose less risk.

Renal function also is determined by gestational and chronologic age.[7] The glomerular clearance of drugs in neonates is slow compared with that in older children and adults. Aminoglycosides and glycopeptide antibiotics are almost exclusively eliminated by the renal route, and adjusted gestational age is the best predictor of their clearance. The glomerular filtration rate increases during infancy to approach an adult rate by 6 months of age.[8,9] Antibiotic dosing in neonates is further complicated because neonates have larger total-body-water content and a higher proportion of extracellular fluid compared with older children, which translates into a larger volume of distribution.

Although age correlates with body weight as the child grows, pharmacokinetic parameters do not necessarily follow. In many cases, body-weight-normalized drug clearance in children exceeds that of adults; therefore, a higher dosage based on body weight may be necessary. Maximum-body-weight dosages prevent overdosing in adolescents and overweight children. Adjusting dosages based on body surface area may help to avoid overdosing of certain antibiotics, especially in older children. Monitoring of antibiotic serum concentrations is sometimes indicated to assess both efficacy and toxicity.

In addition, adherence to oral antibiotic therapy is another relevant issue to consider in children. For those who can only take liquid formulations, palatability plays an important role in compliance with therapy (**Table 1**).[10–14]

PHARMACODYNAMICS

Pharmacodynamics describes the effects, activity, or toxicity of a pharmaceutical agent within the body. When selecting an antibiotic for pediatric use, knowledge about

Table 1 Comparative palatability of selected antibiotic suspensions used in pediatrics[10–14]		
Pleasant Taste	**Inconsistent Preference**	**Unpleasant Taste**
Amoxacillin	Amoxacillin/clavulanic acid	Cefpodoxime
Cefdinir	Azithromycin	Cefuroxime
Cefixime	Ciprofloxacin	Clarithromycin
Cephalexin	Erythromycin	Clindamycin
Loracarbef/rifampin	Trimethoprim/sulfamethoxazole	Linezolid

the specific causative organism and its susceptibility to different antibiotics is crucial. Early isolation of the organism by obtaining appropriate clinical samples for laboratory testing before beginning antibiotic therapy is ideal, although sometimes empiric selection of an antibiotic is necessary. The site of infection is another factor to consider when choosing a particular agent because antibiotic concentrations vary in different compartments.

The minimum inhibitory concentration (MIC) determines the susceptibility of a particular pathogen to a specific antibiotic. The MIC is the lowest concentration of the antibiotic that inhibits the growth of the pathogen in vitro. Not all isolates of a pathogen have the same MIC for a given antibiotic.[15]

Resistance to antibiotics varies greatly depending on the specific bacterial mechanisms of resistance and host factors. Local epidemiologic data are key to assessing the prevalent patterns of resistance in a community and are helpful in selecting the most appropriate initial empiric antibiotic therapy.

Two main patterns of bactericidal activity exist. Antibiotics such as penicillins and cephalosporins demonstrate time-dependent killing, that is, the duration that the concentration of the drug is greater than the MIC of the target organism is directly related to bacterial killing.[16] Vancomycin, clindamycin, and the macrolides also show time-dependent antibacterial activity. Bacterial killing by such antibiotics as the aminoglycosides and fluoroquinolones, on the other hand, is concentration dependent, that is, a higher drug concentration leads to a greater rate and extent of bacterial killing.

The duration of therapy is determined in many cases by common practice and general experience because critical evaluations of therapy duration have been performed for only a few diseases. In general, a longer duration of therapy should be used (1) for tissues in which antibiotic concentrations may not be high (eg, bone), (2) when the organisms are less susceptible to antibiotic therapy, (3) when a relapse of infection is unacceptable (eg, CNS infections), or (4) when the host is immunocompromised in some way.[17]

BETA-LACTAMS

Penicillin was discovered more than 5 decades ago, and the beta-lactam antibiotics have been synthetically modified. They continue to be widely used in pediatrics. Despite the development of resistance by several organisms, this group of antibiotics continues to be used against a variety of infections in children.

Penicillins

Penicillins are the most frequently prescribed antibacterials in the United States and many other parts of the world. Amoxicillin accounts for ~50% of all oral liquid antibacterials and ~75% of all oral liquid penicillins prescribed in primary care settings in England.[18]

In the 1950s, the entire beta-lactam family of antibiotics included only penicillin G and penicillin V. Today, these antibiotics remain the first-line therapy for infections caused by susceptible streptococci, including group A streptococcal pharyngitis. They are also the drugs of choice in syphilis, meningococcal, *Listeria*, and neonatal group B streptococcal infections.

Broad-spectrum penicillins, the aminopenicillins, were developed in the 1960s. Ampicillin, and later amoxicillin, provided activity against gram-negative bacteria and enterococci.[19] Amoxicillin is structurally related to ampicillin and has the same spectrum of activity and potency. It is much better absorbed when given orally, achieving blood concentrations approximately twice as high as those obtained with ampicillin. Initially, aminopenicillins were active against many gram-negative strains of bacteria, including *Escherichia coli*, *Proteus* spp, *Salmonella* spp, and beta-lacta-mase–negative *Haemophilus influenzae*. Unfortunately, these organisms have developed various mechanisms of resistance, and the aminopenicillins no longer remain the first choice for many of these infections, although they continue to be used against susceptible isolates. *Streptococcus pneumoniae,* the most common etiologic agent of otitis media, is another example of the development of bacterial resistance to penicillins. Through selection of strains producing penicillin-binding proteins with decreased affinity for penicillins, the resistance of many strains of *S pneumoniae* has progressively increased. However, because the mutations in the penicillin-binding proteins usually result in only modestly reduced susceptibility, higher doses of aminopenicillins result in serum concentrations that exceed the MIC for a greater portion of the dosing interval, thus allowing effective killing.[20] Therefore, the currently recommended dosage of amoxicillin is 80 to 90 mg/kg/d instead of 40 mg/kg/d when treating otitis media caused by some penicillin-nonsusceptible *S pneumoniae* isolates.[21]

Another mechanism of resistance became evident in the mid-1960s with the identification of bacteria-producing beta-lactamases. The first semisynthetic penicillin that was stable to staphylococcal penicillinase was methicillin. This was followed by other semisynthetic penicillins that had increased activity and the option of oral administration, such as cloxacillin, flucloxacillin, and dicloxacillin. Dicloxacillin has excellent bioavailability as an oral agent, but is poorly palatable, and for treating infections caused by beta-lactamase–producing organisms in children, it has been replaced by other antibiotics. Penicillinase-resistant parenteral semisynthetic penicillins that are more commonly used than methicillin include nafcillin and oxacillin. These antibiotics are effective for treating methicillin-susceptible *Staphylococcus aureus* (MSSA) infections in children. The emergence of methicillin-resistant *S aureus* (MRSA) in the pediatric population has caused a decrease in their use in children.

A different approach to counteract beta-lactamase has been the development of beta-lactamase inhibitors such as clavulanic acid.[22] The combination of amoxacillin and clavulanic acid became available in 1980, and it has been widely used in children to treat otitis media, community-acquired pneumonia, sinusitis, infections of the skin and subcutaneous tissues, urinary tract infections, and animal and human bites. This combination has an expanded activity to include MSSA, beta-lactamase–positive *H influenzae*, and many anaerobes as well. Sulbactam is another beta-lactamase inhibitor. In combination with ampicillin for IV administration, it is FDA-approved for use in children aged 1 year and older for treatment of skin and subcutaneous tissue infections. Its spectrum of activity is similar to that of amoxicillin/clavulanic acid, and there is evidence that it is an effective therapy for intra-abdominal infections and meningitis caused by susceptible organisms.[23]

Extended-spectrum penicillins were also developed with the goal of treating infections caused by *Pseudomonas aeruginosa*. These penicillins include the carboxypenicillins and ureidopenicillins. Side effects unique to these two groups include hypokalemia and hypernatremia. The carboxypenicillins consist of carbenicillin and ticarcillin. Compared with ampicillin, both have enhanced activity against *P aeruginosa* and other gram-negative bacteria. Ticarcillin has greater antipseudomonal activity compared with carbenicillin in vitro. However, the aminopenicillins continue to have superior activity against enterococci compared with the carboxypenicillins. Ticarcillin is approved for use in pediatrics to provide treatment for intra-abdominal infections, skin and subcutaneous tissue infections, respiratory tract infections, septicemia, and urinary tract infections caused by susceptible organisms. The combination of ticarcillin and clavulanic acid is also approved for use in children older than 3 months of age for similar indications, there is also evidence for its efficacy as an empiric therapy in febrile neutropenic pediatric patients.[24] The ureidopenicillins have enhanced aerobic gram-negative activity, including antipseudomonal activity. They have a decreased frequency of side effects and are active against *Enterococcus* spp. Included in this group are mezlocillin, azlocillin, and piperacillin. Piperacillin is the ureidopenicillin most commonly used in pediatrics, and its combination with tazobactam, another penicillinase inhibitor, has been approved to provide therapy for appendicitis and peritonitis in children aged 2 months and older.[25] Evidence supports its efficacy as an empiric therapy for febrile episodes in pediatric neutropenic patients.[26]

Cephalosporins

Cephalosporins are among the most commonly used beta-lactam antibiotics in children. Various cephalosporins are derived by doing modifications of the prototype molecule, cephalosporin C, which is produced by the fungus *Cephalosporium acremonium*. These antimicrobials are routinely classified into "generations," based mainly on their spectrum of activity. Both oral and parenteral agents are available within each category (**Table 2**).[27] In general, first-generation cephalosporins are most active against aerobic gram-positive cocci. Second-generation cephalosporins are more active against selected gram-negative organisms; additionally, cefoxitin and cefotetan (both cephamycins, the latter not FDA-approved for use in children) are active against anaerobic bacteria. Third-generation cephalosporins are the most active against gram-negative organisms, including some with activity against *P aeruginosa* (ceftazidime and, to a lesser extent, cefoperazone). Fourth-generation cephalosporins include cefepime and cefpirome, the latter not FDA-approved for use in adults or children.

Some organisms, including all enterococci, *Listeria* monocytogenes, and atypical pneumonia organisms such as *Legionella*, *Mycoplasma*, and *Chlamydia* spp, are always resistant to all cephalosporins.

Cephalosporins are generally well tolerated. Orally administered cephalosporins may cause gastrointestinal complaints such as nausea, vomiting, or diarrhea. Thrombophlebitis occurs in about 1% to 2% of patients who receive cephalosporins intravenously. Hypersensitivity or allergic reactions occur in 1% to 3% of patients who receive cephalosporin drugs, and skin testing helps confirm such reactions.[28] The rate of cross-reactive cephalosporin allergy in patients who have known penicillin allergy is poorly defined, but it appears to be low.[29,30] Other side effects include occasional leukopenia and thrombocytopenia; eosinophilia may occur. Cephalosporins can also cause hypoprothrombinemia and transient elevation of transaminases; they are rarely nephrotoxic or neurotoxic.

Table 2 FDA-approved cephalosporins for use in children		
Generation	Oral	Parenteral[b]
First generation	Cefadroxil	Cefazolin[a]
	Cephalexin[a]	Cephalothin
	Cephradine	Cephradine
Second generation	Cefaclor	Cefoxitin
	Cefprozil	Cefuroxime
	Cefuroxime	
Third generation	Cefditoren	Cefotaxime[a]
	Cefixime[a]	Ceftazidime[a]
	Cefpodoxime	Ceftizoxime
	Ceftibuten	Ceftriaxone[a]
	Cefdinir[a]	
Fourth generation	—	Cefepime

[a] Most commonly used in pediatrics.
[b] All parenterally administered cephalosporins are available in intramuscular and IV forms.

Newer cephalosporins under investigation and with broader activity, including activity against MRSA, are ceftobiprole[31] and ceftaroline.[32]

First-generation oral cephalosporins are mainly used to treat skin and soft-tissue infections caused by susceptible organisms (they are not active against MRSA), streptococcal tonsillopharyngitis, and urinary tract infections. Cephalexin is most commonly used for these indications. At higher doses, oral cephalosporins are useful to treat bone and joint infections in children. The most common side effects include skin reactions and gastrointestinal upset.

Parenteral first-generation cephalosporins are for the most part used to treat bone, urinary tract, respiratory tract, and skin and soft-tissue infections, and for preoperative prophylaxis when indicated.

Cefuroxime is the most commonly used *second-generation* cephalosporin used in children. It is available for oral and parenteral administration. Cefuroxime is the only cephalosporin of this group that has demonstrable penetration into the CNS. However, its use for treatment of bacterial meningitis was associated with delayed sterilization and a higher incidence of hearing loss.[33] Other indications include pharyngitis, otitis media, lower respiratory tract infections, soft-tissue infections, and urinary tract infections. Other oral second-generation cephalosporins include cefaclor and cefprozil, both with a spectrum of activity similar to cefuroxime axetil. Cefaclor has been associated with serum sickness–like reactions that have limited its use in this patient population. Cefprozil is better tolerated and is more palatable. Loracarbef and cefamandole are second-generation cephalosporins that are no longer available in the United States.

Oral *third-generation* cephalosporins used commonly in pediatrics include cefixime, cefpodoxime, ceftibuten, and cefdinir. Cefixime is FDA-approved for use in children older than 6 months of age and is commonly used in urinary tract infections and for the treatment of *Salmonella* infections. Cefpodoxime may be dosed once or twice daily and is approved for use in children older than 2 months of age, but it is poorly palatable. Ceftibuten has similar coverage to cefpodoxime, and is approved only for treatment of respiratory tract infections, sinusitis, and otitis media in children aged 6 months and older. Cefdinir has a broader spectrum of activity, with activity against MSSA and streptococci that is comparable with that of the first-generation agents. It may be dosed once or twice daily, and it has a favorable taste.

The most widely used parenteral third-generation cephalosporins in children are ceftriaxone, cefotaxime and ceftazidime. These agents have enhanced activity compared with second-generation agents against Enterobacteriaceae. In general, they have activity against penicillin nonsusceptible *S pneumoniae* and *Haemophilus, Neisseria*, and *Moraxella* spp. Third-generation parenteral cephalosporins are the drugs of choice for the treatment of many types of bacterial meningitis. Ceftriaxone has the convenience of dosing once daily for the treatment of most infections. It can be given either intravenously or intramuscularly. Its affinity to bind albumin can cause displacement of bilirubin; therefore, it is not recommended for use in neonates, particularly for those who have hyperbilirubinemia. Ceftriaxone achieves excellent peak serum concentrations and efficacy against resistant nonmeningeal *S pneumoniae* infections. However, with the increase in the number of nonsusceptible isolates, the use of vancomycin plus a third-generation cephalosporin is recommended when initiating antibiotic therapy for bacterial meningitis, until culture and susceptibility results are available. Cefotaxime has equivalent coverage to that of ceftriaxone, and has no restrictions for use during the newborn period. Ceftazidime is the only third-generation agent that has activity against susceptible strains of *P aeruginosa*. Overall, these agents are well tolerated. They, like other beta-lactams, can be associated with agranulocytosis, thrombocytopenia, pseudomembranous colitis, and hypersensitivity reactions. Ceftriaxone has been associated with reversible pseudocholelithiasis. Its administration with any calcium-containing IV solutions should be avoided.[34]

Cefepime is a parenterally administered *fourth-generation* cephalosporin that was first approved by the FDA in 1997. It has good activity against gram-positive bacteria, including MSSA and α-hemolytic streptococci. Also, it has the best activity against penicillin-resistant pneumococcus among the cephalosporins. In addition, its gram-negative activity against *H influenzae, Neisseria* spp, and *Pseudomonas* spp is excellent. It is also more active against Enterobacteriaceae, including strains that produce extended-spectrum beta-lactamases, than third-generation cephalosporins are.[35] Cefepime is FDA-approved for use in children older than 2 months of age for empiric therapy of febrile neutropenia, and to treat skin and soft-tissue infections, moderate to severe pneumonia, and urinary tract infections. Adverse effects associated with cefepime use include headache, gastrointestinal upset, local reactions, and rash that occur in less than 2% of individuals. More serious adverse effects include encephalopathy and seizures.

Carbapenems and Monobactams

Carbapenems are a class of antibiotics that have one of the broadest spectra of antimicrobial activity for use in pediatrics. The chemical structure of the carbapenems is very similar to that of the penicillin ring, with the side chain providing resistance to most beta-lactamase enzymes. Imipenem, meropenem and ertapenem have activity against most gram-negative and gram-positive organisms, with differences in activity that depend on the particular beta-lactamase produced by the pathogen. Meropenem is less active against gram-positive organisms and more active against gram-negative organisms than imipenem. Ertapenem has decreased activity against *Pseudomonas* isolates compared with imipenem and meropenem. Carbapenems are not active against MRSA, *Enterococcus faecium, Burkholderia cepacia, Stenotrophomonas maltophilia, Chlamydia* spp, and *Mycoplasma* spp.

Imipenem is approved for use in pediatrics to treat endocarditis, septicemia, and intra-abdominal, bone, and urinary tract infections. Meropenem is approved for use in children older than 3 months of age to provide therapy for meningitis (recommended dose for this indication of 120 mg/kg/day, maximum dose of 6 g/day), complicated skin and soft-tissue infections, and intra-abdominal infections. Ertapenem is approved for use in children older than 3 months of age to provide therapy for severe pneumonia, complicated skin and soft-tissue infections, and intra-abdominal and pelvic infections.

Carbapenems are administered parenterally, and their excretion is predominantly by glomerular filtration. Imipenem must be administered with cilastatin to avoid hydrolysis and to reduce nephrotoxicity. In general, tolerability to carbapenems is good.[36] Seizures are a well-known side effect of imipenem/cilastatin, especially in patients who have meningitis. Seizures occur in approximately 3% of patients who are treated with imipenem and who do not have CNS infections, but the incidence of seizures can be as high as 33% in patients who have bacterial meningitis.[37]

Despite their broad-spectrum activity, resistance to carbapenems, especially by gram-negative organisms, has been reported.[38]

Aztreonam is the only monobactam approved for pediatric use. Its spectrum of activity resembles that of the aminoglycosides, and it has activity against most aerobic gram-negative bacilli, including *P aeruginosa*. When used for empiric therapy, aztreonam must be given in combination with other antimicrobial agents that are active against gram-positive and anaerobic species.[39] It is approved for use in children 9 months of age and older to provide therapy for lower respiratory tract infections, urinary tract infections, septicemia, and intra-abdominal infections caused by susceptible organisms. Aztreonam may be administered intramuscularly or intravenously; the primary route of elimination is by urinary excretion. The drug is not nephrotoxic and has not been associated with disorders of coagulation. Anaphylactic reactions have been reported in less than 1% of individuals who receive the drug.

AMINOGLYCOSIDES

Aminoglycosides are one of the oldest groups of antibiotics still in use. Streptomycin, the first aminoglycoside available, was discovered in the mid-1940s and was used to treat tuberculosis. The aminoglycosides are bactericidal inhibitors of protein synthesis. They are not available for oral administration, so they are mainly used in parenteral form, although inhaled tobramycin is FDA-approved for use in children older than 6 years of age who have cystic fibrosis.[40,41]

Aminoglycosides are predominantly used to treat gram-negative bacillary infections. They have some activity against *S aureus* and are synergistic against *Enterococcus* spp, but their gram-positive activity as single agents is very limited. In pediatrics, they remain key agents to treat gram-negative bacteria, including *E coli*, *Salmonella* spp, *Shigella* spp, *Enterobacter* spp, *Citrobacter* spp, *Acinetobacter* spp, *Proteus* spp, *Klebsiella* spp, *Serratia* spp, *Morganella* spp, *Pseudomonas* spp, and mycobacteria. Therefore, they are useful in the treatment of urinary tract infections, intra-abdominal infections, neonatal sepsis, complicated infections in cystic fibrosis, and as empiric therapy for febrile neutropenic patients. They are also used to treat plague, tularemia, and brucellosis.

The three most commonly used aminoglycosides in children are gentamicin, tobramycin, and amikacin. In general, tobramycin has greater antipseudomonal activity, and amikacin is more active against resistant gram-negative bacilli.

Because the aminoglycosides are concentration-dependent antibiotics, their bactericidal effect depends on an adequate peak concentration. Adult studies have shown enhanced bactericidal effect and minimized toxicity using once-daily dosing of aminoglycosides. Pediatric studies of once-daily dosing have been conducted and also support this dosing regimen.[42]

Ototoxicity and nephrotoxicity are the most notable adverse effects. However, studies have failed to demonstrate a consistent correlation between aminoglycosides and hearing loss in pediatric patients[43]; the risk for nephrotoxicity in pediatric patients also has rarely been demonstrated.

MACROLIDES

Macrolides inhibit RNA-dependent protein synthesis by reversibly binding to the 50S ribosomal subunit of susceptible microorganisms. Besides their direct antimicrobial activity, clinical trials in patients who have chronic inflammatory lung diseases have suggested an anti-inflammatory effect by documenting significant improvement in lung function and quality of life along with fewer exacerbations when macrolides are used.[44] The mechanism of action mediating these effects is currently under investigation.[45]

Erythromycin is the oldest agent in this group; it has been available since the mid-1950s. The antimicrobial activity of erythromycin includes various gram-positive organisms, and *Legionella, Mycoplasma*, and *Chlamydia* spp. Its disadvantages include poor gastrointestinal tolerance and a short half-life. Erythromycin was commonly used as an alternative therapy for penicillin-allergic children who were afflicted with streptococcal pharyngitis, sinusitis, or acute otitis media; however, recent increases in macrolide-resistant *S pneumoniae* and *H influenzae* have decreased its utility in children.[46–48] Macrolide resistance is mainly due to either an alteration of the drug-binding site on the ribosome that is caused by methylation (macrolide-lincosamide-streptogramin B resistance) or to active drug efflux. Macrolide hydrolysis caused by esterases is a resistance mechanism in Enterobacteriaceae.

Newer macrolides for use in children include azithromycin and clarithromycin. They are used for the treatment of respiratory tract infections, sexually transmitted diseases, and infections caused by *Helicobacter* or *Mycobacterium avium* complex. The bioavailability of the azithromycin suspension is not affected by meals, and its half-life allows once-daily administration. Azithromycin is also available for IV dosing. Clarithromycin possesses increased acid stability, which results in improved oral bioavailability and reduced gastrointestinal intolerance.[49]

Ketolides are semisynthetic derivatives of the 14-membered ring macrolide antibiotics that have an expanded spectrum of activity.[50] Telithromycin, a member of this group, is approved for the treatment of mild to moderate pneumonia in adults, but its safety and efficacy in children have not yet been established.

Side effects of macrolides include alteration of gastrointestinal motility, potential for cardiac arrythmia, and inhibition of drug metabolism that leads to clinically relevant drug–drug interactions.[51] Erythromycin stimulates gastric motility more so than clarithromycin and azithromycin do. The association of erythromycin with increased risk for hypertrophic pyloric stenosis in newborns has prompted some clinicians to use azithromycin instead to treat pertussis and chlamydia infections in these patients.[52]

LINCOSAMIDES

Lincomycin and clindamycin are clinically useful lincosamide antibiotics. They are bacteriostatic and act by inhibiting protein synthesis.[53] Clindamycin is usually more active than lincomycin in the treatment of bacterial infections, particularly those caused by anaerobic species. Among aerobic gram-positive bacteria, it is active against most strains of pneumococcus, group A *Streptococcus*, *Streptococcus viridans*, and many *Staphylococcus* strains. Clindamycin also inhibits the production of exotoxin associated with toxic shock syndromes, and it also affects some protozoa. Clindamycin is available for oral, intramuscular, and IV administration.

Clindamycin use is on the increase in pediatrics because of the increase in community-acquired MRSA infections. Evidence to support the use of clindamycin to provide therapy for community-acquired MRSA in children is limited,[54] and there is currently no specific indication by the FDA for the use of clindamycin to treat MRSA infections in children.

The most common adverse effect of clindamycin is diarrhea, which is reported in 2% to 20% of patients. Antibiotic-associated pseudomembranous colitis is possible as well. Hypersensitivity reactions are also common, presenting as a morbilliform rash; erythema multiforme and Stevens-Johnson syndrome are rare.[55] Less common adverse effects include liver toxicity, bone marrow suppression, and muscle weakness, all of which are reversible after drug discontinuation. Clindamycin can prolong the effect of neuromuscular blocking agents.

GLYCOPEPTIDES

Vancomycin and teicoplanin are the two glycopeptides that have been used clinically for the treatment of multidrug-resistant infections that are caused by gram-positive organisms. Vancomycin is more widely used in pediatrics.

Vancomycin is a glycopeptide that inhibits synthesis of the bacterial cell wall. It is commonly used for infections that are caused by MRSA, coagulase-negative staphylococci, ampicillin-resistant enterococci, and Bacillus and Corynebacterium spp. It has become an important agent used in combination with other antibiotics when initiating therapy for biologic hardware infections (eg, central venous catheters, ventriculoperitoneal shunts) because of its activity against coagulase-negative staphylococci. It is also used in bacterial meningitis because of its activity against penicillin-nonsusceptible S pneumoniae, and in selected episodes of febrile neutropenia because of the possibility of resistant viridans streptococci.[56] Oral vancomycin is used to treat pseudomembranous colitis caused by Clostridium difficile. This use carries the potential risk for the development of vancomycin-resistant enterococci (VRE).[57,58]

Unfortunately, resistance to vancomycin by several organisms, including S aureus and enterococci, continues to increase. Although the incidence of strains that have a reduced susceptibility to vancomycin seems low, the true incidence may be much higher because of technical difficulties with common methods of detection. Current methods for testing vancomycin are not completely reliable in many laboratories. One concern is that vancomycin treatment failures are related to the presence of vancomycin-resistant subpopulations of MRSA strains that seem to be vancomycin susceptible in the laboratory.[59] Reduced clinical efficacy of vancomycin has been reported in patients who have clinical isolates that have a MIC of more than 1 μg/mL, even though the MIC is still within the susceptible range (MIC $\leq$ 2 μg/mL).[60]

In general, vancomycin is well tolerated, but reported adverse effects include gastrointestinal, hypotension, and cardiovascular effects after rapid infusion; drug-mediated skin reactions; thrombophlebitis; and rarely, ototoxicity. Also, previous preparations of vancomycin were associated with nephrotoxicity, but this occurrence is infrequent with the newer preparation. Red man syndrome is probably histamine-mediated and responds to antihistamine or corticosteroid administration and a slowing of the infusion rate.

Dalbavancin and telavancin are new lipoglycopeptides that are undergoing clinical trials, but the FDA has not yet granted approval for their use in adults or children.[61,62]

OXAZOLIDINONES, STREPTOGRAMINS, AND LIPOPEPTIDES

Linezolid is the first oxazolidinone approved for use in the United States, including use in children. The drug is predominately bacteriostatic, and it has antimicrobial activity against gram-positive organisms such as streptococci, staphylococci, and entero-cocci, including species that are resistant to conventional antibacterials.[63] Linezolid has activity against rapidly growing mycobacterial species, multiple *Nocardia* spp, and *Mycobacterium tuberculosis*. It has excellent bioavailability, both intravenously and orally, and a very good safety profile in children.[64] There is also evidence for its safety in neonates.[65,66] It is approved for use in adults and children for the treatment of serious infections caused by *Enterococcus faecium* or *E fecalis*, including VRE; *S aureus*, including MRSA; coagulase-negative staphylococci; and streptococci, including penicillin-resistant *S pneumoniae*. It is used for complicated soft-tissue and skin-structure infections caused by MRSA, nosocomial pneumonia caused by MRSA, bacteremia caused by VRE, and bacteremic community-acquired pneumonia caused by penicillin-resistant *S pneumoniae*. Its most common adverse reactions are diarrhea, headache, vomiting, nausea, elevated serum transaminase concentrations, and rash. Thrombocytopenia is common in adults, so it is recommended to monitor blood counts in children weekly while they are receiving therapy with linezolid.

Dalfopristin/quinupristin is a streptogramin combination approved for use in patients aged 16 years and older for treatment of complicated skin and soft-tissue infections and VRE infections.[67] This antibiotic is active against MRSA, coagulase-negative staphylococci, resistant pneumococcus, and vancomycin-resistant *Enterococcus faecium*. However, it has no activity against vancomycin-resistant *E faecalis*. It is available for parenteral use. Adverse effects include infusion site reactions (eg, pain, edema), nausea and vomiting, diarrhea, headache, mylagias, and arthralgias.[68]

Daptomycin is a novel cyclic lipopeptide, approved for use in the United States in 2003, that is bactericidal against gram-positive bacteria, including MRSA and VRE. Daptomycin kills gram-positive bacteria by the disruption of multiple bacterial plasma membrane functions, without penetrating the cytoplasm.[69] Daptomycin is also effective against a variety of streptococci, such as beta-hemolytic streptococci and other *Streptococcus* spp. Synergy with daptomycin has been described in vitro for amino-glycosides such as gentamicin, oxacillin, other beta-lactams, and rifampicin.[70] The drug is highly protein bound (92%); excretion is primarily renal. Daptomycin is approved to treat skin and soft-tissue infections,[71] *S aureus* bacteremia, and right-sided endocarditis in adults. It is not approved for the treatment of pneumonia. Its safety and efficacy in patients younger than 18 is under study.

SULFONAMIDES

The combination of trimethoprim/sulfamethoxazole (TMP/SMX) is one of the most commonly used antibiotics within this group in pediatrics. The antibiotics act by inhib-iting folic acid synthesis in bacteria at two different enzymatic steps.[72] After oral administration, 85% of the drug is absorbed readily, regardless of the presence of food or other medications; there is also an IV form available.

TMP/SMX is approved for use in children older than 2 months of age to provide therapy for urinary tract infections, selected gastrointestinal infections caused by gram-negative organisms, acute otitis media (not as a first line agent for this indica-tion), and *Pneumocystis jiroveci* pneumonia. TMP/SMX is also an alternative to treat *Listeria* meningitis in penicillin-allergic patients.

The rapid emergence of community-acquired MRSA in children has changed the empiric choice for outpatient antibiotic therapy, especially in cases of localized infections such as cellulitis and abscesses.[73] In these cases, and although it is not FDA approved for this specific indication, TMP/SMX may be the antibiotic of choice, especially if the rate of inducible clindamycin resistance is high in the community (>15%).[74] TMP/SMX may not be active against group A streptococci; therefore, when this organism is suspected as a copathogen, other effective therapies need to be considered. The rates of TMP/SMX resistance for community-acquired MRSA in the United States have remained low; however, in Europe the TMP/SMX resistance rates to MRSA in general have been reported to be between 53% and 76%.[75] Most of the experience with using TMP/SMX to provide therapy for S aureus infection in children is anecdotal; therefore, more studies are needed to ascertain its efficacy as a first-line therapy in this population.[76]

Adverse effects for TMP/SMX include mild to severe dermatologic conditions and various gastrointestinal symptoms. Bone marrow suppression can occur with prolonged use. Aseptic meningitis has occurred as well. TMP/SMX competes with bilirubin for plasma protein-binding sites, thereby increasing the risk for kernicterus, particularly in preterm or already jaundiced neonates. Patients who have glucose 6-phosphate-dehydorgenase (G-6-PD) deficiency, including fetuses and preterm neonates, may develop dose-related acute hemolytic anemia if treated with TMP/SMX.

QUINOLONES

The fluoroquinolones are bactericidal agents that are derivatives of nalidixic acid. They are inhibitors of DNA replication by binding to the topoisomerases of their target bacteria. They are broad-spectrum agents that have activity against gram-positive organisms, including some penicillin-nonsusceptible pneumococci and MRSA. They exhibit excellent activity against gram-negative bacteria, including the Enterobacteriaceae, Moraxella catarrhalis, beta-lactamase–producing H influenzae, and Shigella, Salmonella, and Neisseria spp. In addition, they have activity against P aeruginosa, with ciprofloxacin being most active. Atypical organisms, including Mycoplasma and Chlamydia spp, Legionella pneumophila, Ureaplasma urealyticum, and strains of Mycobacterium are also susceptible.

Ciprofloxacin is the only quinolone approved for use in children, and it is only approved to provide therapy for complicated urinary tract infections, pyelonephritis, and postexposure treatment of inhalation anthrax. Other older quinolones that are approved for use in adults include levofloxacion, ofloxacin, and norfloxacin. Newer agents include gatifloxacin, gemifloxacin, and moxifloxacin.

Early in their development, fluoroquinolones were found to affect cartilage in juvenile animals, resulting in arthropathy. Although the pathogenesis remains unknown, the potential for arthropathy in children is a concern that has limited the use of these drugs in pediatrics. Case reports and retrospective cohort studies, mostly in children who have cystic fibrosis, have failed to demonstrate an association with irreversible arthropathy; however, although the association between quinolones and pediatric arthropathy is weak, it is prudent to use these antibiotics only when safer alternatives are not available.[77]

Despite their limited approval for use in children, it is estimated that more than one-half million prescriptions for quinolones are written in the United States every year for patients younger than 18 years of age.

The use of fluoroquinolones in children should be limited to patients who have cystic fibrosis and life-endangering infections, resistant gram-negative neonatal meningitis, Salmonella and Shigella spp infections, chronic suppurative otitis media, and some cases of complicated acute otitis media.[78] The unskilled use of fluoroquinolones in children, particularly in community-acquired lower respiratory infections, could accelerate the problem of pneumococcal resistance.[79]

SUMMARY

Many antibacterial agents are safe and effective in pediatrics. Unfortunately, microbial pathogens have continued to develop new mechanisms of resistance that limit the treatment options for infections in children. Reducing antibiotic overuse in pediatrics by prescribing antibiotics responsibly and by encouraging people to follow their physician's instructions about dosing and duration would likely delay the development of resistance. Research on antibiotic development and the clinical applications in children will continue to meet the need for better therapeutic options in this population.

REFERENCES

1. Rossignoli A, Clavenna A, Bonati M. Antibiotic prescription and prevalence rate in the outpatient paediatric population: analysis of surveys published during 2000–2005. Eur J Clin Pharmacol 2007;63:1099–106.
2. Mangione-Smith R, Wong L, Elliott MN, et al. Measuring the quality of antibiotic prescribing for upper respiratory infections and bronchitis in 5 US health plans. Arch Pediatr Adolesc Med 2005;159:751–7.
3. Bartelink IH, Rademaker CM, Schobben AF, et al. Guidelines on paediatric dosing on the basis of developmental physiology and pharmacokinetic considerations. Clin Pharmacokinet 2006;45:1077–97.
4. Alcorn J, McNamara PJ. Ontogeny of hepatic and renal systemic clearance pathways in infants: part I. Clin Pharmacokinet 2002;41:959–98.
5. Strolin Benedetti M, Baltes EL. Drug metabolism and disposition in children. Fundam Clin Pharmacol 2003;17:281–99.
6. Kearns GL. Impact of developmental pharmacology on pediatric study design: overcoming the challenges. J Allergy Clin Immunol 2000;106:S128–38.
7. Allegaert K, Anderson BJ, van den Anker JN, et al. Renal drug clearance in preterm neonates: relation to prenatal growth. Ther Drug Monit 2007;29:284–91.
8. van der Heijden AJ, Grose WF, Ambagtsheer JJ, et al. Glomerular filtration rate in the preterm infant: the relation to gestational and postnatal age. Eur J Pediatr 1988;148:24–8.
9. Sonntag J, Prankel B, Waltz S. Serum creatinine concentration, urinary creatinine excretion and creatinine clearance during the first 9 weeks in preterm infants with a birth weight below 1500 g. Eur J Pediatr 1996;155:815–9.
10. Angelilli ML, Toscani M, Matsui DM, et al. Palatability of oral antibiotics among children in an urban primary care center. Arch Pediatr Adolesc Med 2000;154:267–70.
11. Steele RW, Blumer JL, Kalish GH. Patient, physician, and nurse satisfaction with antibiotics. Clin Pediatr (Phila) 2002;41:285–99.
12. Matsui D, Barron A, Rieder MJ. Assessment of the palatability of antistaphylococcal antibiotics in pediatric volunteers. Ann Pharmacother 1996;30:586–8.
13. Pichichero ME. Empiric antibiotic selection criteria for respiratory infections in pediatric practice. Pediatr Infect Dis J 1997;16:S60–4.
14. Steele RW, Russo TM, Thomas MP. Adherence issues related to the selection of antistaphylococcal or antifungal antibiotic suspensions for children. Clin Pediatr (Phila) 2006;45:245–50.
15. Pong AL, Bradley JS. Guidelines for the selection of antibacterial therapy in children. Pediatr Clin North Am 2005;52:869–94, viii.

16. Craig WA. The hidden impact of antibacterial resistance in respiratory tract infection. Re-evaluating current antibiotic therapy. Respir Med 2001;95(Suppl A): S12–9 [discussion S26–7].

17. Bradley JS, Nelson JD. 2006–2007 Nelson's pocket book of pediatrics antimicrobial therapy. 16th edition. Buenos Aires, Argentina: Alliance for World Wide Editing; 2006.

18. Sharland M. The use of antibacterials in children: a report of the Specialist Advisory Committee on Antimicrobial Resistance (SACAR) paediatric subgroup. J Antimicrob Chemother 2007;60(Suppl 1):15–26.

19. Rolinson GN, Geddes AM. The 50th anniversary of the discovery of 6-aminopenicillanic acid (6-APA). Int J Antimicrob Agents 2007;29:3–8.

20. Craig WA, Andes D. Pharmacokinetics and pharmacodynamics of antibiotics in otitis media. Pediatr Infect Dis J 1996;15:255–9.

21. Subcommittee on Management of Acute Otitis Media. Diagnosis and management of acute otitis media. Pediatrics 2004;113:1451–65.

22. Geddes AM, Klugman KP, Rolinson GN. Introduction: historical perspective and development of amoxicillin/clavulanic. Int J Antimicrob Agents 2007;30(Suppl 2): S109–12.

23. Lode HM. Rational antibiotic therapy and the position of ampicillin/sulbactam. Int J Antimicrob Agents 2008;32:10–28.

24. Yu LC, Shaneyfelt T, Warrier R, et al. The efficacy of ticarcillin-clavulanic and gentamicin as empiric treatment for febrile neutropenic pediatric patients with cancer. Pediatr Hematol Oncol 1994;11:181–7.

25. Tornoe CW, Tworzyanski JJ, Imoisili MA, et al. Optimising piperacillin/tazobactam dosing in paediatrics. Int J Antimicrob Agents 2007;30:320–4.

26. Corapcioglu F, Sarper N, Zengin E. Monotherapy with piperacillin/tazobactam versus cefepime as empirical therapy for febrile neutropenia in pediatric cancer patients: a randomized comparison. Pediatr Hematol Oncol 2006;23:177–86.

27. Marshall WF, Blair JE. The cephalosporins. Mayo Clin Proc 1999;74:187–95.

28. Romano A, Gaeta F, Valluzzi RL, et al. Diagnosing hypersensitivity reactions to cephalosporins in children. Pediatrics 2008;122:521–7.

29. Pichichero ME. Use of selected cephalosporins in penicillin-allergic patients: a paradigm shift. Diagn Microbiol Infect Dis 2007;57:13S–8S.

30. DePestel DD, Benninger MS, Danziger L, et al. Cephalosporin use in treatment of patients with penicillin allergies. (2003). J Am Pharm Assoc 2008;48:530–40.

31. Murthy B, Schmitt-Hoffmann A. Pharmacokinetics and pharmacodynamics of ceftobiprole, an anti-MRSA cephalosporin with broad-spectrum activity. Clin Pharmacokinet 2008;47:21–33.

32. Ge Y, Biek D, Talbot GH, et al. In vitro profiling of ceftaroline against a collection of recent bacterial clinical isolates from across the United States. Antimicrobial Agents Chemother 2008;52:3398–407.

33. Schaad UB, Suter S, Gianella-Borradori A, et al. A comparison of ceftriaxone and cefuroxime for the treatment of bacterial meningitis in children. N Engl J Med 1990;322:141–7.

34. Monte SV, Prescott WA, Johnson KK, et al. Safety of ceftriaxone sodium at extremes of age. Expert Opin Drug Saf 2008;7:515–23.

35. Kessler RE. Cefepime microbiologic profile and update. Pediatr Infect Dis J 2001; 20:331–6.

36. Ayalew K, Nambiar S, Yasinskaya Y, et al. Carbapenems in pediatrics. Ther Drug Monit 2003;25:593–9.

37. Wong VK, Wright HT Jr, Ross LA, et al. Imipenem/cilastatin treatment of bacterial meningitis in children. Pediatr Infect Dis J 1991;10:122–5.
38. Shah PM. Parenteral carbapenems. Clin Microbiol Infect 2008;14(Suppl 1):175–80.
39. Hellinger WC, Brewer NS. Carbapenems and monobactams: imipenem, meropenem, and aztreonam. Mayo Clin Proc 1999;74:420–34.
40. Pai VB, Nahata MC. Efficacy and safety of aerosolized tobramycin in cystic fibrosis. Pediatr Pulmonol 2001;32:314–27.
41. Cheer SM, Waugh J, Noble S. Inhaled tobramycin (TOBI): a review of its use in the management of *Pseudomonas aeruginosa* infections in patients with cystic fibrosis. Drugs 2003;63:2501–20.
42. Contopoulos-Ioannidis DG, Giotis ND, Baliatsa DV, et al. Extended-interval aminoglycoside administration for children: a meta-analysis. Pediatrics 2004;114:e111–8.
43. McCracken GH Jr. Aminoglycoside toxicity in infants and children. Am J Med 1986;80:172–8.
44. Equi A, Balfour-Lynn IM, Bush A, et al. Long term azithromycin in children with cystic fibrosis: a randomised, placebo-controlled crossover trial. Lancet 2002; 360:978–84.
45. Shinkai M, Rubin BK. Macrolides and airway inflammation in children. Paediatr Respir Rev 2005;6:227–35.
46. Jacobs MR, Johnson CE. Macrolide resistance: an increasing concern for treatment failure in children. Pediatr Infect Dis J 2003;22:S131–8.
47. Richter SS, Heilmann KP, Beekmann SE, et al. Macrolide-resistant *Streptococcus pyogenes* in the United States, 2002–2003. Clin Infect Dis 2005;41:599–608.
48. Doern GV. Macrolide and ketolide resistance with *Streptococcus pneumoniae*. Med Clin North Am 2006;90:1109–24.
49. Zuckerman JM. Macrolides and ketolides: azithromycin, clarithromycin, telithromycin. Infect Dis Clin North Am 2004;18:621–49, xi.
50. Nguyen M, Chung EP. Telithromycin: the first ketolide antimicrobial. Clin Ther 2005;27:1144–63.
51. Abu-Gharbieh E, Vasina V, Poluzzi E, et al. Antibacterial macrolides: a drug class with a complex pharmacological profile. Pharm Res 2004;50:211–22.
52. Cooper WO, Griffin MR, Arbogast P, et al. Very early exposure to erythromycin and infantile hypertrophic pyloric stenosis. Arch Pediatr Adolesc Med 2002; 156:647–50.
53. Spizek J, Novotna J, Rezanka T. Lincosamides: chemical structure, biosynthesis, mechanism of action, resistance, and applications. Adv Appl Microbiol 2004;56: 121–54.
54. Frank AL, Marcinak JF, Mangat PD, et al. Clindamycin treatment of methicillin-resistant *Staphylococcus aureus* infections in children. Pediatr Infect Dis J 2002;21:530–4.
55. Kasten MJ. Clindamycin, metronidazole, and chloramphenicol. Mayo Clin Proc 1999;74:825–33.
56. Tunkel AR, Sepkowitz KA. Infections caused by viridans streptococci in patients with neutropenia. Clin Infect Dis 2002;34:1524–9.
57. Bartlett JG. The case for vancomycin as the preferred drug for treatment of *Clostridium difficile* infection. Clin Infect Dis 2008;46:1489–92.
58. Brook I. Pseudomembranous colitis in children. J Gastroenterol Hepatol 2005;20:182–6.
59. Moore MR, Perdreau-Remington F, Chambers HF. Vancomycin treatment failure associated with heterogeneous vancomycin-intermediate *Staphylococcus aureus* in a patient with endocarditis and in the rabbit model of endocarditis. Antimicrobial Agents Chemother 2003;47:1262–6.

60. Sakoulas G, Moise-Broder PA, Schentag J, et al. Relationship of MIC and bactericidal activity to efficacy of vancomycin for treatment of methicillin-resistant *Staphylococcus aureus* bacteremia. J Clin Microbiol 2004;42:2398–402.

61. Billeter M, Zervos MJ, Chen AY, et al. Dalbavancin: a novel once-weekly lipoglycopeptide antibiotic. Clin Infect Dis 2008;46:577–83.

62. Stryjewski ME, Graham DR, Wilson SE, et al. Telavancin versus vancomycin for the treatment of complicated skin and skin-structure infections caused by gram-positive organisms. Clin Infect Dis 2008;46:1683–93.

63. Stalker DJ, Jungbluth GL. Clinical pharmacokinetics of linezolid, a novel oxazolidinone antibacterial. Clin Pharmacokinet 2003;42:1129–40.

64. Tan TQ. Update on the use of linezolid: a pediatric perspective. Pediatr Infect Dis J 2004;23:955–6.

65. Deville JG, Adler S, Azimi PH, et al. Linezolid versus vancomycin in the treatment of known or suspected resistant gram-positive infections in neonates. Pediatr Infect Dis J 2003;22:S158–63.

66. Weisman LE. Coagulase-negative staphylococcal disease: emerging therapies for the neonatal and pediatric patient. Curr Opin Infect Dis 2004;17:237–41.

67. Loeffler AM, Drew RH, Perfect JR, et al. Safety and efficacy of quinupristin/dalfopristin for treatment of invasive gram-positive infections in pediatric patients. Pediatr Infect Dis J 2002;21:950–6.

68. Gupte G, Jyothi S, Beath SV, et al. Quinupristin-dalfopristin use in children is associated with arthralgias and myalgias [letter]. Pediatr Infect Dis J 2006;25:281.

69. Woodworth JR, Nyhart EH Jr, Brier GL, et al. Single-dose pharmacokinetics and antibacterial activity of daptomycin, a new lipopeptide antibiotic, in healthy volunteers. Antimicrobial Agents Chemother 1992;36:318–25.

70. Credito K, Lin G, Appelbaum PC. Activity of daptomycin alone and in combination with rifampin and gentamicin against *Staphylococcus aureus* assessed by time-kill methodology. Antimicrobial Agents Chemother 2007;51:1504–7.

71. Seaton RA. Daptomycin: rationale and role in the management of skin and soft tissue infections. J Antimicrob Chemother 2008;62(Suppl 3):15–23, iii.

72. Masters PA, O'Bryan TA, Zurlo J, et al. Trimethoprim-sulfamethoxazole revisited. Arch Intern Med 2003;163:402–10.

73. Grim SA, Rapp RP, Martin CA, et al. Trimethoprim-sulfamethoxazole as a viable treatment option for infections caused by methicillin-resistant *Staphylococcus aureus*. Pharmacotherapy 2005;25:253–64.

74. Paintsil E. Pediatric community-acquired methicillin-resistant *Staphylococcus aureus* infection and colonization: trends and management. Curr Opin Pediatr 2007;19:75–82.

75. Gemmell CG, Edwards DI, Fraise AP, et al. Guidelines for the prophylaxis and treatment of methicillin-resistant *Staphylococcus aureus* (MRSA) infections in the UK. J Antimicrob Chemother 2006;57:589–608.

76. Proctor RA. Role of folate antagonists in the treatment of methicillin-resistant *Staphylococcus aureus* infection. Clin Infect Dis 2008;46:584–93.

77. Forsythe CT, Ernst ME. Do fluoroquinolones commonly cause arthropathy in children? CJEM 2007;9:459–62.

78. Committee on Infectious Diseases. The use of systemic fluoroquinolones. Pediatrics 2006;118:1287–92.

79. Leibovitz E. The use of fluoroquinolones in children. Curr Opin Pediatr 2006;18:64–70.

Antibacterial Agents in the Elderly

Stephen Weber, MD, MS[a],*, Emily Mawdsley, MD[a], Donald Kaye, MD[b]

KEYWORDS

- Infection • Aged • Aged, 80 and over • Agents • Antimicrobial

Older patients (defined here as persons aged 65 and older) unduly suffer the burden of infectious diseases in the United States. In this vulnerable population, the incidence of community-acquired and health care–associated infections exceeds that observed in younger adult populations.[1,2] Among older patients, the consequences of infection are also more severe. For example, there is an increased risk of mortality among older individuals with community-acquired pneumonia and other common but serious infections that occur outside of the hospital.[3] The increased risk of death is even more pronounced for infections that occur as a complication of medical care. The risk of mortality for hospitalized older patients with central line–related bloodstream infections is significantly greater than for younger adults with the same infections.[4] For older patients who survive their infection, the clinical sequelae are also more severe. Infections in older patients are associated with prolonged length of hospital stay, increased risk of complications, and significant and sustained declines from baseline functional status (an important but underutilized metric for evaluating the effects of infection on this population).[5]

The significance of the substantial impact of infection on older patients is magnified by the ever-increasing size of this segment of the US population. It is estimated that by the year 2030, 20% of the US population will be over the age of 65. More significantly, the proportion of individuals living beyond the age of 85 (the oldest old) is also expected to grow.[6] This group is at particularly high risk for infections and associated morbidity and mortality. The net effect is that all adult clinicians—not just specialists in geriatric medicine and infectious diseases—need to achieve proficiency, if not mastery, of the use of antimicrobial agents in older patients.

Because of these evolving demographic trends and the distinct clinical implications of the frequency and impact of infection among older patients, it is incumbent upon physicians and other prescribers to ensure that the use of antimicrobial agents for known or suspected infection in this population is rational and appropriate. An

[a] Section of Infectious Diseases and Global Health, University of Chicago Medical Center, 5841 South Maryland Avenue, MC 5065, Chicago, IL 60637, USA
[b] Department of Medicine, Drexel University College of Medicine, 1535 Sweet Briar Road, Gladwyne, Philadelphia, PA 19035, USA
* Corresponding author.
E-mail address: sgweber@medicine.bsd.uchicago.edu (S. Weber).

Infect Dis Clin N Am 23 (2009) 881–898
doi:10.1016/j.idc.2009.06.012
0891-5520/09/$ – see front matter © 2009 Elsevier Inc. All rights reserved.

understanding of the immunologic, pharmacologic, epidemiologic, and microbiologic underpinnings that drive a sophisticated approach to antibiotic therapy for older patients is essential and should lead to an effective and consistent strategy for the management of infection in this group by all clinicians, no matter their area of specialization or level of experience.

This article continues with a detailed overview of the unique factors that should influence the approach to antimicrobial therapy for older patients. The impact of these factors is specifically discussed in the context in which they inform decisions about the selection of specific antimicrobial agents, route of administration, dose, and duration of anti-infective therapy. After this introduction, these tenets are applied to the formulation of appropriate antimicrobial strategies for older patients who suffer from an array of common but potentially life-threatening infections.

FACTORS THAT INFLUENCE THE CHOICE OF ANTIMICROBIAL THERAPY FOR OLDER PATIENTS
Immunity

Changes in quantitative and qualitative immune function greatly hinder the ability of older patients to evade infection and ensure a rapid and complete recovery once infected. Taken together, these changes are generally referred to as the phenomenon of immunosenescence.[7–9] In terms of humoral immunity, there is a decline in the absolute immunoglobulin levels and the number of naïve immunoglobulin-producing cells among elderly subjects.[10–12] B cells from older patients demonstrate significant impairment in activation and subsequent proliferation.[13] The net effect on older patients is a unique susceptibility to infections, particularly those caused by encapsulated bacterial pathogens (eg, Streptococcus pneumoniae) and impaired response to vaccine administration.[14]

The situation is similar in the case of cell-mediated immunity. As they age, older patients typically experience a decline in the absolute number of CD8$^+$ naïve T cells available to respond to new infectious challenges.[15] The relative activity of these cells also tends to be less effective than for the same cells in younger adult patients, particularly in terms of dysregulation with other components of cellular immunity.[16] Although the decline in cellular immunity affects the older host's response to nearly all pathogens, this immunologic impairment may render these individuals especially susceptible to infection with fungal and viral pathogens.

Perhaps the most significant, although frequently overlooked, aspect of vulnerability in older patients relates to the compromise of physical barriers to infection. Specifically, impairment at anatomic sites at which the human host routinely interacts with microbes leaves older patients less able to avoid the impact of the potential pathogens to which all individuals are exposed. The integument of older patients becomes frailer with aging, which permits easier entry of colonizing flora that can cause superficial skin and soft tissue infections and more serious and disseminated deep infections.[17] In the lung, anatomic barriers to the establishment of lower respiratory infection are especially compromised in this group. Ciliary function is impaired, and the cough reflex and swallowing mechanism are typically weakened compared to younger adults.[18–20]

In short, for older individuals the capacity to fight infection is more rapidly and more easily overwhelmed. The product is the increased morbidity and mortality observed among infected older patients. For clinicians who treat such individuals, it is important to support the patient's weakened immune system by aggressively treating infection as early as possible, before host defenses are overwhelmed and infection can progress. In this context, the most appropriate approach might include the use of agents with a broader spectrum of antimicrobial coverage (while confirmatory microbiological diagnosis and susceptibility testing are pending). Theoretically, the approach might even favor the use of bactericidal agents because of the possibility that these agents would be superior to bacteriostatic agents in the elderly population with impaired host immunity.

Pharmacologic Considerations

There are a multitude of changes in the manner in which antimicrobial drugs and other pharmaceutical agents are absorbed, distributed, and metabolized by older patients as compared to younger adults (**Table 1**). All of these factors could potentially influence clinicians in the selection, dose, and route of administration of antimicrobial therapy for this group. Despite the complexity of all of these changes, however, the singular impairment that most significantly influences the medical management of infection in older patients is the decline in renal function commonly observed in this group.[21] To compound matters, not only does impairment of renal function accompany normal aging but also the decline is exacerbated in the context of other comorbid medical conditions and the intensive (and frequently nephrotoxic) therapy required when treating these conditions in older patients.[22]

The complex influence of pharmacodynamic and pharmacokinetic considerations (and particularly the influence of impaired renal function) has the net effect of demanding extreme caution in prescribing antibiotics for older patients.[23–25] Specifically, the use of nomograms and dosing strategies that are not at least age-adjusted is ill advised and may result in an increased risk of toxicity and hypersensitivity. This is especially true for antimicrobial agents with a narrow therapeutic index, such as the aminoglycosides. The need for careful and standardized therapeutic drug monitoring is also crucial in this population and must be accounted for in considering any antibiotic regimen for an older patient, whether institutionalized or at home.[26,27] The need for such close monitoring (including frequent assessment of end organ function for evidence of toxicity) necessarily increases the costs associated with antibiotic therapy in this population.

Table 1
Changes in pharmacokinetic factors associated with aging and potential effects on antimicrobial dosing

Elimination	Decreased renal function	Impaired clearance of specific drugs
Absorption	Decreased gastric acidity	Decreased absorption
	Decreased gastric motility	Decreased absorption
	Decreased small bowel surface area	Decreased absorption
	Decreased splanchnic blood flow	Decreased absorption
Metabolism	Decreased hepatic blood flow	Impaired metabolism of specific agents
	Decreased enzyme activity	Increased half-life of drugs metabolized by P-450 cascade
Distribution	Decreased lean body mass	Increased half-life of lipid-soluble drugs
	Variation of total body water	Increased or decreased concentration of water-soluble drugs
	Malnutrition	Increased concentration of free drugs

Arguably, the most important pharmacologic consideration in the prescription of antimicrobial therapy for older patients is the concern for drug hypersensitivity and drug-drug interactions. In the latter case, older patients are frequently already required to take multiple pharmaceutical agents to manage other comorbid conditions prior to needing antimicrobial therapy.[25] In these cases, clinicians must be careful to ensure that the resulting polypharmacy does not unduly affect drug levels to either reduce efficacy or potentiate toxicity to one or more agents. Another underappreciated consequence of polypharmacy in older patients is the challenge of adherence to complicated pharmacologic regimens reported in this population.[28–30] Fortunately, several tools and strategies have been described to assist older patients in this regard.[31]

Epidemiologic Factors

An array of factors, categorized together in this article as epidemiologic in nature, influence the likelihood of infection, the breadth of infecting pathogens, and the severity and consequences of infection among older patients. Some of these factors are inherent to the physiology of older patients themselves, whereas others are related to the manner and intensity with which these patients are managed in the health care setting. All factors influence the selection, route, dose, and duration of antibiotic therapy prescribed for older patients, however. The influence of these factors is partly mediated through alteration of either the native or infecting bacterial flora of older patients, whether in or out of the hospital.

Comorbid conditions can make antimicrobial management especially challenging in older patients. Not only can some prevalent medical conditions increase the risk of infection among older patients (such as diabetes mellitus and chronic leukemia) but comorbid disease also can complicate the administration of antimicrobial agents by affecting pharmacodynamic and pharmacokinetic parameters and increase the risk of toxicity or drug-drug interactions.[32] Specific examples include baseline renal insufficiency increasing the risk of nephrotoxicity and congestive heart failure altering the volume of distribution for some antimicrobial agents.

Because of the increased likelihood of residence in a nursing home or other long-term nonacute care facility, older patients may be exposed to an increased risk of colonization and infection with multidrug-resistant organisms (MDRO), such as methicillin-resistant Staphylococcus aureus (MRSA), and may in general be more susceptible to infection. Although some of this effect may be mediated through the poor functional status of these patients, increasing attention is being applied to inconsistent application of basic infection prevention strategies in nonacute health care settings, an area in which more research to define best practices is needed.[33] Frequent contact with acute care hospitals and the associated intensity of medical care administered in such settings also may leave older patients at risk for complicated infections, such as those associated with medical devices (eg, indwelling catheters).

Microbiology

Although the "normal flora" of older patients is likely different from that of younger adults, one of the most critical considerations influencing antimicrobial management is the frequency and impact of antimicrobial resistant pathogens among older patients. For certain MDRO, particularly MRSA, the incidence and consequences of infection seem to be higher in older versus younger patients.[4] Although evidence for a similar association between older age and other MDRO is currently lacking, comorbid medical illnesses and frequent exposure to antimicrobial therapy, both of which are more common among older patients, predict a greater risk for MDRO colonization and infection. Even a relatively small increase in the proportion of resistant strains in older patients would be significant because of the overall increased risk of infection in this population and their poor physiologic reserve. Because at least some of the increased mortality and morbidity associated with MDRO infection may be attributed to the failure to initiate appropriately broad antibiotic coverage in a timely fashion,[34,35] it is imperative that clinicians who manage infection in older patients carefully consider the possibility that an MDRO is involved and broaden empirical coverage when appropriate.

Although the relationship between older age and antimicrobial resistance remains to be completely elucidated, several specific pathogens have been strongly linked to particular infectious syndromes in this population through careful investigation and extensive experience. For example, bacterial meningitis among older patients is much more commonly attributed to *Listeria moncytogenes* than in younger adult patients.[36] Additional unique epidemiologic associations are addressed at greater length in the later discussion of specific infectious syndromes.

Clinicians whose practice specifically focuses on the management of older patients must be familiar with the most up-to-date information regarding the most likely etiologic cause of the infectious syndromes that they encounter most frequently in practice. In addition to keeping abreast of the medical literature, clinicians also should carefully follow local trends and patterns of antimicrobial resistance. One of the most valuable tools may be the institutional antibiotic susceptibility report (antibiogram), which is generally compiled and disseminated regularly at most US hospitals. A more sophisticated approach might be to develop a similar resource specifically addressing the microbiologic flora of older patients.

SPECIFIC INFECTIOUS SYNDROMES AND CLINICAL SCENARIOS
Pneumonia and Other Respiratory Infections

Lower respiratory infections, including pneumonia, are among the most common infectious syndromes observed in older patients.[2,37] The accompanying morbidity and mortality are high in this population.[38] Older patients may be more likely to experience anatomic complications of lung infection, including empyema and lung abscess. The pathogens observed to cause pneumonia in older patients are fairly comparable to those commonly associated with lung infection in younger adult patients. Most prominent among these are *S pneumoniae* and the influenza virus (during the appropriate season). More difficult to quantify among older patients are infections caused by the so-called atypical bacteria, including *Mycoplasma pneumoniae* and *Chlamydia pneumoniae*,[39] which are common among younger patients.

The expected etiologic agent that causes pneumonia is greatly influenced by the epidemiologic setting in which older patients contract the infection. Among residents of long-term care facilities (LTCFs), infection caused by pathogens such as *S aureus* and *Pseudomonas aeruginosa* are increased in frequency.[40] Older patients are at greater risk for aspiration pneumonia (as a result of altered mental status or instrumentation of the upper airways), and oral anaerobic pathogens may be more common after aspiration at home.[40]

No matter the specific clinical setting, the most appropriate antimicrobial coverage for older patients with known or suspected pneumonia must include reliable coverage for the most common pathogens. For example, for cases with onset in the community, it is crucial to ensure maximal efficacy against *S pneumoniae*. Additional coverage for atypical pathogens (such as *Mycoplasma* and *Chlamydia spp*) is also appropriate.[41] An overview of appropriate antimicrobial therapy for older patients with pneumonia is summarized in **Table 2**. In each setting, the most common pathogens are highlighted.

For all cases of pneumonia in older patients, clinicians should be prepared to refine and intensify the coverage based on epidemiologic clues. There should be a lower threshold for initiation of drugs with activity against *P aeruginosa*, especially for individuals domiciled in LTCF and for patients with chronic structural lung disease (such as bronchiectasis).[41] Severely ill older patients (and especially those admitted to the intensive care unit) should be treated empirically for legionellosis pending the results of diagnostic testing.[41,42] Recently, several tools have been formulated and disseminated to assist clinicians in stratifying patients with pneumonia according to the expected risk for complications and mortality. Clinical scoring tools have been specifically designed for application to older patients.[43,44]

Dosing antimicrobial agents for older patients with lower respiratory tract infection is comparable to that for younger adult patients. Recent evidence suggests that early switch to oral therapy should be the rule and that inpatient observation for hospitalized patients is not necessary after the conversion to oral antibiotics.[42] As is the case for younger patients, the optimal duration of therapy for pneumonia in older patients has not yet been adequately established. The usual duration applied is 7 to 10 days for most cases and 3 weeks in cases of confirmed legionellosis.[41,42] A growing amount of evidence suggests that hospital-acquired pneumonia may be adequately treated with as little as 7 to 8 days of antibiotic therapy.[41]

Patients should be monitored while on therapy for toxicity and evidence of local complication of infection, including empyema and lung abscess. Any older patient under treatment for pneumonia who experiences persistent fever (>72 hours after the initiation of antibiotic therapy) or other worsening symptoms should be evaluated for evidence of complication, usually through radiographic examination and drainage if a new focus is identified.

Skin and Soft Tissue Infections

Cormorbid conditions and the relatively frail skin of older patients leave them especially vulnerable to infection.[45,46] As a result, older patients frequently experience an array of infectious syndromes of the skin and soft tissue, including cellulitis and furunculosis, necrotizing fasciitis (NF), diabetic foot infection (discussed in the section on bone and joint infections) and decubitus ulcers. Streptococci and staphylococci dominate as the most common pathogens associated with skin and soft tissue infection among older patients, as is also the case for younger adults. Among older patients with comorbid disease, however, including longstanding diabetes and liver disease, an increased incidence of skin infection with gram-negative pathogens has been reported.[47,48]

The emergence of strains of *S aureus* that are resistant to methicillin (MRSA) in the community among individuals without extensive prior contact with the health care system is arguably the single most important epidemiologic phenomenon that has been described to impact the management of bacterial infections over the past quarter century.[49–51] These so-called community-associated MRSA (CA-MRSA) strains have an apparent predilection to cause complicated skin and soft tissue infection.[52] In some patients, these infections may be especially aggressive and even recurrent.[53,54] Unlike MRSA strains that have been well described as a complication of hospital therapy, CA-MRSA strains tend to have preserved susceptibility to non–β -lactam antibiotics, particularly clindamycin, trimethoprim/sulfamethoxazole, and doxycycline. Increasingly, the use of one of these three agents is becoming the standard approach to management of affected patients, especially in the outpatient setting. A large multicenter study is currently underway to determine the optimal

Table 2
Approach to antimicrobial therapy for the older patient with pneumonia

Clinical Setting	Common Pathogens	Recommended Empirical Regimen	Notes
Community-acquired, not hospitalized	S pneumoniae, atypical bacteria (M pneumonia, C pneumoniae), viral pathogens	Respiratory fluoroquinolone (levofloxacin or moxifloxacin), OR azithromycin plus high-dose amoxicillin (1g, 3 times daily)	If influenza is suspected and symptoms have been present for <48 hours, consider early therapy with oseltamivir
Community-acquired, hospitalized	S pneumoniae, atypical bacteria (M pneumoniae, C pneumoniae)	Third-generation cephalosporin (eg, ceftriaxone) plus azithromycin, OR respiratory fluoroquinolone (moxifloxacin or levofloxacin)	If influenza is suspected and symptoms have been present for <48 hours, consider early therapy with oseltamivir
Community-acquired, hospitalized in ICU	S pneumoniae, Legionella spp	Third-generation cephalosporin (eg, ceftriaxone) plus respiratory fluoroquinolone (levofloxacin or moxifloxacin)	If P aeruginosa is suspected: antipseudomonal β-lactam (cefepime, imipenem, piperacillin/tazobactam) plus antipseudomonal fluoroquinolone (ciprofloxacin)
Community-acquired, LTCF resident	S pneumoniae, influenza, Enterobacteriaceae, P aeruginosa, S aureus (including MRSA)	Third-generation cephalosporin plus respiratory fluoroquinolone plus vancomycin (if S aureus or MRSA suspected)	If P aeruginosa is suspected: antipseudomonal β-lactam (cefepime, imipenem, piperacillin/tazobactam) plus antipseudomonal fluoroquinolone plus vancomycin
Hospital-acquired	P aeruginosa, Enterobacteriaceae, S aureus (including MRSA)	Cefepime, imipenem, or piperacillin/tazobactam plus respiratory fluoroquinolone plus vancomycin or linezolid (if S aureus or MRSA suspected)	—

approach to patients infected with these pathogens. An additional controversial but as yet unresolved consideration in managing these patients is the benefit of therapy with topical agents, such as mupirocin and chlorhexidine gluconate, in order to eradicate nasal and skin colonization, respectively, because colonization may be associated with an increased risk of relapse or dissemination to others.[55]

In the case of the most superficial infections, including cellulitis, a definitive etiologic diagnosis is generally not possible. There is no clinical presentation sufficiently characteristic to presume a single pathogen as the sole cause, and confirmatory microbiologic diagnosis is generally not possible in this setting.[56,57] Optimal empirical antimicrobial therapy generally requires coverage for streptococci and staphylococci. Typical regimens have generally included antistaphylococcal penicillins (eg, dicloxacillin) and first-generation cephalosporins (eg, cephelexin and cefazolin) and, for patients with a severe β-lactam allergy, clindamycin. This approach needs to be re-evaluated, however, because of the emergence of MRSA as a significant pathogen in the community and in LTCFs. If one of these regimens is used, the patient must be followed closely to ensure clinical improvement. The better course, especially where MRSA is a high possibility, is to use an agent active against MRSA and group A streptococci, such as clindamycin for community-acquired disease and linezolid for LTCF-acquired disease. The usual duration of therapy for cellulitis in an older patient is generally 10 days; however, limited evidence supports this standard, and less severe cases may be managed with a shorter course.[58]

For patients with superficial skin abscesses (including furunculosis), antibiotic therapy should be undertaken only in conjunction with adjunctive surgical intervention. For many older patients, even persons with multiple boils or skin abscesses, incision and drainage alone may be sufficient to resolve the infection. In the setting of accompanying cellulitis or evidence of systemic signs of infection (eg, fever, hypotension, or tachycardia), however, a period of systemic antibiotic therapy is prudent. Older outpatients with cellulitis and superficial skin abscesses generally can be managed with oral antibiotics (provided adherence and gastrointestinal absorption can be assured). Patients whose infection is sufficiently serious to warrant hospital admission probably should receive at least several days of parenteral therapy until treating clinicians are assured that the infection is resolving.

Fortunately, NF is an unusual infection in young and old patients; however, the per-case mortality rate remains exceedingly high in all groups.[59] The urgency with which this syndrome must be recognized to ensure timely and potentially curative medical and surgical therapy warrants discussion. It is crucial to remember that one of the most common skin injuries to predispose patients to NF in the United States is actually surgery or other clinical procedure (including incisions for laparoscopic procedures and intravascular devices). The most important bedside clinical findings to distinguish NF from other serious skin and soft tissue infection are severe pain and toxemia and rapid progression of the infection over a short period of time.[60] As soon as the diagnosis is suspected, immediate surgical consultation is essential for exploration for diagnostic purposes and definitive therapy. Operative intervention has been definitively associated with improved outcomes for these patients.[61] It is strongly advised that treating clinicians carefully demarcate the periphery of the area of involvement using a marker or pen. If the area of inflammation extends beyond this margin within 1 to 2 hours, it is suggestive of the diagnosis.

There are two main types of NF: the type caused by group A streptococci and the type caused by various combinations of mixed aerobic and anaerobic flora (including streptococci, staphylococci, Enterobacteriaceae, and gram-positive and -negative anaerobes). The second type is most likely in patients with skin and soft tissue infection of the perineum or after open abdominal surgery. The most appropriate initial antibiotic therapy for patients with known or suspected NF should cover all of the previously mentioned organisms. Increasingly, consideration must be given to the possible involvement of MRSA and other MDRO.[62,63] For rapidly progressive infections (especially caused by group A streptococci), one key addition is the inclusion of antimicrobial agents with activity against protein synthesis, most often clindamycin. The theoretical basis for this recommendation is that attenuation of toxin synthesis may promote clinical improvement even before the antimicrobial agents take their full effect in killing microbes.[64]

Pressure ulcers represent a debilitating and frequently preventable complication of acute medical management and long-term care. The best strategy for addressing this complication is prevention, a topic that is beyond the scope of this article. Once an ulcer has developed, it is important for clinicians to appreciate that not every ulcer—no matter how severe in terms of size or depth of tissue involvement—specifically warrants intervention with systemic antimicrobial agents. Avoiding unnecessary antibiotic therapy protects the patient from the complications of toxicity, drug-drug interactions, and emerging antimicrobial resistance. When there is evidence of infection of an existing ulcer (eg, fever, leukocytosis, worsening purulent drainage), antimicrobial therapy is appropriate.[65]

The typical initial antimicrobial regimen for a patient with a pressure ulcer that is known or suspected to be infected is generally broad. Until definitive culture results are available, the inclusion of agents active against MRSA, highly-resistant gram-negative bacteria, and even anaerobes may be appropriate depending on local epidemiology. Typical regimens might include a carbapenem (imipenem or meropenem) or a β-lactam/β-lactamase inhibitor combination (piperacillin/tazobactam) with vancomycin added to either agent. Confirmatory microbiologic diagnosis is elusive for these patients in that only deep tissue or bone specimens are reliably predictive. Organisms isolated only from superficial swab or drainage specimens lack specificity and could prompt clinicians to prescribe an overly aggressive (and potentially toxic) regimen. The duration of therapy for infected pressure ulcers depends on the state and clinical improvement of the wound over time and generally requires 4 or more weeks of treatment. Particular attention should be given to the likelihood of underlying bone involvement because osteomyelitis would warrant an exceptionally long period of therapy (6–12 weeks).

Urinary Tract Infections

Infections of the urologic system are the most common type of infection observed among older men and women.[66] The high incidence of urinary tract infection affects older patients in the community, LTCF, and hospital. Although bacteriuria (and urinary infections) are many more times likely in younger women than younger men, this gender gap closes among older patients, and older men seem to be equally vulnerable to these infections.[67] The microbiology of urinary tract infections is not substantively different in older versus younger patients.[68] *Escherichia coli* is the most common pathogen identified from urine cultures of both groups.[68] As is the case for infection at other sites, however, the spectrum of pathogens responsible for infection of the bladder and urologic system among older patients tends to be broader.[69] There is, for example, an increased incidence of infections caused by other gram-negative pathogens, including *Proteus mirabilis* (especially among older men), *Klebsiella spp,* and *Enterobacter spp.* Among the gram-positive pathogens that cause urinary infection among older patients, enterococci and coagulase-negative staphylococci are particularly common.

Although the spectrum of possible etiologic pathogens determines the selection of the most appropriate breadth of antimicrobial coverage, it is the degree of involvement of the urinary system that dictates the intensity and duration of antimicrobial therapy for this group. Most serious are infections that involve the upper urologic system (including the renal calyces and parenchyma). These infections are frequently complicated by accompanying bacteremia, and may result in other anatomic complications of infection, including renal and perinephric abscesses.[66] Nephrolithiasis and obstruction also may complicate upper urologic tract infections. In all cases of suspected severe upper urinary tract infection in older patients, early broad-spectrum empirical therapy should be initiated with intent to narrow coverage on the basis of culture results.

Less severe, but more common, are infections of the lower urinary tract, including those involving the bladder and the urethra. These infections are only rarely complicated by anatomic extension and are frequently amenable to therapy with short courses of antibiotic therapy. Specific recommendations regarding antimicrobial regimens to treat upper versus lower urinary tract infection among older patients are summarized in **Table 3**.

The management of asymptomatic bacteriuria remains a point of some confusion for many clinicians. Extensive study in a variety of older populations convincingly demonstrates that there is no benefit to the treatment of asymptomatic bacteriuria among women or men.[70] To treat this otherwise harmless condition is to needlessly

Table 3
Variation in the approach to upper versus lower urinary tract infection in older adults

	Upper Urinary Tract Infection	Lower Urinary Tract Infection
Determinants of initial therapy	Urine Gram stain results and overall clinical status	Previously prescribed regimens and prevalence of community/facility resistance to commonly prescribed agents
Typical empirical regimens	Piperacillin/tazobactam ± aminoglycoside if gram-negative suspected and severely ill/septic Ampicillin or vancomycin if enterococci are suspected	Ciprofloxacin or trimethoprim/sulfamethoxazole For LTCF residents or hospitalized patients, local susceptibility data should guide empirical therapy
Follow-up	Narrow coverage to single effective agent once susceptibility results are available If no clinical improvement in 72 hours, evaluate for anatomic complication (abscess or obstruction)	—
Typical duration of therapy	14 days for men and women or 7 days if a quinolone is used and good clinical response is achieved	3 days for women; 7–10 days for men

expose the older patient to the potential for drug toxicity, hypersensitivity reactions, drug-drug interactions, and the promotion of antimicrobial resistance. The sole exception is in the setting of a planned urologic procedure (including cystoscopy).[71] In this context, periprocedural antimicrobial therapy has been demonstrated to reduce the incidence of bacteremia. The briefest regimen with the narrowest spectrum of activity is appropriate in this setting. Similarly, treatment of asymptomatic candiduria, even when an indwelling urinary catheter is in place or has been removed recently, is unwarranted.[72]

Gastrointestinal Infections

In addition to the most common gastrointestinal pathogens (including norovirus and domestic food-borne pathogens), older individuals are increasingly likely to endure the symptoms of upper and lower gastrointestinal tract infection because of a broader array of microbes. The active lifestyle of many older individuals increasingly brings them into contact with more unusual bacteria and parasites as a consequence of travel outside of North America. Immunosenescence and intensive medical therapy renders older patients susceptible to infection with opportunistic pathogens, including cryptosporidium.[73] Most gastrointestinal infections in older patients tend to be self-limited in nature and require only symptomatic treatment (hydration and judicious use of antimotility agents). Older patients need to be closely monitored, however, even in the outpatient setting, because the potential sequelae of intestinal infection (electrolyte derangements, dehydration, and subsequent falls) may be especially severe.

Perhaps the most important etiologic cause of diarrhea in older patients is *Clostridium difficile* infection (CDI), which is the primary focus of this section.[74] In recent years, there has been proliferation of a virulent, toxin hyperproducing epidemic strain in the United States, Canada, the United Kingdom, and Europe. Overall, the incidence of CDI and its severity and attributable mortality have increased dramatically.[75,76] Although metronidazole (250 mg every 6 hours or 500 mg every 8 hours) is appropriate for mild or moderate CDI, therapy with oral vancomycin (125 mg every 6 hours) should be used for patients with severe CDI, including persons who are hospitalized for their symptoms.[77] Therapy of mild or moderate CDI should be changed to oral vancomycin if there is unsatisfactory response to metronidazole. In all cases, precipitating systemic antibiotic therapy should be discontinued if feasible. The most appropriate duration of therapy for CDI is probably between 10 and 14 days.

The antimicrobial management for older patients with recrudescent CDI is more complex, and there is considerably less evidence or fewer authoritative recommendations to guide clinicians at the bedside. Most experts recommend that a patient who fails first-line therapy for CDI be treated with a second course of antimicrobial therapy, generally with the same agent.[78] In extreme cases, success has been reported with the use of unconventional dosing regimens, including prolonged tapering and pulse dosing of oral vancomycin.[78] Well-controlled evidence to support the use of these strategies remains lacking, however. Similarly, there is as yet insufficient information to recommend or guide the use of probiotic products in the management of CDI among older patients.[78]

Bone and Joint Infections

Two specific clinical syndromes demand considerably different approaches to the management of bone and joint infections among older patients. The underlying concepts discussed at the outset of this article still govern the approach to patients with prosthetic joint infections and diabetic foot ulcers.

The proportion of older patients living with orthopedic prosthetic devices, predominantly artificial hips and knees, continues to grow. Despite advances in surgical technique and implant technology, a small fraction of these procedures and these implants are complicated by infection. The microbiology of prosthetic hip and knee infections most often involves gram-positive pathogens, with staphylococcal species (including S aureus and coagulase-negative staphylococci) being most common.[79] With the increasing prevalence of staphylococcal strains resistant to methicillin on the rise in the health care setting and in the community, MRSA always must be considered a potential pathogen in an infected prosthetic joint.[80,81]

Medical therapy alone is generally suboptimal for the management of prosthetic joint infections. Several retrospective reviews, prospective studies, and decision analyses have pointed to the advantage of combined medical-surgical therapy.[82–84] Most typically, it involves a two-stage surgical procedure. At the first operation, the infected hardware is completely removed and tissue and fluid cultures are obtained to confirm the microbiologic diagnosis and direct subsequent antimicrobial treatment. An inert spacer (often impregnated with antimicrobial agents such as an aminoglycoside or vancomycin) may be left in place.[85]

After the first procedure, a parenteral antibiotic regimen is selected based on the results of the intraoperative culture results. If the culture results are negative (generally as a result of antibiotic administration before the first surgery), broad coverage to include MRSA and gram-negative pathogens is appropriate. In view of the extended duration of intensive therapy required, a premium is placed on the selection of parenteral antimicrobial agents with limited toxicity and the greatest convenience of dosing. Typical regimens include vancomycin plus the choice of piperacillin/tazobactam, a carbapenem (ertapenem, as long as P aeruginosa is not suspected because just once daily dosing is needed), or a fluoroquinolone (depending on local susceptibility patterns). Generally, after 6 to 8 weeks of therapy (depending on the clinical response), the patient can be returned to the operating room for replacement of the hardware.

In contrast to this fairly regimented strategy for the treatment of prosthetic joint infection, the approach to management of the diverse population of patients with diabetic foot infections is more heterogeneous. Generally resulting from neuropathic injury to the distal lower extremities, these infections can be difficult to manage with medical therapy, and patients frequently require aggressive debridement and even amputation.[86] Even if such radical interventions are not anticipated, early consultation with a surgeon is appropriate. Bone or other deep tissue biopsy with culture is the most specific means by which to direct the broad-spectrum antimicrobial coverage generally required to manage these patients. In as much as these intensive (typically parenteral) antibiotic combinations require close monitoring to avoid frequent toxicity, a specific microbiologic diagnosis is crucial. Revascularization procedures, historically through the use of peripheral vascular bypass procedures, also may be essential to promote the resolution of the infection.

A diverse range of pathogens have been associated with the cause of diabetic foot infection. The most common contributors are gram-positive cocci, particularly staphylococci (including MRSA). In older patients with comorbid medical conditions (and presumably more frequent and intense contact with the health care system), highly resistant gram-negative bacteria and even anaerobic pathogens may be involved. In general, the use of agents that specifically target gram-positive organisms may be sufficient for less severe wounds in patients with few or no comorbid conditions. Where broader coverage is deemed necessary for these lower risk patients, the combination of oral ciprofloxacin plus clindamycin offers a reasonable alternative to intravenous therapy. For higher risk patients (individuals with multiple comorbid conditions, high suspicion for MDRO, or deeper wounds), more intensive therapy may be required, including the use of long-term intravenous agents. For most such patients, the duration of therapy is at least 2 to 4 weeks and often longer, depending on the status of the wound and the results of adjunctive surgical procedures. Patients with known or suspected osteomyelitis require a more prolonged course of antibiotics.[87] For many patients with bone and joint infection, monitoring of the C-reactive protein or erythrocyte sedimentation rate may be useful to gauge the response to treatment and help to determine the length of antimicrobial therapy.

Infections at the End of Life

One of the most complicated settings in which to make rational recommendations for the use of antimicrobial therapy comes at the end of life. Increasingly, older patients are being appropriately referred to end-of-life care programs (including hospice) in which the primary goal of care focuses on the comfort and dignity of the patient. Clinicians, especially those with less experience in the management of terminally ill patients, often struggle to determine the appropriate use of antimicrobial therapy in this setting.

A fundamental concern in this circumstance is whether antibiotics contribute significantly to the goals of therapy in the setting of hospice or comfort care. Put another way: is the possibility of improving or avoiding the symptomatic discomfort of infection (fever, chills, malaise, site-specific pain) outweighed by the possibility of unintended extension of life through the resolution of infection? Several recent studies suggested that antimicrobial therapy may alleviate some (but not all) of the symptoms of infection among patients undergoing hospice care. Simultaneously, the administration of antibiotics did not seem to extend life in this group of patients.[88,89]

Another potential downside of antibiotic therapy for any patient, including those in hospice programs, relates to the unintended consequences of antibiotic administration: specifically toxicity (including hypersensitivity and drug-drug interactions) and the promotion of resistance.

SUMMARY

The management of infection among older patients is complicated and should be undertaken with great caution. The most rational approach to antibiotic therapy for older patients relies on an understanding and appreciation of the complicated immunologic, epidemiologic, pharmacologic, and microbiologic factors that influence the susceptibility, presentation, and consequences of infection in this group. This knowledge, paired with an understanding of local susceptibility patterns and access to expert consultation in geriatric medicine, infectious diseases, and clinical pharmacy, ensures the best outcomes when treating these vulnerable patients.

REFERENCES

1. Gavazzi G, Krause KH. Ageing and infection. Lancet Infect Dis 2002;2(11): 659–66.
2. Yoshikawa TT. Epidemiology and unique aspects of aging and infectious diseases. Clin Infect Dis 2000;30(6):931–3.
3. Ochoa-Gondar O, Vila-Corcoles A, de Diego C, et al. The burden of community-acquired pneumonia in the elderly: the Spanish EVAN-65 study. BMC Public Health 2008;8:222.

4. Malani PN, Rana MM, Banerjee M, et al. *Staphylococcus aureus* bloodstream infections: the association between age and mortality and functional status. J Am Geriatr Soc 2008;56(8):1485–9.
5. High K, Bradley S, Loeb M, et al. A new paradigm for clinical investigation of infectious syndromes in older adults: assessing functional status as a risk factor and outcome measure. J Am Geriatr Soc 2005;53(3):528–35.
6. Bureau USC. U.S. Interim Projections by age, sex, race and Hispanic origin. Available at: www.census.gov/population/www/projections/usinterimproj. Accessed November 11, 2008.
7. Castle SC, Uyemura K, Fulop T, et al. Host resistance and immune responses in advanced age. Clin Geriatr Med 2007;23(3):463–79, v.
8. Aw D, Silva AB, Palmer DB. Immunosenescence: emerging challenges for an ageing population. Immunology 2007;120(4):435–46.
9. Hakim FT, Gress RE. Immunosenescence: deficits in adaptive immunity in the elderly. Tissue Antigens 2007;70(3):179–89.
10. Listi F, Candore G, Modica MA, et al. A study of serum immunoglobulin levels in elderly persons that provides new insights into B cell immunosenescence. Ann N Y Acad Sci 2006;1089:487–95.
11. Lock RJ, Unsworth DJ. Immunoglobulins and immunoglobulin subclasses in the elderly. Ann Clin Biochem 2003;40(Pt 2):143–8.
12. Ginaldi L, De Martinis M, D'Ostilio A, et al. The immune system in the elderly: I. Specific humoral immunity. Immunol Res 1999;20(2):101–8.
13. Burns EA, Goodwin JS. Immunodeficiency of aging. Drugs Aging 1997;11(5): 374–97.
14. Kumar R, Burns EA. Age-related decline in immunity: implications for vaccine responsiveness. Expert Rev Vaccines 2008;7(4):467–79.
15. Pfister G, Weiskopf D, Lazuardi L, et al. Naive T cells in the elderly: are they still there? Ann N Y Acad Sci 2006;1067:152–7.
16. Lazuardi L, Jenewein B, Wolf AM, et al. Age-related loss of naive T cells and dys-regulation of T-cell/B-cell interactions in human lymph nodes. Immunology 2005; 114(1):37–43.
17. Sunderkotter C, Kalden H, Luger TA. Aging and the skin immune system. Arch Dermatol 1997;133(10):1256–62.
18. Marik PE, Kaplan D. Aspiration pneumonia and dysphagia in the elderly. Chest 2003;124(1):328–36.
19. Newnham DM, Hamilton SJ. Sensitivity of the cough reflex in young and elderly subjects. Age Ageing 1997;26(3):185–8.
20. Ho JC, Chan KN, Hu WH, et al. The effect of aging on nasal mucociliary clear-ance, beat frequency, and ultrastructure of respiratory cilia. Am J Respir Crit Care Med 2001;163(4):983–8.
21. Turnheim K. Drug dosage in the elderly: is it rational? Drugs Aging 1998;13(5): 357–79.
22. Tedla FM, Friedman EA. The trend toward geriatric nephrology. Prim Care 2008; 35(3):515–30, vii.
23. Noreddin AM, El-Khatib W, Haynes V. Optimal dosing design for antibiotic therapy in the elderly: a pharmacokinetic and pharmacodynamic perspective. Recent Pat Antiinfect Drug Discov 2008;3(1):45–52.
24. Noreddin AM, Haynes V. Use of pharmacodynamic principles to optimise dosage regimens for antibacterial agents in the elderly. Drugs Aging 2007; 24(4):275–92.

25. Faulkner CM, Cox HL, Williamson JC. Unique aspects of antimicrobial use in older adults. Clin Infect Dis 2005;40(7):997–1004.
26. Begg EJ, Barclay ML, Kirkpatrick CM. The therapeutic monitoring of antimicrobial agents. Br J Clin Pharmacol 2001;52(Suppl 1):35S–43S.
27. Cox AM, Malani PN, Wiseman SW, et al. Home intravenous antimicrobial infusion therapy: a viable option in older adults. J Am Geriatr Soc 2007;55(5):645–50.
28. Cockburn J, Gibberd RW, Reid AL, et al. Determinants of non-compliance with short term antibiotic regimens. Br Med J (Clin Res Ed) 1987;295(6602): 814–8.
29. Cockburn J, Reid AL, Bowman JA, et al. Effects of intervention on antibiotic compliance in patients in general practice. Med J Aust 1987;147(7):324–8.
30. Claesson S, Morrison A, Wertheimer AI, et al. Compliance with prescribed drugs: challenges for the elderly population. Pharm World Sci 1999;21(6):256–9.
31. George J, Elliott RA, Stewart DC. A systematic review of interventions to improve medication taking in elderly patients prescribed multiple medications. Drugs Aging 2008;25(4):307–24.
32. Beyth RJ, Shorr RI. Epidemiology of adverse drug reactions in the elderly by drug class. Drugs Aging 1999;14(3):231–9.
33. Smith PW, Bennett G, Bradley S, et al. SHEA/APIC guideline: infection prevention and control in the long-term care facility, July 2008. Infect Control Hosp Epidemiol 2008;29(9):785–814.
34. Deal EN, Micek ST, Ritchie DJ, et al. Predictors of in-hospital mortality for bloodstream infections caused by *Enterobacter* species or *Citrobacter freundii*. Pharmacotherapy 2007;27(2):191–9.
35. Marcos M, Inurrieta A, Soriano A, et al. Effect of antimicrobial therapy on mortality in 377 episodes of *Enterobacter* spp. bacteraemia. J Antimicrob Chemother 2008;62(2):397–403.
36. Gellin BG, Broome CV, Bibb WF, et al. The epidemiology of listeriosis in the United States–1986. Listeriosis Study Group. Am J Epidemiol 1991;133(4):392–401.
37. Jackson ML, Neuzil KM, Thompson WW, et al. The burden of community-acquired pneumonia in seniors: results of a population-based study. Clin Infect Dis 2004;39(11):1642–50.
38. Kothe H, Bauer T, Marre R, et al. Outcome of community-acquired pneumonia: influence of age, residence status and antimicrobial treatment. Eur Respir J 2008;32(1):139–46.
39. El-Solh AA, Sikka P, Ramadan F, et al. Etiology of severe pneumonia in the very elderly. Am J Respir Crit Care Med 2001;163(3 Pt 1):645–51.
40. Marrie TJ. Pneumonia in the long-term-care facility. Infect Control Hosp Epidemiol 2002;23(3):159–64.
41. Guidelines for the management of adults with hospital-acquired, ventilator-associated, and healthcare-associated pneumonia. Am J Respir Crit Care Med 2005;171(4):388–416.
42. Mandell LA, Bartlett JG, Dowell SF, et al. Update of practice guidelines for the management of community-acquired pneumonia in immunocompetent adults. Clin Infect Dis 2003;37(11):1405–33.
43. Neill AM, Martin IR, Weir R, et al. Community acquired pneumonia: aetiology and usefulness of severity criteria on admission. Thorax 1996;51(10):1010–6.
44. Bont J, Hak E, Hoes AW, et al. Predicting death in elderly patients with community-acquired pneumonia: a prospective validation study reevaluating the CRB-65 severity assessment tool. Arch Intern Med 2008;168(13):1465–8.
45. Laube S. Skin infections and ageing. Ageing Res Rev 2004;3(1):69–89.

46. Farage MA, Miller KW, Elsner P, et al. Functional and physiological characteristics of the aging skin. Aging Clin Exp Res 2008;20(3):195–200.
47. Horowitz Y, Sperber AD, Almog Y. Gram-negative cellulitis complicating cirrhosis. Mayo Clin Proc 2004;79(2):247–50.
48. Brook I, Frazier EH. Clinical features and aerobic and anaerobic microbiological characteristics of cellulitis. Arch Surg 1995;130(7):786–92.
49. Herold BC, Immergluck LC, Maranan MC, et al. Community-acquired methicillin-resistant Staphylococcus aureus in children with no identified predisposing risk. JAMA 1998;279(8):593–8.
50. Hersh AL, Chambers HF, Maselli JH, et al. National trends in ambulatory visits and antibiotic prescribing for skin and soft-tissue infections. Arch Intern Med 2008;168(14):1585–91.
51. Klevens RM, Morrison MA, Nadle J, et al. Invasive methicillin-resistant Staphylococcus aureus infections in the United States. JAMA 2007;298(15):1763–71.
52. Stryjewski ME, Chambers HF. Skin and soft-tissue infections caused by community-acquired methicillin-resistant Staphylococcus aureus. Clin Infect Dis 2008; 46(Suppl 5):S368–77.
53. David MZ, Mennella C, Mansour M, et al. Predominance of methicillin-resistant Staphylococcus aureus among pathogens causing skin and soft tissue infections in a large urban jail: risk factors and recurrence rates. J Clin Microbiol 2008; 46(10):3222–7.
54. Skiest DJ, Cooper TW. High recurrence rate of CA-MRSA skin and soft tissue infections. Arch Intern Med 2007;167(22):2527 [author reply 2527].
55. Ellis MW, Griffith ME, Dooley DP, et al. Targeted intranasal mupirocin to prevent colonization and infection by community-associated methicillin-resistant Staphylococcus aureus strains in soldiers: a cluster randomized controlled trial. Antimicrob Agents Chemother 2007;51(10):3591–8.
56. Perl B, Gottehrer NP, Raveh D, et al. Cost-effectiveness of blood cultures for adult patients with cellulitis. Clin Infect Dis 1999;29(6):1483–8.
57. Kielhofner MA, Brown B, Dall L. Influence of underlying disease process on the utility of cellulitis needle aspirates. Arch Intern Med 1988;148(11):2451–2.
58. Hepburn MJ, Dooley DP, Skidmore PJ, et al. Comparison of short-course (5 days) and standard (10 days) treatment for uncomplicated cellulitis. Arch Intern Med 2004;164(15):1669–74.
59. Gabillot-Carre M, Roujeau JC. Acute bacterial skin infections and cellulitis. Curr Opin Infect Dis 2007;20(2):118–23.
60. Levine EG, Manders SM. Life-threatening necrotizing fasciitis. Clin Dermatol 2005;23(2):144–7.
61. Wong CH, Chang HC, Pasupathy S, et al. Necrotizing fasciitis: clinical presentation, microbiology, and determinants of mortality. J Bone Joint Surg Am 2003; 85(8):1454–60.
62. Young LM, Price CS. Community-acquired methicillin-resistant Staphylococcus aureus emerging as an important cause of necrotizing fasciitis. Surg Infect (Larchmt) 2008;9(4):469–74.
63. Charnot-Katsikas A, Dorafshar AH, Aycock JK, et al. Two cases of necrotizing fasciitis due to Acinetobacter baumannii. J Clin Microbiol 2008;47:258–63.
64. Hidalgo-Grass C, Dan-Goor M, Maly A, et al. Effect of a bacterial pheromone peptide on host chemokine degradation in group A streptococcal necrotising soft-tissue infections. Lancet 2004;363(9410):696–703.
65. EPUAP. Pressure ulcer treatment guidelines. Oxford: EPUAP; 1999.

66. Sobel J, Kaye D. Urinary tract infection. In: Mandell GL, Bennett JE, Dolin R, editors. Principles and practice of infectious diseases, vol. 2. Philadelphia: Elsevier; 2005. p. 875–905.
67. Baldassarre JS, Kaye D. Special problems of urinary tract infection in the elderly. Med Clin North Am 1991;75(2):375–90.
68. Ronald A. The etiology of urinary tract infection: traditional and emerging pathogens. Dis Mon 2003;49(2):71–82.
69. Nicolle LE. Urinary tract infections in long-term-care facilities. Infect Control Hosp Epidemiol 2001;22(3):167–75.
70. Nicolle LE, Bradley S, Colgan R, et al. Infectious Diseases Society of America guidelines for the diagnosis and treatment of asymptomatic bacteriuria in adults. Clin Infect Dis 2005;40(5):643–54.
71. Olson ES, Cookson BD. Do antimicrobials have a role in preventing septicaemia following instrumentation of the urinary tract? J Hosp Infect 2000;45(2): 85–97.
72. Sobel JD, Kauffman CA, McKinsey D, et al. Candiduria: a randomized, double-blind study of treatment with fluconazole and placebo. The National Institute of Allergy and Infectious Diseases (NIAID) Mycoses Study Group. Clin Infect Dis 2000;30(1):19–24.
73. Gomez Morales MA, Pozio E. Humoral and cellular immunity against Cryptosporidium infection. Curr Drug Targets Immune Endocr Metabol Disord 2002;2(3): 291–301.
74. Simor AE, Bradley SF, Strausbaugh LJ, et al. *Clostridium difficile* in long-term-care facilities for the elderly. Infect Control Hosp Epidemiol 2002;23(11): 696–703.
75. McDonald LC, Killgore GE, Thompson A, et al. An epidemic, toxin gene-variant strain of *Clostridium difficile*. N Engl J Med 2005;353(23):2433–41.
76. McDonald LC, Owings M, Jernigan DB. *Clostridium difficile* infection in patients discharged from US short-stay hospitals, 1996–2003. Emerg Infect Dis 2006; 12(3):409–15.
77. Zar FA, Bakkanagari SR, Moorthi KM, et al. A comparison of vancomycin and metronidazole for the treatment of *Clostridium difficile*-associated diarrhea, stratified by disease severity. Clin Infect Dis 2007;45(3):302–7.
78. Gerding DN, Muto CA, Owens RC Jr. Treatment of *Clostridium difficile* infection. Clin Infect Dis 2008;46(Suppl 1):S32–42.
79. Moran E, Masters S, Berendt AR, et al. Guiding empirical antibiotic therapy in orthopaedics: the microbiology of prosthetic joint infection managed by debridement, irrigation and prosthesis retention. J Infect 2007;55(1):1–7.
80. Tai CC, Nirvani AA, Holmes A, et al. Methicillin-resistant *Staphylococcus aureus* in orthopaedic surgery. Int Orthop 2004;28(1):32–5.
81. Shams WE, Rapp RP. Methicillin-resistant staphylococcal infections: an important consideration for orthopedic surgeons. Orthopedics 2004;27(6): 565–8.
82. Betsch BY, Eggli S, Siebenrock KA, et al. Treatment of joint prosthesis infection in accordance with current recommendations improves outcome. Clin Infect Dis 2008;46(8):1221–6.
83. Toulson C, Walcott-Sapp S, Hur J, et al. Treatment of infected total hip arthroplasty with a 2-stage reimplantation protocol update on "our institution's" experience from 1989 to 2003. J Arthroplasty 2008 [Epub ahead of print].

84. Lieberman JR, Callaway GH, Salvati EA, et al. Treatment of the infected total hip arthroplasty with a two-stage reimplantation protocol. Clin Orthop Relat Res 1994;(301):205–12.

85. Parvizi J, Saleh KJ, Ragland PS, et al. Efficacy of antibiotic-impregnated cement in total hip replacement. Acta Orthop 2008;79(3):335–41.

86. Dalla Paola L, Faglia E. Treatment of diabetic foot ulcer: an overview strategy for clinical approach. Curr Diabetes Rev 2006;2(4):431–47.

87. Lipsky BA, Berendt AR, Deery HG, et al. Diagnosis and treatment of diabetic foot infections. Clin Infect Dis 2004;39(7):885–910.

88. White PH, Kuhlenschmidt HL, Vancura BG, et al. Antimicrobial use in patients with advanced cancer receiving hospice care. J Pain Symptom Manage 2003;25(5): 438–43.

89. Reinbolt RE, Shenk AM, White PH, et al. Symptomatic treatment of infections in patients with advanced cancer receiving hospice care. J Pain Symptom Manage 2005;30(2):175–82.

Use of Antibacterial Agents in Renal Failure

Brett Gilbert, DO, FACOI[a],*, Paul Robbins, DO[b],
Lawrence L. Livornese, Jr, MD, FACP, FIDSA[c]

KEYWORDS

- Antibiotics • Renal failure • Volume of distribution • MDRD
- Dosing antibiotics with dialysis • Pharmacokinetics
- Dosing antibiotics with continuous renal replacement therapy
- Serum levels

The kidney is the major organ for maintaining fluid and electrolyte homeostasis. Changes in renal function, whether associated with normal aging or disease, can have profound effects on the pharmacology of antibacterial agents. It is imperative that clinicians have a basic understanding of these consequences to effectively prescribe antibacterial agents in the face of impaired or changing renal function.

This article reviews the pharmacokinetics of antibacterial agents in patients who have normal and decreased renal function. The concepts of volume of distribution, rate of elimination, loading and maintenance doses, and therapeutic drug monitoring are delineated. The recent controversy in the literature regarding proper vancomycin levels is reviewed. An updated formula to determine the glomerular filtration rate (GFR) is discussed. Comment is made about the use of intermittent dosing of cefazolin for patients who are receiving high-flux hemodialysis. The utility of once-daily aminoglycoside administration is reviewed. Newer and traditional methods of extracorporeal circulation and the resultant changes in the pharmacokinetics of antibacterial agents are discussed.

PHARMACOKINETICS
Bioavailability and Metabolism

Bioavailability refers to the degree that a drug is absorbed into the systemic circulation after extravascular administration. Relatively few studies have addressed this issue in patients who have renal failure. In chronic renal failure, numerous factors, such as nausea, vomiting, diabetic gastroparesis, and intestinal edema, may decrease

B.G. is on the speakers' bureaus for Merck and Wyeth. No other potential conflicts of interest exist.

[a] Division of Infectious Diseases, Department of Medicine, Thomas, Jefferson University Hospital, Lankenau Hospital, Lankenau Medical Building, Suite 164, Wynnewood, PA 19096, USA
[b] Division of Nephrology, Department of Medicine, Lankenau Hospital, Lankenau Medical Building, Suite 130, Wynnewood, PA 19096, USA
[c] Division of Infectious Diseases, Department of Medicine, Drexel University College of Medicine, Lankenau Hospital, Lankenau Medical Building, Suite 164, Wynnewood, PA 19096, USA
* Corresponding author.
E-mail address: santorow@mlhs.org (B. Gilbert).

Infect Dis Clin N Am 23 (2009) 899–924
doi:10.1016/j.idc.2009.06.009
0891-5520/09/$ – see front matter © 2009 Elsevier Inc. All rights reserved.

id.theclinics.com

gastrointestinal absorption. The conversion of urea to ammonia by gastric urease, antacids, or the use of alkalating agents such as bicarbonate and citrate increases gastric pH, thereby reducing the levels of drugs that require an acidic milieu for absorption.[1] Some drugs are bound by antacids and phosphate binders, which are commonly used in renal failure.[2] In chronic renal failure, bioavailability is further reduced as the result of decreased small bowel absorption.[3] First-pass hepatic metabolism may also be diminished in uremia, leading to increased serum levels of oral antibacterial agents. Impaired plasma protein binding increases the level of free drug; this permits more of a drug to bind to the site of action and, conversely, increases the amount of a drug available for elimination by dialysis or hepatic metabolism. Of note, the rates of glucuronidation, sulfated conjugation, and oxidation are generally unchanged in the presence of uremia.[4]

Distribution and Elimination

Plasma levels for a given drug are a function of the dose, bioavailability, volume of distribution, and rate of metabolism and excretion. The volume of distribution (V_d) is calculated by dividing the amount of drug in the body by the plasma concentration. In general, drugs that are highly protein bound are found mainly in the vascular space and have a small V_d. Those agents that are highly lipid soluble have a large V_d because they are able to penetrate body tissues more easily. Volumes of distribution can exceed the total volume of body water because the V_d is a mathematical construct that does not necessarily correspond to a distinct physiologic space. (This is why the term "apparent V_d" is often used.) The V_d is important in calculating the plasma half-life $(T_{1/2})$ of a drug and may also be used to determine the loading dose. The major routes of elimination of antibacterial agents and their metabolites are by way of the kidney and the liver. Small, generally inconsequential amounts are lost in sweat, saliva, expired air, and breast milk. The rate of elimination of most antibacterial agents follows first-order kinetics, that is, the rate of elimination is proportional to the amount of a drug in the body, and as the amount of a drug increases, so does the rate of elimination.

There is an elimination constant (K), such that:

Rate of elimination $= K \times$ amount of drug in body

Because the amount of a drug in the body can be calculated by multiplying the plasma concentration by the V_d, one can restate the equation:

Rate of elimination $= K \times V_d \times$ plasma concentration

Plasma drug clearance is calculated by dividing the rate of elimination by the plasma concentration. Therefore:

Plasma drug clearance $= K \times V_d$

It is traditional that the rate of plasma clearance is expressed as the time required for the concentration of a drug to decline by 50%, which is the $T_{1/2}$. The $T_{1/2}$ remains constant at all times for all drugs that follow first-order kinetics because as the concentration decreases, so does the rate of plasma clearance. Additionally, the $T_{1/2}$ is independent of the initial plasma concentration; it is purely a function of the elimination constant (K). Therefore:

$$T_{1/2} = \ln 2 / K = 0.693 / K$$

By substituting for K from plasma drug clearance $= K \times V_d$:

$T_{1/2} = (0.693)(V_d)/$plasma drug clearance

Therefore, the $T_{1/2}$ is determined by using only the V_d and the plasma clearance. Any process that alters these will change the $T_{1/2}$. In renal insufficiency, the presence of edema or ascites will increase the V_d of highly protein-bound or water-soluble drugs, resulting in lower than expected plasma levels. However, muscle loss and dehydration can decrease V_d and lead to higher than expected concentrations of these same agents.

Renal Clearance

The rate of elimination of drugs by the kidneys depends on the GFR, a measure of kidney function that represents the filtration rates of all of the functioning nephrons and is a function of cardiac output. The renal clearance of antibiotics and other agents is determined by glomerular filtration along with renal tubular secretion and reabsorption. The glomerular filtration of a drug is influenced by its molecular size and protein-binding characteristics. When an increase in protein binding reduces glomerular filtration, elimination by way of renal tubular secretion may be enhanced. The proximal tubules have active transport systems that can secrete and reabsorb drugs. Beta-lactams are actively secreted by this system. In the setting of impaired renal function, whether as the result of normal aging or intrinsic renal disease, a reduction in both glomerular filtration and tubular secretion of drugs may occur, resulting in higher serum concentrations of these agents.

When considering the administration of an antibacterial agent that is excreted by the kidneys, determining the appropriate dosage requires that renal function be assessed. A 24-hour urine collection allows for accurate determination of the endogenous creatinine clearance, which is a close approximation of the GFR. (A small amount of creatinine is secreted in the proximal tubules.) In practice, it is often too time consuming or impractical to obtain a 24-hour urine collection to determine the GFR. The equation of Cockcroft and Gault[5] can be used to estimate creatinine clearance:

$$\text{Creatinine clearance in males} = \frac{(140 - \text{age}) \times \text{total body weight in KG}}{(72 \times \text{serum creatinine in mg/dl})}$$

In women, the clearance is 85% of this value.

Pesola and colleagues[6] suggest using ideal body weight (IBW) instead of total body weight. IBW can be calculated using height and gender, as stated by Devine.[7]

Male IBW $= 50$kg $+ 2.3$kg for each inch of height more than 5 ft

Female IBW $= 45.5$kg $+ 2.3$kg for each inch of height more than 5 ft

The above calculations are only valid when the renal function is stable and the serum creatinine is constant. When the patient is oliguric or the serum creatinine is rapidly rising, the creatinine clearance should be assumed to be less than 10 mL/min.

A newer equation has been developed as a method to estimate GFR based on data from the Modification of Diet in Renal Disease (MDRD) Study that uses six clinical and demographic variables, including serum creatinine.[8] The equation takes into account body-surface area and eliminates weight as a variable. In 2005, the MDRD equation was reformulated to use four variables rather than six for ease of clinical use, and it is used by many clinical laboratories to report estimated GFR.[9] This modification results in a 5% decrease in estimated GFR compared with the previous formula. The new formula is:

$$GFR = 175 \times standardized \ (serum \ creatinine) - 1 \cdot 154 \times (age) - 0 \cdot 203$$
$$\times \ 0.742 \ (if \ female) \ and \times 1.212 \ (if \ black)$$

The MDRD formula[10,11] is probably most useful to assist the clinician for drug adjustment dosing decisions in patients who have relatively stable kidney function.[9] The formula, however, has not been validated for use in dosing all antibiotics, and many clinicians prefer the Cockcroft-Gault formula for its ease of use and because of their longer experience in using it for antibiotic dosing. In addition, one needs to keep in mind that when a patient is critically ill, elderly, malnourished, or obese and potentially nephrotoxic drugs are concurrently being used, so that the above equations used to estimate the GFR may be inaccurate, and an alternative method may need to be used to correctly adjust drug dosages.[12] A 24-hour urine collection should be obtained in this setting, using the midpoint between the creatinine and urea clearance.

Serum creatinine alone is not a reliable measure of creatinine clearance because it is a function of the GFR and muscle mass. In an elderly or debilitated patient, the serum creatinine may appear normal, even in the presence of significant renal insufficiency.

Trimethoprim and cimetidine compete with creatinine for secretory pathways in the proximal tubule and may cause an increase in serum creatinine without a change in the GFR.[13,14] A false elevation in serum creatinine, which is caused by interference with certain creatinine assays,[15,16] has been reported when using cefoxitin and cephalothin.

DOSING OF ANTIBACTERIAL AGENTS IN RENAL FAILURE
Initial Dose

The loading, or initial, dose is based on the extracellular fluid volume and is not altered in the presence of decreased renal function. The presence of ascites or edema may necessitate a larger dose, whereas dehydration may require a reduction in the dose. When a loading dose is not used, four maintenance doses are required to achieve a steady state. When antibacterial agents that have a short $T_{1/2}$ are used, each maintenance dose acts as a loading dose, and therefore no separate initial dose is used. A loading dose is generally used when it is necessary to achieve therapeutic plasma levels rapidly.

Maintenance Dose

After the loading dose, subsequent maintenance doses frequently require modification in patients who have decreased renal function.

Table 1 outlines specific dosing guidelines for the use of antibiotics in patients that are in renal failure. The classification is based on chemical class and then subdivided alphabetically.

The second through fifth columns indicate the percentage of drug excreted unchanged, the $T_{1/2}$ of each agent in normal patients and those who have end-stage renal disease, and the percentage of protein binding and V_d, respectively. The columns to the right provide recommendations for dosing schedules based on renal function. Modifications of doses are dictated by the severity of renal impairment as determined by the estimated GFR. The adjustments are labeled either "D" for dose reduction or "I" for interval extension. In the dose reduction method (D), a percentage of the usual dose of an antibacterial is given at the standard interval. In the interval extension method (I), the dose of an individual antibacterial agent remains constant, but the interval between doses is extended. Additional dosing requirements for various dialysis modalities, if available, are found in the last column to the right. If available, supplemental information for hemodialysis, continuous ambulatory peritoneal dialysis (CAPD), and continuous arteriovenous hemofiltration (CAVH) is indicated as well.

Once-Daily Aminoglycosides

In the era of antibiotic resistance, aminoglycoside antibiotics continue to play a critical role in the treatment of certain gram-negative bacterial infections. Because of the aminoglycosides' high side-effect profile and their prolonged postantibiotic effect, novel treatment approaches and dosing schedules have been implemented in an attempt to limit toxicity.[17,18] In the last 10 years, once-daily aminoglycoside therapy has been introduced to take advantage of aminoglycoside pharmacodynamics while attempting to reduce nephrotoxicity and ototoxicity.[19] Credence for this concept was supported by early animal studies that suggested that the incidence of acute renal failure could be reduced by using once-daily administration.[20] Nephrotoxicity in this class of antibiotics depends on the cumulative dose or concentrations that are greater than a critical level, so achieving the therapeutic goal quickly may allow for a shorter course of therapy.[21] Achieving increased periods of time in which the patient has a negligible serum concentration will reduce renal cortical and auditory exposure, potentially decreasing toxicity.[22] A meta-analysis performed by Hatala and colleagues[23] reviewed 13 studies, and the authors concluded that standard and once-daily regimens had similar bacteriologic cure rates and that once-daily dosing showed a trend toward reduced toxicity and mortality. Other benefits of once-daily dosing include reduced costs and prolonged postantibiotic effect. Lab draws will also be reduced because serum levels will have to be monitored less frequently.

Patient selection is important when considering a once-daily regimen. Only certain patient populations are appropriate for once-daily dosing; these include patients who have pelvic inflammatory disease, gram-negative bacteremia, urinary tract infections, febrile neutropenia, gynecologic infections, and respiratory infections.[24] Once-daily aminoglycoside dosing should not be used in cases for which little apparent benefit is expected, or for cases in which clinical evidence is lacking. There is little data for using once-daily aminoglycosides in the following situations: pregnancy, creatinine clearance less then 20 mL/min, bone and joint infections, central nervous system infections, infective endocarditis, obesity, burns, and solid organ transplantation.

Initial dosing for once-daily aminoglycosides should be based on creatinine clearance. **Table 2** provides dosage adjustments for patients who have renal insufficiency. Serum drug levels for patients who are receiving once-daily doses of gentamicin or tobramycin should achieve a peak concentration of 15 to 20 μg/mL. The trough concentration should be kept to less than 1 μg/ml.[25,26] Finally, the clinician should be comfortable using amikacin as a single daily dose. Fifteen mg/kg of amikacin should yield a peak of about 60 μg/mL. In the last five years, multidrug-resistant gram-negative organisms have become increasingly prevalent. These organisms often remain susceptible to amikacin as a result of the presence of different aminoglycoside modifying enzymes that render gentamicin and tobramycin resistant; therefore, amikacin is often the aminoglycoside of choice in many gram-negative infections.

Intermittent-Dosing of Cefazolin with Hemodialysis

In hemodialysis patients who have suspected bloodstream or vascular infections, vancomycin and gentamicin are frequently given as empiric therapy. Often, when an isolate such as methicillin-susceptible *Staphylococcus aureus* (MSSA) is recovered,

Table 1
Recommended drug dosages and adjustments for patients in renal failure

Drug	Excreted, Unchanged %	T1/2 (Normal/ ESRD; Hours)	Plasma Protein Binding (%)	Vd (L/kg)	Dose for Normal Renal Function	Method	>50	10–50	<10	Supplement for Dialysis		
Aminoglycoside antibiotics												
Amikacin	95	1.4–2.3/ 17–150	<5	0.22–0.29	5 mg/kg q8h	D and I	60%–90% q12h	30%–70% q12–18h	20%–30% q24–48h	IHD	2/3 normal dose after dialysis	
										CAPD	15–20 mg/L	
										CRRT	Dose for GFR 10–50 and measure levels	
Gentamicin	95	1.8/ 20–60	<5	0.23–0.26	1–1.7 mg/kg q8h	D and I	60%–90% q8–12h	30%–70% q12h	20%–30% q24–48h	IHD	2/3 normal dose after dialysis	
										CAPD	3–4 mg/L	
										CRRT	Dose for GFR 10–50 and measure levels	
Netilmicin	95	1–3/ 35–72	<5	0.19–0.23	2 mg/kg q8h	D and I	50%–90% q8–12h	20%–60% q12h	10%–20% q24–48h	IHD	2/3 normal dose after dialysis	
										CAPD	3–4 mg/L	
										CRRT	Dose for GFR 10–50 and measure levels	
Streptomycin	70	2.5/100	35	0.26	15 mg/kg q24h; 1 g max daily	I	q24h	q24–72h	q72–96h	IHD	1/2 normal dose after dialysis	
										CAPD	20–40 mg/L	
										CRRT	Dose for GFR 10–50 and measure levels	
Tobramycin	95	2.5/ 27–60	<5	0.22–0.33	1–1.7 mg/kg q8h	D and I	60%–90% q8–12h	30%–70% q12h	20%–30% q24–48	IHD	2/3 normal dose after dialysis	
										CAPD	3–4 mg/L	
										CRRT	Dose for GFR 10–50 and measure levels	
Carbapenems												
Doripenem	70	1/18	8.1	16.8	500 mg q8h	D and I	100%	250 mg q8–12	No data	IHD	No data	
										CAPD	No data	
										CRRT	No data	

Drug				Dose for normal renal function	Method	GFR >50	GFR 10–50	GFR <10	Supplement for dialysis
Ertapenem	38	4/6	85–95	8.2	1 g q24h	D	100%	100%	50%	IHD 150 mg after dialysis CAPD No data CRRT No data
Imipenem	20–70	1.0/4.0	13–21	0.17–0.30	0.25–1.0 g q6h	D	100%	50%	25%	IHD Dose after dialysis CAPD Dose for GFR <10 CRRT Dose for GFR 10–50
Meropenem	65	1.1/6–8	Low	0.35	0.5–1.0 g q6h	D and I	500 mg q6h	250–500 mg q12h	250–500 mg q24h	IHD Dose after dialysis CAPD Dose for GFR <10 CRRT Dose for GFR 10–50
Cephalosporin antibiotics									
Cefaclor	70	1/3	25	0.24–0.35	250–500 mg q8h	D	100%	50%–100%	50%	IHD 250 mg after dialysis CAPD 250 mg q8–12h CRRT Not applicable
Cefadroxil	70–90	1.4/22	20	0.31	0.5–1.0 g q12h	I	q12h	q12–24h	q24–48h	IHD 0.5–1.0 g after dialysis CAPD 0.5 g/d CRRT Not applicable
Cefazolin	75–95	2/40–70	80	0.13–0.22	0.5–2.0 g q8h	I	q8h	q12h	q24–48h	IHD 0.5–1 g after dialysis[a] CAPD 0.5 g q12h CRRT Dose for GFR 10–50
Cefdinir	18	1.7/16	60–70	0.35	300 mg q12h	I	q12h	q12h	q24h	IHD 300 mg after dialysis CAPD Not applicable CRRT Not applicable
Cefditoren	99	1.6/4.7	88	0.35	200–400 mg q12h	D and I	100%	50%	50% q24h	IHD No data CAPD No data CRRT No data
Cefepime	85	2.2/18	16	0.3	0.25–2.0 g q8h	I	q12h	q16–24h	q24–48h	IHD 1 g after dialysis CAPD Dose for GFR <10 CRRT Not recommended

(continued on next page)

Table 1
(continued)

Drug	Excreted, Unchanged %	T1/2 (Normal/ESRD; Hours)	Plasma Protein Binding (%)	Vd (L/kg)	Dose for Normal Renal Function	Adjustment for Renal Function GFR, mL/min				Supplement for Dialysis
						Method	>50	10–50	<10	
Cefixime	18–50	3.1/12	50	0.6–1.1	250 mg q12h	D	100%	75%	50%	IHD 300 mg after dialysis CAPD 200 mg/day CRRT Not applicable
Cefotaxime	60	1/15	37	0.15–0.50	1 g q6h	I	q6h	q 8–12h	q24h	IHD 1 g after dialysis CAPD 1 g q24h CRRT 1 g q12h
Cefotetan	75	3.5/13–25	85	0.15	1–2 g q12h	D	100%	50%	25%	IHD 1 g after dialysis CAPD 1 g/d CRRT 750 mg q12h
Cefoxitin	80	1/13–23	41–75	0.2	1–2 g q6–8h	I	q8h	q8–12h	q24–48h	IHD 1 g after dialysis CAPD 1 g/d CRRT Dose for GFR 10–50
Cefpodoxime	30	2.5/26		0.6–1.2	200 mg q12h	I	q12h	q16h	q24–48h	IHD 200 mg after dialysis only CAPD Dose for GFR <10 CRRT Not applicable
Cefprozil	65	1.7/6		0.65	500 mg q12h	D and I	250 mg q12h	250 mg q12–16h	250 mg q24	IHD 250 mg after dialysis CAPD Dose for GFR <10 CRRT Dose for GFR <10
Ceftazidime	60–85	1.2/13–25	17	0.28–0.40	1–2 g q8h	I	q8–12h	q24–48h	q48h	IHD 1 g after dialysis CAPD 0.5 g q24h CRRT Dose for GFR 10–50
Ceftibuten	56	2/22	65	0.21	400 mg q24h	D	100%	50%	25%	IHD 400 mg after dialysis CAPD Not applicable CRRT Not applicable

					Dose					Supplement
Ceftizoxime	57–100	1.4/35	28–50	0.26–0.42	1–2 g q8–12h	I	q8–12h	q12–24h	q24h	IHD 1 g after dialysis CAPD 0.5–1.0 g q24h CRRT Dose for GFR 10–50
Ceftriaxone	30–65	7–9/12–24	90	0.12–0.18	1–2 g q12–24h	—	100%	100%	100%	IHD None CAPD 750 mg q12h CRRT Dose for GFR 10–50
Ceftobiprole	?	3–4/no data ?	?	?	500 mg q8–12h	I	q8–12h	q12h	—	IHD ? CAPD No data for GFR <30 CRRT ?
Cefuroxime axetil	90	1.2/17	35–50	0.13–1.8	250–500 mg q12h	—	100%	100%	100%	IHD Dose after dialysis CAPD Dose for GFR <10 CRRT Not applicable
Cefuroxime sodium	90	1.2/17	33	0.13–1.8	0.75–1.5 g q8h	I	q8h	q8–12h	q24h	IHD Dose after dialysis CAPD Dose for GFR <10 CRRT 1 g q12h
Cephalexin	98	0.7/16	20	0.35	250–500 mg q6h	I	q8h	q12h	q12h	IHD Dose after dialysis CAPD Dose for GFR <10 CRRT Not applicable
Macrolide antibiotics										
Azithromycin	6–12	10–60/?	10–50	18	250–500 mg q24h	—	100%	100%	100%	IHD None CAPD None CRRT None
Clarithromycin	15	2.3–6/22	70	2.4	500 mg q12h	D	100%	75%	50%–75%	IHD Dose after dialysis CAPD None CRRT None
Erythromycin	15	1.4/5.6	60–95	0.78	250–500 mg q6–12h	D	100%	100%	50%–75%	IHD None CAPD None CRRT None
Miscellaneous antibacterials										
Aztreonam	75	1.7–2.9/6–8	55	0.1–2.0	1–2 g q8–12h	D	100%	50%–75%	25%	IHD 0.5g after dialysis CAPD Dose for GFR <10 CRRT Dose for GFR 10–50

(continued on next page)

Table 1
(continued)

Drug	Excreted, Unchanged %	T1/2 (Normal/ESRD; Hours)	Plasma Protein Binding (%)	Vd (L/kg)	Dose for Normal Renal Function	Adjustment for Renal Function GFR, mL/min				Supplement for Dialysis
						Method	>50	10–50	<10	
Chloramphenicol	10	1.6–3.3/3–7	45–60	0.5–1.0	12.5 mg/kg q6h	—	100%	100%	100%	IHD None / CAPD None / CRRT None
Cilastin	60	1/12	44	0.22	With imipenem	D	100%	50%	Avoid	IHD Avoid / CAPD Avoid / CRRT Avoid
Clavulanic acid	40	1/3–4	30	0.3	100 mg q4–6h	D	100%	100%	50%–75%	IHD Dose after dialysis / CAPD Dose for GFR <10 / CRRT Dose for GFR 10–50
Clindamycin	10	2–4/3–5	60–95	0.6–1.2	150–900 mg q6–8h	—	100%	100%	100%	IHD None / CAPD None / CRRT None
Colistin	?	2–3/>48	Low	?	160mg q12h	D	100%	q24h	q36h	IHD 80 mg after dialysis
Daptomycin	78	9/28	92	0.1	4–6 mg/kg q24h	I	q24h	q24h	q48h	IHD Give after HD on HD days / CAPD 4 mg/kg q48h / CRRT 4 mg/kg q48h
Linezolid	30, 20	4.5/?	31	40–50	400–600 mg q12h	—	100%	100%	100%	IHD No data / CAPD No data / CRRT No data
Metronidazole	20	6–14/7–21	20	0.25–0.85	7.5 mg/kg q6–12h	D	100%	100%	75%	IHD Dose after dialysis / CAPD Dose for GFR <10 / CRRT Dose for GFR 10–50
Nitrofurantoin	30–40	0.5/1	20–60	0.3–0.7	50–100 mg q6h	D	100%	Avoid	Avoid	IHD Not applicable / CAPD Not applicable / CRRT Not applicable

Drug					Dose	Method	>50	10–50	<10	Supplement for dialysis
Sulbactam	50–80	1/10–21	30	0.25–0.50	0.75–1.5 g q6–8h	I	q6–8h	q12–24h	q12–48h	IHD Dose after dialysis CAPD 0.75–1.5 g/d CRRT 750 mg q12h
Sulfamethoxazole	70	10/20–50	50	0.28–0.38	1.0 g q8h	I	q12h	q18h	q24h	IHD 1 g after dialysis CAPD 1 g q24 CRRT Dose for GFR 10–50
Sulfisoxazole	70	3–7/6–12	85	0.14–0.28	1–2 g q6h	I	q6h	q8–12h	q12–24h	IHD 2g after dialysis CAPD 3 g/d CRRT Not applicable
Synercid										
Quinupristin	15	0.9/?	55–78	1	7.5 mg/kg q8–12h	—	100%	100%	100%	IHD None CAPD None CRRT None
Dalfopristin	19	0.75/?	11–26	1		—	—	—	—	
Tazobactam	65	1/17	22	0.21	1.5–2.25 g/d	D	100%	75%	50%	IHD 1/3 dose after dialysis CAPD Dose for GFR <10 CRRT Dose for GFR 10–50
Teicoplanin	40–60	33–190/62–230	60–90	0.5–1.2	6 mg/kg q24h	I	q24h	q48h	q72h	IHD Dose for GFR <10 CAPD Dose for GFR <10 CRRT Dose for GFR 10–50
Tigecycline	22	42	71–89	7–9	100 mg; then 50 mg q12h	—	100%	100%	100%	IHD None
Trimethoprim	40–70	9–13/20–49	30–70	1–2.2	100–200 mg q12h	I	q12h	q18h	q24h	IHD Dose after dialysis CAPD q24h
Vancomycin	90–100	6–8/200–250	10–50	0.47–1.1	1 g q12h	D and I	500 mg q6–12h	500 mg q24–48 h	500 mg q48–96 h	IHD Dose for GFR <10 CAPD Dose for GFR <10 CRRT Dose for GFR 10–50

(continued on next page)

Table 1
(continued)

Drug	Excreted, Unchanged %	T1/2 (Normal/ESRD; Hours)	Plasma Protein Binding (%)	Vd (L/kg)	Dose for Normal Renal Function	Adjustment for Renal Function				Supplement for Dialysis	
						Method	GFR, mL/min				
							>50	10–50	<10		
Penicillins											
Amoxicillin	50–70	0.9–23/5–20	15–25	0.26	250–500 mg q8h	I	q8h	q8–12h	q24h	IHD CAPD CRRT	Dose after dialysis 250 mg q12h Not applicable
Ampicillin	30–90	0.8–1.5/7–20	20	0.17–0.31	250 mg–2 g q6h	I	q6h	q6–12h	q12–24h	IHD CAPD CRRT	Dose after dialysis 250 mg q12h Dose for GFR 10–50
Dicloxacillin	35–70	0.7/1–2	95	0.16	250–500 mg q6h	—	100%	100%	100%	IHD CAPD CRRT	None None Not applicable
Nafcillin	35	0.5/1.2	85	0.35	1–2 g q4–6h	—	100%	100%	100%	IHD CAPD CRRT	None None None
Penicillin G	60–85	0.5/6–20	50	0.30–0.42	0.5–4 million U q4h	D	100%	75%	50%	IHD CAPD CRRT	Dose after dialysis Dose for GFR <10 Dose for GFR 10–50
Penicillin VK	60–90	0.6/4.1	50–80	0.5	250 mg q6h	—	100%	100%	100%	IHD CAPD CRRT	Dose after dialysis Dose for GFR <10 Not applicable
Piperacillin	75–90	0.8–1.5/3.3–5.1	30	0.18–0.30	3–4 g q4h	I	q4–6h	q6–8h	q8h	IHD CAPD CRRT	Dose after dialysis Dose for GFR <10 Dose for GFR 10–50
Ticarcillin	85	1.2/11–16	45–60	0.14–0.21	3 g q4h	D and I	1–2 g q4h	1–2 g q8h	1–2 g q12h	IHD CAPD CRRT	3 g after dialysis Dose for GFR <10 Dose for GFR 10–50

Quinolone antibacterials

					Dose	Method	GFR >50	GFR 10–50	GFR <10	Supplement
Ciprofloxacin	50–70	3–6/6–9	20–40	2.5	400 mg IV or 500 mg orally	D	100%	50%–75%	50%	IHD 50% q12h CAPD 50% q8h CRRT 50% q12h
Levaquin	87	7	24–38	74–122	250–750 mg q24	D and I	100%	50% q24h	50% q48h	IHD Dose for GFR <10 CAPD Dose for GFR <10 CRRT 500 mg q48h
Moxifloxacin	96	12/14.5–16.2	40	2.0–3.5	400 mg q24h		100%	100%	100%	IHD No data CAPD No data CRRT No data
Norfloxacin	30	3.5–6.5/8	14	<0.5	400 mg q12h	I	q12h	q12–24h	Avoid	IHD Not applicable CAPD Not applicable CRRT Not applicable
Ofloxacin	68–80	5–8/28–37	25	1.5–2.5	400 mg q12h	D	100%	200 mg q12h	25%–50% q24h	IHD 100 mg q12h CAPD Dose for GFR <10 CRRT 300 mg q24h

Tetracycline antibacterials

					Dose	Method	GFR >50	GFR 10–50	GFR <10	Supplement
Doxycycline	33–45	15–24/18–25	80–93	0.75	100 mg q12h	—	100%	100%	100%	IHD None CAPD None CRRT None
Minocycline	6–10	12–16/12–18	70	1.0–1.5	100 mg q12h	—	100%	100%	100%	IHD None CAPD None CRRT None
Tetracycline	48–60	6–10/57–108	55–90	>0.7	250–500 mg qid	I	q8–12h	q12–24h	q24h	IHD None CAPD None CRRT None

Abbreviations: CRRT, continuous renal replacement therapy; D, dose reduction; ESRD, end-stage renal disease; HD, hemodialysis; I, interval increase; IHD, intermittent hemodialysis.

a See text for additional dosing comments.

Table 2
Suggested single daily dosage requirements of aminoglycosides adjustment for renal insufficiency

Estimated CRCL (mL/min)	Dosage Interval (h)	Dose (mg/kg)	Estimated Level (µg/mL) at Time Interval		
			1h	18h	24h
Gentamicin/tobramycin					
>80	24	5.0	20	<1	<1
70	24	4.0	16	<1	<1
60	24	4.0	16	1.5	<1
50	24	3.5	14	1.0	<1
40	24	2.5	10	1.5	<1
30	24	2.5	10	2.5	1.5
20	48	4.0	16	2.0	1.0
10	48	3.0	12	3.0	2.0
Hemodialysis[a]	48	2.0	8.0	6.0	5.0
Amikacin, kanamycin, streptomycin					
>80	24	15	60	<1	<1
70	24	12	48	2.5	<1
50	24	7.5	30	3.5	1.0
30	24	4.0	20	5.0	3.0
20	48	7.5	30	3.3	1.0
10	48	4.0	16	5.0	3.0
Hemodialysis[a]	48	3.0	20	15	12
Netilmicin					
>80	24	6.5	15	<1	<1
70	24	5.0	—	—	—
50	24	4.0	—	—	—
30	24	2.0	—	—	—
20	48	3.0	—	—	—
10	48	2.5	—	—	—
Hemodialysis[a]	48	2.0	—	—	—

Abbreviation: CRCL, creatinine clearance.
[a] Dose posthemodialysis.
Data from Gilbert DW, Bennett WM. Use of antimicrobial agents in renal failure. Infect Dis Clin North Am 1989;3:517–31; *Data from* Gilbert DN, Mollering RC, Sande MA. The Sanford guide to antimicrobial therapy 2008. Sperryville (VA): Antimicrobial Therapy Inc; 2008.

vancomycin is continued because doses of this drug may be given to patients who are undergoing hemodialysis, and there is no need for additional intravenous access. However, the emergence of vancomycin-resistant enterococcus and concerns about the increasing resistance of *S aureus* to glycopeptides has led to recommendations to limit the use of vancomycin when possible.[27] Stryjewski and colleagues[28] studied a group of long-term hemodialysis patients who had MSSA bacteremia and who were treated using either cefazolin or vancomycin over an 84-month period. Treatment failure, as defined by death or relapse of infection, was significantly higher in the vancomycin group, with an odds ratio of 3.53. The authors concluded that vancomycin was inferior to cefazolin for the treatment of MSSA bacteremia in hemodialysis patients and should not be continued after susceptibilities are known unless a patient has a beta-lactam allergy. This result is consistent with data from other clinical scenarios, demonstrating the superior efficacy of beta-lactam antibiotics compared with vancomycin when treating MSSA infections.

Sowinski and colleagues[29] studied the pharmacokinetics and clearance of cefazolin in 25 uninfected subjects undergoing thrice-weekly hemodialysis. Fifteen subjects underwent hemodialysis using high-efficiency hemodialyzers, and 10 using high-flux hemodialyzers. The subjects were given an intravenous dose of 15 mg/kg of cefazolin immediately after hemodialysis; both groups maintained cefazolin levels that were greater than the breakpoint for sensitive organisms (8 µg/mL), even with a 3-day inter-dialytic period.

In a previous study, Fogel and colleagues[30] concluded that for anuric hemodialysis patients, cefazolin can be effectively used at a dose of 1 g intravenously after each hemodialysis session. A number of nonanuric subjects were included in the study by Sowinski and colleagues. A total of 10 subjects produced enough urine to calculate cefazolin renal clearance, although only three could be considered nonoliguric (urine output >400 mL/day). All 25 subjects in this study maintained adequate cefazolin levels, despite the production of variable amounts of urine.

Kuypers and colleagues[31] used a fixed, postdialysis, 2-g dose of intravenous cefazolin in 15 uninfected hemodialysis patients, 14 of whom received dialysis using high-flux membranes. The weight-based range of doses for this group was from 19.2 to 37.7 mg/kg. Trough levels of cefazolin were obtained before subsequent dialysis sessions, and remained much greater than the MIC for susceptible organisms. However, a higher incidence of adverse effects was seen in this study than in the studies previously discussed, raising the concern that the higher serum levels of cefazolin achieved in this study led to undesirable side effects. The previously discussed studies demonstrated clearly that cefazolin can be administered on either a weight-based or fixed-dose schedule after each dialysis session and can provide a safe and effective alternative to vancomycin for susceptible organisms.

SERUM LEVELS

Because of potential toxicity, especially when vancomycin and aminoglycosides are combined, antimicrobial serum levels are most useful, and are generally obtained, when using either of these drugs. There is an increased incidence of nephrotoxicity when these agents are combined. Appropriate dosing requires the consideration of multiple factors, including patient weight, extracellular fluid shifts, renal function, hypoalbuminemia, location and severity of infection, and potential for toxicity. When administering aminoglycosides, it is even more important to establish safe serum levels in patients who have underlying renal failure because the potential for toxicity is greater.

Vancomycin drug levels have been reviewed extensively and are based on early reports of clinical observation and toxicity.[32] Vancomycin exhibits concentration-independent killing action in vitro, and its pharmacokinetics are affected by inoculum size. However, serum levels do not always correlate with a favorable microbiologic response.[33] In 2006, the Clinical and Laboratory Standards Institute modified vancomycin breakpoints for susceptible isolates to 2 µg/ml or less because of an increase of reports in the literature of vancomycin failures when the minimum inhibitory concentration approached 4 µg/ml. This modification was intended to increase detection of difficult-to-identify, heterogeneously resistant isolates that often result in clinical failure of vancomycin.[34] A significant number of vancomycin failures have been seen in the setting of methicillin-resistant *S aureus* pneumonia. This issue was addressed in a consensus statement by the American Society of Health-System Pharmacists, the Infectious Disease Society of America, and the Society of Infectious Disease Pharmacists.[35] They recommend that vancomycin serum-trough concentrations always be maintained at levels greater than 10 mg/L and that peak serum concentrations need not be checked. Additionally, they recommend that serum trough concentrations be maintained at between 15 and 20 mg/L for patients being treated for complicated infections such as endocarditis, osteomyelitis, meningitis, and hospital-acquired pneumonia. In contrast to aminoglycosides, vancomycin levels have not consistently been correlated with toxicity, and their utility continues to be debated in the literature.[36–39] Unlike vancomycin, aminoglycosides exhibit concentration-dependent killing action. This is important clinically because bactericidal activity is directly proportional to concentration levels.[18] Nevertheless, levels must be followed closely when using aminoglycosides because increased trough levels have been correlated with nephrotoxicity.[40]

Peak and trough concentrations are measured after achieving steady-state concentration. The latter correlates with the fourth dose in patients who have normal renal function, assuming that a loading dose has not been given. The peak concentration is measured approximately 30 to 60 min after completion of the infusion, rather than immediately following the dose, to allow for rapid-phase distribution to occur; otherwise, the measurement will reflect only the plasma volume and not the extracellular compartment. Trough levels are obtained immediately before the next scheduled dose. Random levels are obtained in patients who have underlying renal disease in cases in which the $T_{1/2}$ is sufficiently prolonged and intermittent dosing is being used.

DIALYSIS

When renal failure progresses to the point of uremia or inadequate urine output (oliguria), dialytic intervention is indicated. Typically, dialysis is begun when the GFR is less than 15 mL/min for patients who have diabetes or less than 10 mL/min for patients who do not have diabetes. There are a number of dialytic modalities used in both acute and chronic renal failure.

Hemodialysis

Standard, thrice-weekly, intermittent hemodialysis is the mainstay therapy for end-stage renal failure.[41] **Box 1** summarizes the factors affecting drug clearance by using hemodialysis. The clearance of low-molecular-weight antibiotics (<500 daltons [Da]) depends on blood flow rates, dialysate flow rates, and dialyzer surface area. As a rule, higher-molecular-weight drugs (>500–5,000 Da) are poorly dialyzed by conventional dialyzers. However, there is a trend toward using larger, more permeable (high-flux) membranes. These membranes have been shown to enhance the clearance of middle molecules, recently defined as being compounds that have a molecular weight of 500 to 12,000 Da, and to increase the removal of both low- and high-molecular-weight antibiotics.[29,42–44] To reduce the clearance of antibiotics during high-flux hemodialysis and avoid subtherapeutic drug levels, the administration of antibiotics at the end of a dialysis session or the use of higher intradialytic doses have been recommended.[43,45–47] For situations in which the transport properties of a drug or antibiotic are not known, Maher[48,49] proposed that the hemodialysis clearance of unbound drug can be estimated by multiplying the urea clearance by the ratio of the molecular weight of urea (60 Da) to the antibiotic's molecular weight (MW) (in which K = clearance and X is the antibiotic involved).

Box 1
Factors affecting hemodialysis drug clearance
Drug properties
Molecular weight
Charge
Lipid or water solubility
V_d (tissue binding)
Protein binding
Other forms of steric hindrance
Membrane binding
Rapid excretion by another pathway
Red blood cell partitioning
Hemodialyzer properties
Blood flow
Surface area
Membrane permeability
Pore size
Fluid films (membrane geometry)
Dialysate properties
Flow rate
Solute concentration
pH
Temperature
Miscellaneous properties
Convective transports during ultrafiltration
Data from Golper TA, Bennett WM. Drug usage in dialysis patients. In: Nissenson R, Fine RN, Gentile DE, editors. Clinical dialysis. 2nd edition. Norwalk (CT): Appleton and Lange; 1990, p. 608–30.

$$KX = Kurea \times 60/MWx$$

The nephrologist administering the dialysis therapy should be able to provide an estimate of the urea clearance for a given treatment. Fortunately, the clearance by dialysis of many antibiotics and postdialysis supplement requirements have been established for some time.[48–50] **Table 1** summarizes the data for those agents along with more recent additions.

Intermittent hemodialysis also remains the mainstay treatment of acute renal failure. In such a setting, however, it may be performed more or less often than thrice weekly. It therefore becomes very important to be aware of the dialysis schedule and to monitor antibiotic levels. Unfortunately, unless the laboratory's determination of the antibiotic level is performed and reported quickly, the next dose of antibiotic is likely to have been administered before the trough level is known. In fact, the trough level obtained prior to dialysis is obviously higher than the level at the end of dialysis, when the next dose is typically administered. Therefore, it is important to know when the trough level was obtained. If it was taken at the end of dialysis, there is no realistic opportunity for the level to be known by the time of dosing, unless administration is delayed.

Continuous Renal Replacement Therapy

Increasingly in acute renal failure, continuous methods of renal replacement therapy (CRRT) are being used. These include continuous arteriovenous hemofiltration (CAVH), continuous venovenous hemofiltration (CVVH), continuous arteriovenous hemodialysis (CAVHD), and continuous venovenous hemodialysis (CVVHD).

Hemofiltration (CAVH, CVVH) refers to the removal of an ultrafiltrate of plasma in which there is the solute loss only by convection or solvent drag, not diffusion. The plasma is filtered, but no dialysate is used, so the solute only moves along with plasma water. The efficiency of drug (or any solute) removal is related to the sieving coefficient (SC), which is the mathematical expression of the ability of a solute to cross a membrane convectively. The SC is determined by the ratio of the concentration of the substance in the ultrafiltrate to the plasma. When the patient is on CAVH, the concentration of the substance may be different in arterial and venous samples. For practical purposes of antibiotic or drug administration, the arterial and venous samples can be assumed to be equal, and therefore: SC = [UF]/[A], in which [UF] is the concentration of the antibiotic in the ultrafiltrate and A is arterial concentration. An SC of 1.0 means that a substance freely crosses the membrane and is removed in the same concentration as it exists in the plasma. An SC of zero means there is no removal (typically as the result of extensive size or protein-binding factors).

The rate of antibiotic clearance = SC × UFR (ultrafiltration rate)

Table 3 lists the SC for intravenous antibacterials commonly used to treat serious infections. Because CRRT is by definition continuous, antibiotic levels in this setting more accurately reflect true, real-time estimates of patient antibiotic levels than do levels for intermittent hemodialysis. The first of the two formulae used to determine the amount of antibiotic removed is: Amount antibiotic removed (in mg) = ultrafiltrate concentration (mg/L) × UFR (L/min) × time of procedure (min). This method depends on being able to obtain antibiotic levels in the ultrafiltrate. The second method is to extrapolate the ultrafiltrate concentration from the plasma sample, whereby: ultrafiltrate concentration = [plasma] × unbound fraction (because only the unbound fraction is filtered). The protein-bound fraction for commonly used antibiotics in the critical care setting is provided in **Table 1**. It should be noted that these protein-binding data are for healthy people and may be less reliable in critically ill patients. Nonetheless: amount of antibiotic removed (in mg) = [plasma] (mg/L) × unbound fraction × UFR (L/min) × time of procedure (min). Note that the plasma sample should reflect a steady-state level halfway between maintenance doses and after at least three $T_{1/2}s$.[41,51–53]

Continuous Hemodialysis

Removal of antibiotics during CAVHD or CVVHD occurs largely by diffusion across the dialyzer membrane into the drug-free dialysate on the other side of the membrane. Convective clearance, or solvent drag, is a less significant factor in drug removal in this modality. The two major limiting factors to antibiotic removal by diffusion are protein binding and molecular size. The type of membrane and its permeability characteristics are important determinants of antibiotic and drug removal. As a rule, the membranes used in CRRT are at least as permeable (and often more so) than those used in intermittent hemodialysis. Dosing for maintenance and additional or loading doses can be

Table 3 Sieving coefficient	
Antibacterials	SC
Amikacin	0.9
Amphotericin B	0.3
Amphotericin B, liposomal	0.10
Ampicillin	0.7
Cefoxitin	0.6
Ceftazidime	0.9
Ceftriaxone	0.2
Ciprofloxacin	0.8
Gentamicin	0.8
Imipenem	1.0
Levaquin	0.8
Linezolid	0.8
Metronidazole	0.8
Mezlocillin	0.7
Oxacillin	0.02
Penicillin	0.7
Piperacillin	0.7
Sulfamethoxazole	0.9
Vancomycin	0.8

There is usually a close correlation between the SC and unbound fraction because only the free or unbound drug is available for removal by hemofiltration.
Adapted from Nephrology UpToDate, vol. 16. Wellesley (MA): 2008. p. 3.

calculated when the desired plasma concentration of the antibiotic is known. The presently observed level is subtracted from the desired level. The difference in concentrations (in mg/L) $\times$ V_d (in L/kg) $\times$ body weight (kg) represents the amount of antibiotic necessary to achieve the desired antibiotic plasma level. This formula can be applied when the amount of antibiotic removal has not been directly measured or calculated.[41,52,54,55]

Peritoneal Dialysis in End-Stage Renal Failure

Peritoneal dialysis as a chronic modality is performed with less than 15% of the end-stage renal disease population. The most common variety has been CAPD, in which the patient receives four exchanges per day (draining 2 L of dialysate, then instilling 2 L of fresh dialysate into the peritoneal cavity, where it dwells for 4–6 hours). The use of continuous-cycler peritoneal dialysis or automated peritoneal dialysis (APD) is becoming more prevalent. These modalities perform a number of exchanges using shorter dwell times during the night, allowing the patient to be free during the day. Often, the patient will receive an extra exchange during the day to enhance the adequacy of dialysis. For peritoneal dialysis, intraperitoneal (IP) antibiotic administration can be used to load, maintain, or reduce plasma levels. Dosing of IP antibiotics can be done once daily (intermittent dosing) or in each exchange (continuous dosing). For intermittent dosing, the dialysis solution that has the antibiotic added must dwell for at least 6 hours to insure adequate systemic absorption. Data support the contention that intermittent dosing is as effective as continuous dosing.[56] Heparin and insulin, which are common IP additives, do not affect the activity or stability of IP antibiotics.[57] The factors affecting peritoneal drug clearance are listed in **Box 2**. IP dosing guidelines for commonly used antibiotics used in CAPD are found in **Table 4**, and IV dosing and supplementation are described in **Table 1**.[41,57,58] In treating peritonitis, IP dosing is often preferred to IV dosing because IP absorption is increased when using many antibiotics for patients who have peritonitis, and higher IP antibiotic levels are achieved.[59] In contrast to CAPD, antibiotic dosing in APD has been less well studied. The use of shorter, more frequent exchanges in APD raises the concern of inadequate time for absorption to achieve therapeutic levels when using IP administration. Based on a randomized study that included children on APD, intermittent dosing of vancomycin in

---

Box 2
Factors affecting peritoneal dialysis drug clearance

Drug properties

   Molecular weight

   Charge

   Lipid or water solubility

   V_d (tissue binding)

   Protein binding

   Other forms of steric hindrance

   Rapid excretion by another pathway

   Red cell partitioning

Intrinsic peritoneal membrane properties

   Surface blood flow

   Surface area

   Location

   Sclerosis

   Pore size

   Vascular disease

   Fluid films

Dialysate properties

   Flow rate

   Volume

   Chemical composition

   Distribution

   Temperature

Miscellaneous properties

   Ultrafiltration

   Clearance-raising additives

Data from Golper TA. Drugs and peritoneal dialysis. Dial Transplant 1979;8:41–3.

a long dwell is as effective as when it is administered in CAPD.[60] However a shorter dosing interval of 4 to 5 days is recommended to maintain serum trough levels that are greater than 15 μg/mL. Monitoring levels more frequently may be appropriate in the presence of residual renal function.

There is an inverse semilogarithmic relationship between peritoneal clearance and molecular weight. For most drugs, the peritoneal clearance of the unbound drug can be calculated by multiplying the urea clearance (20 mL/min) by the ratio of the square root of the weight of urea (60 Da) over the square root of the antibiotic's molecular weight. Charged antibiotics diffuse more slowly than neutral ones. As a rule, drugs that are not removed by hemodialysis are also not cleared by peritoneal dialysis.[61]

PERITONEAL DIALYSIS IN ACUTE RENAL FAILURE

Acute peritoneal dialysis may have variable dwell times, from no dwell time to 6 hours (similar to CAPD). In the setting of long dwell times (4–6 hours), the guidelines in **Table 4** cited should be appropriate for determining antibiotic dosing. In the setting of short dwell times, IP dosing may not be cost effective or as predictable in delivering or removing the antibiotic from the blood. In the critical care setting, multiple factors, such as hypotension or hypoperfusion of the mesenteric circulation, ileus, peristalsis, and dialysate temperature, may adversely affect clearance.[62,63] In patients receiving acute peritoneal dialysis with short dwells, it is recommended to administer antibiotics intravenously and exploit the peritoneal dialysis as a means of clearing the drug to allow trough levels to develop. As with any CRRT, continuous administration, whether IV or IP, can result in the absence of safe trough levels, with potential antibiotic-related toxicity. Because the number of exchanges per day (and hence, the degree of antibiotic clearance achieved) may change frequently in the critical care setting, it is important to communicate closely with the nephrologist to appropriately adjust antibiotic loading, maintenance, and removal based on the amount of dialysis being prescribed.

ADVERSE EFFECTS OF ANTIBACTERIAL AGENTS IN RENAL FAILURE

Numerous adverse effects have been reported as resulting from the use of antibacterial agents in patients who have renal failure. Many of these effects are related to inappropriate dosing, whereas others stem from pathologic changes associated with uremia. A review of this topic has been published by Manian and colleagues.[64]

Neurologic toxicity, including psychosis, visual and auditory hallucinations, myoclonus, and seizures has been reported as the result of the use of penicillin, imipenem, beta-lactams, acyclovir, amantadine, and quinolones.[65–68] Ototoxicity in the form of reversible auditory dysfunction can result from high dosages of erythromycin.[69] It remains unclear whether renal failure is an independent risk factor for aminoglycoside- or vancomycin-induced ototoxicity. Sulfonamide-induced hypoglycemia is believed to be the result of the structural similarity of sulfamethoxazole and hypoglycemic agents. Sulfamethoxazole may stimulate insulin secretion and can displace oral hypoglycemic agents from serum proteins, making more free drug available.[70,71] This interaction can be further exacerbated by the decreased clearance and protein binding of sulfamethoxazole in uremia. Platelet aggregation abnormalities induced by high doses of penicillins exacerbate the platelet dysfunction of uremia and vitamin K deficiency, and augment the effect of heparin when patients are on hemodialysis.[72–74] Renal failure does not appear to be an independent risk factor for the coagulopathy associated with cephalosporins containing the N-methyl-thiotetrazole side chain; vitamin K deficiency, which is

Table 4
Intraperitoneal antibiotic dosing guidelines for CAPD. Dosing of drugs with renal clearance in patients with residual renal function (defined as >100 mL/day urine output): dose should be empirically increased by 25%

Antibiotic	Intermittent (per Exchange, Once Daily)	Continuous (mg/L, All Exchanges)
Aminoglycosides		
Amikacin	2 mg/kg	LD 25, MD 12
Gentamicin	0.6 mg/kg	LD 8, MD4
Netilmicin	0.6 mg/kg	LD 8, MD 4
Tobramycin	0.6 mg/kg	LD 8, MD 4
Cephalosporins		
Cefazolin	15 mg/kg	LD 500, MD 125
Cefepime	1 g	LD 500, MD 125
Cephalothin	15 mg/kg	LD 500, MD 125
Cephradine	15 mg/kg	LD 500, MD 125
Ceftazidime	1000–1500 mg	LD 500, MD 125
Ceftizoxime	1000 mg	LD 250, MD 125
Penicillins		
Azlocillin	ND	LD 500, MD 250
Ampicillin	ND	MD 125
Oxacillin	ND	MD 125
Nafcillin	ND	MD 125
Amoxacillin	ND	LD 250–500, MD 50
Penicillin G	ND	LD 50,000 units, MD 25,000 units
Quinolones		
Ciprofloxacin	ND	LD 50, MD 25
Others		
Vancomycin	15–30 mg/kg every 5–7 days	LD 1000, MD 25
Aztreonam	ND	LD 1000, MD 250
Antifungals		
Amphotericin	NA	1.5
Combinations		
Ampicillin/sulbactam	2 g every 12 h	LD 1000, MD 100
Imipenem/cilistatin	1 g b.i.d.	LD 500, MD 200
Quinupristin/dalfopristin	25 mg/L in alternate bags*	

Abbreviations: b.i.d., two times per day; LD, loading dose, in mg; MD, maintenance dose, in mg; NA, not applicable; ND, no data.
  • Given in conjunction with 500 mg intravenous twice daily.
  From Piraino B, Bailie GR, Bernardini J, et al. Peritoneal dialysis-related infections recommendations: 2005 update. Peritoneal Dialysis International 2005;25:107–31; with permission.

often present in renal failure, seems to be the culprit.[75] The fluoroquinolones have been associated with increased risk for spontaneous Achilles tendon rupture in patients who have underlying renal failure.[76] The tetracycline antibiotics (with the exception of doxycyline) should be avoided in patients who have renal insufficiency because there has been an increased incidence of hepatotoxicity. Rarely, acute fatty necrosis of the liver can occur in patients who have underlying renal dysfunction.[77]

REFERENCES

1. Aronoff GR, Abel SR. Principles of administering drugs to patients with renal failure. In: Brenner BM, Stein JH, editors. Contemporary issues in nephrology. New York: Churchill-Livingstone; 1986. p. 77–82.
2. Hurwitz A. Antacid therapy in drug kinetics. Clin Pharm 1977;12:269–80.
3. Aronoff G, Bennett W, Berns J, et al. Drug prescribing in renal failure, dosing guidelines for adults. 5th edition. Philadelphia: American College of Physicians; 2007.
4. Reindenberg MM. The biotransformation of drugs in renal failure. Am J Med 1977; 62:482–5.
5. Cockcroft DW, Gault MH. Prediction of creatinine clearance from serum creatinine. Nephron 1976;16:31–41.
6. Pesola GR, Akhavan I, Madu A, et al. Prediction equation estimates of creatinine clearance in the intensive care unit. Intensive Care Med 1993;19:39–43.
7. Devine BJ. Gentamicin pharmacokinetics. Drug Intell Clin Pharm 1974;8:650–5.
8. Levey AS, Bosch JP, Lewis JB, et al. A more accurate method to estimate glomerular filtration rate from serum creatinine: a new prediction equation. Modification of Diet in Renal Disease Study Group. Ann Intern Med 1999;130:461–70.
9. Levey AS, Coresh J, Greene T, et al. Expressing the MDRD study equation for estimating GFR with IDMS traceable (gold standard) serum creatinine values [abstract]. J Am Soc Nephrol 2005;16:69A.
10. Stevens LA, Coresh J, Greene T, et al. Assessing kidney function—measured and estimated glomerular filtration rate. N Engl J Med 2006;354:2473–83.
11. Mathew TH, Johnson DW, Jones G. Chronic kidney disease and automatic reporting of estimated glomerular filtration rate: revised recommendations. Med J Aust 2007;187:459–63.
12. Froissart M, Rossert J, Jacquot C, et al. Predictive performance of the modification of diet in renal disease and Cockcroft-Gault equations for estimating renal function. J Am Soc Nephrol 2005;16:763–73.
13. Sher PP. Drug interferences with clinical laboratory tests. Drugs 1982;24: 24–63.
14. Sandburg T, Trollfors B. Effect of trimethoprim on serum creatinine in patients with acute cystitis. J Antimicrob Chemother 1986;17:123–4.
15. Harrington D, Drusano G, Smalls V, et al. False elevations of serum creatinine. JAMA 1984;252:2962–4.
16. Sherman RA, Eisenger RP, Weinstein MP, et al. Cefoxitin-induced pseudo acute renal failure. Clin Ther 1981;4:114–7.
17. Demczar DJ, Nafziger AN, Bertino JS. Pharmacokinetics of gentamicin at traditional versus high doses: implications for once-daily aminoglycoside dosing. Antimicrobial Agents Chemother 1997;41:1115–9.
18. Lacy MK, Nicolau DP, Nightingale CH, et al. The pharmacodynamics of aminoglycosides. Clin Infect Dis 1998;27:23–7.
19. Chuck SK, Raber SR, Rodvold KA, et al. National survey of extended-interval aminoglycoside dosing. Clin Infect Dis 2000;30:433–9.
20. Guiliano RA, Verpooten GA, DeBroe ME. The effect of dosing strategy on kidney cortical accumulation of aminoglycosides in rats. Am J Kidney Dis 1986;8:292–6.

21. Tam VH, Kabbara S, Vo G, et al. Comparative pharmacodynamics of gentamicin against *Staphylococcus aureus* and *Pseudomonas aeruginosa*. Antimicrobial Agents Chemother 2006;50:2626–31.
22. Edson RS, Terrell CL. The aminoglycosides. Mayo Clin Proc 1999;74:519–28.
23. Hatala R, Dinh T, CooK DJ. Once-daily aminoglycoside dosing in immunocompetent adults: a meta-analysis. Ann Intern Med 1996;124:717–25.
24. Freeman CD, Nicolau DP, Belliveau PP, et al. Once-daily dosing of aminoglycosides: review and recommendations for clinical practice. J Antimicrob Chemother 1997;39:677–86.
25. Rybak MJ, Abate BJ, Kang SL, et al. Prospective evaluation of the effect of an aminoglycoside dosing regimen on rates of observed nephrotoxicity and ototoxicity. Antimicrobial Agents Chemother 1999;43:1549–55.
26. Nicolau DP, Freeman CD, Belliveau PP, et al. Experience with a once-daily aminoglycoside program administered to 2,184 adult patients. Antimicrobial Agents Chemother 1995;39:650–5.
27. CDC, recommendations for preventing the spread of vancomycin resistance. MMWR 1994;44(RR-12):1–13.
28. Stryjewski ME, Szczech LA, Benjamin DK, et al. Use of vancomycin or first-generation cephalosporins for the treatment of hemodialysis-dependent patients with methicillin susceptible *Staphylococcus aureus* bacteremia. Clin Infect Dis 2007; 44:190–6.
29. Sowinski KM, Mueller BA, Grabe DW, et al. Cefazolin dialytic clearance by high-efficiency and high-flux hemodialyzers. Am J Kidney Dis 2001;37:766–76.
30. Fogel MA, Nussbaum PB, Feintzeig ID, et al. Cefazolin in chronic hemodialysis patients: a safe, effective alternative to vancomycin. Am J Kidney Dis 1998;32:401–9.
31. Kuypers D, Vanwalleghem J, Maes B, et al. Cefazolin serum concentrations with fixed intravenous dosing in patients on chronic hemodialysis treatment. Nephrol Dial Transplant 1999;14:2050–1.
32. Geraci JE, Hermans PE. Vancomycin. Mayo Clin Proc 1983;58:88–91.
33. Ackerman BH, Vannier AM, Eudy EB. Analysis of vancomycin time-kill studies with *Staphylococcus* species by using a curve stripping program to describe the relationship between concentration and pharmacodynamic response. Antimicrobial Agents Chemother 1992;36:1766–9.
34. Tenover FC, Moellering RC. The rationale for revising the Clinical and Laboratory Standards Institute vancomycin minimal inhibitory concentration interpretive criteria for *Staphylococcus aureus*. Clin Infect Dis 2007;44:1208–15.
35. Rybak M, Lomaestro B, Rotschafer JC, et al. Therapeutic monitoring of vancomycin in adult patients: a consensus review of the American Society of Health-System Pharmacists, the Infectious Disease Society of America, and the Society of Infectious Diseases Pharmacists. Am J Health Syst Pharm 2009; 66:82–98.
36. Freeman CD, Quintiliani R, Nightingale CH. Vancomycin therapeutic drug monitoring: is it necessary? Ann Pharmacother 1993;27:594–8.
37. Saunders NJ. Vancomycin administration and monitoring reappraisal. J Antimicrob Chemother 1995;36:279–82.
38. Hammett-Stabler CA, Johns T. Laboratory guidelines for monitoring of antimicrobial drugs. Clin Chem 1998;44:1129–40.
39. Tobin CM, Darville JM, Thomson AH, et al. Vancomycin therapeutic drug monitoring: is there a consensus view? J Antimicrob Chemother 2002;50:713–8.
40. Raveh D, Kopyt M, Hite Y, et al. Risk factors for nephrotoxicity in elderly patients receiving once-daily aminoglycosides. QJM 2002;95:291–7.

41. Golper TA, Bennett WM. Drug usage in dialysis patients. In: Nissenson R, Fine RN, Gentile DE, editors. Clinical dialysis. 2nd edition. 2. Norwalk (CT): Appleton and Lange; 1990. p. 608–30.
42. Vanholder R, DeSmet R, Glorieux G, et al. Review on uremic toxins: classification, concentration, and interindividual variability. Kidney Int 2003;63:1934–43.
43. Marx MA, Frye RF, Matzke GR, et al. Cefazolin as empiric therapy in hemodialysis-related infections: efficacy and blood concentrations. Am J Kidney Dis 1998;32:410–4.
44. Barth RH, DeVincenzo N, Zara AC, et al. Vancomycin pharmacokinetics in high-flux hemodialysis [abstract]. J Am Soc Nephrol 1990;1:348.
45. Barth RH, DeVincenzo N. Use of vancomycin in high-flux hemodialysis: experience with 130 courses of therapy. Kidney Int 1996;50:929–36.
46. Foote EF, Dreitlein WB, Steward CA, et al. Pharmacokinetics of vancomycin when administered during high flux hemodialysis. Clin Nephrol 1998;50:51–5.
47. Mason NA, Neudeck BL, Welage LS, et al. Comparison of 3 vancomycin dosage regimens during hemodialysis with cellulose triacetate dialyzers: post-dialysis versus intradialytic administration. Clin Nephrol 2003;60:96–104.
48. Maher JF. Pharmacokinetics in patients with renal failure. Clin Nephrol 1984;21: 39–46.
49. Maher JF. Principles of dialysis and dialysis of drugs. Am J Med 1977;62: 475–81.
50. Kucers A, Crowe SM, Grayson ML, et al. The use of antibiotics: a clinical review of antibacterial, antifungal and antiviral drugs. London: Hodder Arnold; 1997.
51. Golper TA, Wedel SK, Kaplen AA, et al. Drug removal during continuous arteriovenous hemofiltration: theory and clinical observations. Int J Artif Organs 1985;8: 307–12.
52. Golper TA. Drug removal during continuous renal replacement therapy. In: Rose BD, editor. Nephrology up-to-date, vol.6.3. Wellesley (MA); 1998.
53. Vincent HH, Vos MC, Akcahuseyin E, et al. Drug clearance by continuous hemodialfiltration (CAVHD). Analysis of sieving coefficients of diffusions. Blood Purif 1993;11:99–107.
54. Sigler MH, Teehan BP, Van Valkenbrugh D. Solute transport in continuous hemodialysis. A new treatment for acute renal failure. Kidney Int 1987;32:562–71.
55. Golper TA. Update on drug sieving coefficients and dosing adjustments during continuous renal replacement therapies. Contrib Nephrol 2001;132:349–53.
56. Wiggins KJ, Johnson DW, Craig JC, et al. Treatment of peritoneal dialysis-associated peritonitis: a systematic review of randomized controlled trials. Am J Kidney Dis 2007;50(6):967–88.
57. Sewell DL, Golper TA, Brown SD, et al. Stability of single and combination antimicrobial agents in various peritoneal dialysates in the presence of heparin and insulin. Am J Kidney Dis 1983;3:209–12.
58. Golper TA. Drugs and peritoneal dialysis. Dial Transplant 1979;8:41–3.
59. Piraino B, Bailie GR, Bernardini J, et al. Peritoneal dialysis-related infections recommendations: 2005 update. Perit Dial Int 2005;25(2):107–30.
60. Schaefer F, Klaus G, Muller-Wiefel DE, et al. Intermittent versus continuous intraperitoneal glycopeptide/ceftazidime treatment in children with peritoneal dialysis-associated peritonitis. J Am Soc Nephrol 1999;10(1):136–45.
61. Lasrich M, Maher JM, Hirszel P, et al. Correlation of peritoneal transport rates with molecular weight: a method for predicting clearances. ASAIO J 1979;2:107–13.
62. Gross M, McDonald HP. Effect of dialysate temperature and flow rate of peritoneal clearance. JAMA 1967;202:363–6.

63. Nolph KD, Popovich RP, Ghods AJ, et al. Determinants of low clearances of small solutes during peritoneal dialysis. Kidney Int 1978;13:117–23.
64. Manian F, Stone W, Alford R. Adverse antibiotic effects associated with renal insufficiency. Rev Infect Dis 1990;12:236–49.
65. Calandra G, Lydic E, Carrigan J, et al. Factors predisposing to seizures in seriously ill infected patients receiving antibiotics: experience with imipenem/cilastatin. Am J Med 1988;84:911–8.
66. Ing TS, Daugirdas JT, Soung LS, et al. Toxic effects of amantadine in patients with renal failure. Can Med Assoc J 1979;120:695–8.
67. Oldstone MB, Nelson E. Central nervous system manifestations of penicillin toxicity in man. Neurology 1966;16:693–700.
68. Wright AJ. The penicillins. Mayo Clin Proc 1999;74:290–307.
69. Kroboth PD, McNeil MA, Kreeger A, et al. Hearing loss and erythromycin pharmacokinetics in a patient receiving hemodialysis. Arch Intern Med 1983;143:1263–5.
70. Frankel MC, Leslie BR, Sax FL, et al. Trimethoprim-sulfamethoxazole–related hypoglycemia in a patient with renal failure. N Y State J Med 1984;84:30–1.
71. Lawson DH, Paice BJ. Adverse reactions to trimethoprim-sulfamethoxazole. Rev Infect Dis 1982;4:429–33.
72. Andrassy K, Scherz M, Ritz E, et al. Penicillin-induced coagulation disorder. Lancet 1976;2:1039–41.
73. McClure PD, Casserly JG, Monsier C, et al. Carbenicillin-induced bleeding disorder. Lancet 1970;2:1307–8.
74. Stuart JJ. Ticarcillin-induced hemorrhage in a patient with thrombocytosis. Southampt Med J 1980;73:1084–5.
75. Cohen H, Scott SD, Mackie IJ, et al. The development of hypoprothrombinaemia following antibiotic therapy in malnourished patients with low serum vitamin K1 levels. Br J Haemotol 1988;68:63–6.
76. Linden PD, Sturkenboom MC, Herings RM, et al. Increased risk of achilles tendon rupture with quinolone antibacterial use, especially in elderly patients taking oral corticosteroids. Arch Intern Med 2003;163:1801–7.
77. Smilack JD. The tetracyclines. Mayo Clin Proc 1999;74:727–9.

Strategies and New Developments in the Management of Bacterial Meningitis

Justine Miranda, MD[a], Allan R. Tunkel, MD, PhD[b],*

KEYWORDS

- Bacterial meningitis • Cerebrospinal fluid
- Antimicrobial therapy • Blood-brain barrier
- Antimicrobial resistance

Despite significant advances in the management of bacterial meningitis over the past few decades, the disease continues to have a high mortality rate, with long-term neurologic sequelae developing in many survivors.[1–3] Childhood immunization programs have proved effective in prevention,[4] with declines in the incidence of bacterial meningitis caused by *Haemophilus influenzae* type b and in invasive pneumococcal disease.[5,6] This changing epidemiology and the emergence of resistant organisms present continued challenges to therapy.[7,8] Recent retrospective reviews suggested that despite the widespread decline in invasive pneumococcal disease after use of the heptavalent pneumococcal conjugate vaccine, there is emergence of cases of pneumococcal meningitis caused by serotype strains that are not in the vaccine.[9,10] These challenges drive the need for continuing research and development of new strategies for the management of this devastating disease.

Success in the treatment of patients with bacterial meningitis and the development of improved strategies for disease management rely on knowledge of key pharmacologic principles for use of antimicrobial agents that are efficacious in the unique environment of the cerebrospinal fluid (CSF), including penetration of the drug across the blood-brain barrier (BBB), activity of the drug in purulent CSF, and the intrinsic pharmacodynamic properties of the drug.[11] Our understanding of the efficacy of antimicrobial agents in bacterial meningitis relies largely on their use in experimental animal models, particularly the rabbit model, which uses an intracisternal method of organism inoculation and sampling of CSF.[1,12] In this article, we review the principles of use of

[a] Department of Internal Medicine, Division of Infectious Diseases, Baystate Medical Center, 759 Chestnut Street, Springfield, MA 01199, USA
[b] Department of Internal Medicine, Monmouth Medical Center, 300 Second Avenue, Long Branch, NJ 07740, USA
* Corresponding author.
E-mail address: atunkel@sbhcs.com (A.R. Tunkel).

Infect Dis Clin N Am 23 (2009) 925–943
doi:10.1016/j.idc.2009.06.014
0891-5520/09/$ – see front matter © 2009 Elsevier Inc. All rights reserved.

id.theclinics.com

antimicrobial agents in the therapy of bacterial meningitis and summarize recent experimental and clinical data in the use of new antimicrobial agents.

PRINCIPLES OF ANTIMICROBIAL THERAPY
CSF Penetration

The penetration of antimicrobials across the BBB and into the CSF is the first determinant in the ability of the drug to treat bacterial meningitis effectively. The environment of the CSF is unique, and pharmacokinetic parameters are different in this compartment than in other areas of the body. Antimicrobial agents are generally not significantly metabolized in the CSF, and concentrations of most drugs primarily depend on penetration and elimination through the BBB.[13]

The microanatomy of the central nervous system (CNS) contributes to the distinct nature of the CSF environment. The presence of tight junctions and the absence of intracytoplasmic pinocytic vesicles in the microvascular endothelium of the cerebral capillaries limit the amount of drug transport into the subarachnoid space. An active transport system in the choroid plexus also eliminates compounds (eg, penicillins, cephalosporins, aminoglycosides, and fluoroquinolones) from the CSF and into the blood. A different active transport system that is present in the cerebral capillaries transports penicillins and cephalosporins from the blood to the CSF, although its low drug affinity and capacity limit its ability to transport significant drug concentrations into the CSF.[14,15]

In inflamed meninges, inflammatory cytokines act to damage and separate the tight junctions and increase the number of pinocytotic vesicles in the endothelial cells of the BBB, which enhances drug entry into the CSF.[16] These inflammatory cytokines also inhibit drug elimination by the choroid plexus system, which leads to further accumulation of agents in the CSF. These mechanisms are most important in the penetration of antimicrobial agents, such as vancomycin and β-lactams, that would otherwise not achieve adequate CSF concentrations as a result of dependence on entry through tight junctions.[13] Agents that reduce meningeal inflammation, such as dexamethasone, have been shown to decrease drug permeability into CSF in experimental animal models.[17–19] As meningeal inflammation subsides during treatment of meningitis, antimicrobial entry also decreases, indicating that appropriate antimicrobial dosages should be sustained throughout the course of therapy of meningitis to maintain adequate CSF concentrations.[1]

Intrinsic drug characteristics that determine CSF penetration are as follows:[11,14,20]

1. Lipid solubility. The ability of lipophilic agents, such as the fluoroquinolones, chloramphenicol, rifampin and sulfonamides, to enter the CSF via passive diffusion down a concentration gradient allows them to reach peak CSF concentrations more rapidly, maintain adequate CSF concentrations, and reach CSF half-lives similar to those in serum, regardless of the presence or absence of meningeal inflammation. Hydrophilic agents, such as β-lactams and vancomycin, have poor penetration and delayed onset of peak CSF concentrations because of their dependence on the opening of tight junctions for entry.
2. Molecular weight. The low molecular weight and simple structure of some drugs, such as the fluoroquinolones and rifampin, correlate with improved CSF penetration compared with larger compounds with more complex structures, such as vancomycin.
3. Ionization. In bacterial meningitis, the pH of CSF is lower than that of plasma, and antibiotics with high ionization have poor CSF penetration. β-lactam antibiotics, which are weak acids and highly ionized in the physiologic pH of plasma, have

poor penetration into the CSF and tend to pass from the CSF into the plasma instead of in the reverse direction.

4. Protein binding. Only unbound fractions of antimicrobials enter the CSF; a high degree of protein binding in the serum (eg, with ceftriaxone) limits the degree of CSF penetration.

The percent penetration of individual antimicrobial agents into CSF can be assessed in several ways. Because the concentration time curve of drugs in the CSF lags behind that in the serum, assessment of penetration by simultaneous sampling of serum and CSF concentrations can yield inaccurate results.[21] The ratio of the area under the concentration curve in the CSF to that in serum is a more accurate assessment than measuring peak concentrations in serum and CSF; however, this method is not feasible in human studies because it requires multiple sampling of the CSF and serum.[13] Most available data use concentration ratios, but this method should be considered to provide only an approximation of percent penetration because of differences in drug delivery, timing of sampling, and underlying differences among patients.

Activity in Purulent CSF

The activity of the drugs in the purulent CSF of bacterial meningitis is a second determinant of its efficacy. The following factors contribute to drug activity:[1,11,12,20]

1. CSF pH. Accumulation of lactate in bacterial meningitis decreases CSF pH, which inhibits the activity of certain drugs, such as the aminoglycosides. Clarithromycin, which in one experimental study exhibited good in vitro activity against a pneumococcal strain, was found to have no bactericidal activity in the CSF of test animals, possibly because of a substantial increase in the minimal bactericidal concentration (MBC) of clarithromycin in the acidic environment of CSF.[22]

2. CSF protein concentration. Elevated protein concentrations in purulent CSF may diminish the amount of free drug available for microbial killing.

3. Bacterial growth. A slower bacterial generation time in CSF compared with maximal growth rates in vitro may reduce the bactericidal effects of drugs such as β-lactams, which rely on bacterial growth for optimal bactericidal activity.

4. Metabolism. Some antimicrobial agents undergo metabolism to compounds with different antimicrobial activity. For example, cephalothin is converted in vivo to desacetylcephalothin, which is less active than the parent compound. In contrast, cefotaxime is metabolized in vivo to desacetylcefotaxime, which has equal activity compared with its parent compound.

5. Synergy and antagonism. Some drug combinations may act synergistically when coadministered, such as penicillin or ampicillin with gentamicin in *Listeria monocytogenes* meningitis, ampicillin plus mecillinam in *Escherichia coli* meningitis, and ampicillin plus gentamicin against *Streptococcus agalactiae*. Recent experimental studies also found synergy between levofloxacin and either ceftriaxone or cefotaxime in a rabbit model of pneumococcal meningitis.[23,24] On the other hand, antagonism has been demonstrated when bactericidal agents are coadministered with a bacteriostatic agent, such as chloramphenicol with either penicillin or gentamicin.

6. Inoculum effect. High bacterial loads can be found in the CSF in bacterial meningitis, with bacterial concentrations of 10^8 CFU/mL or more. In this environment, the minimal inhibitory concentration (MIC) of some antimicrobial agents against specific micro-organisms may increase dramatically, a phenomenon called the inoculum effect.[25,26]

Mode of Administration

The third determinant of success for an antimicrobial agent in bacterial meningitis is the mode of administration of the drug, whether by intermittent or continuous intravenous administration.[20] Although the standard clinical practice is intermittent administration, which leads to higher peak CSF concentrations, this method may not maintain concentrations above the MBC for the entire dosing interval. On the other hand, continuous infusion allows maintenance above the MBC during nearly 100% of the dosing interval, although a lower peak CSF concentration is attained.[11] The mode of administration has been a concept of considerable debate, but a recent meta-analysis of randomized controlled trials involving severe infections mainly outside the CNS showed that fewer clinical failures were seen in infections treated with continuous intravenous infusion of antibiotics that act by time-dependent killing (eg, β-lactams) and even with aminoglycosides that exhibit concentration-dependent killing.[27]

Antimicrobial Pharmacodynamics in CSF

The fourth and final determinant of response to antimicrobial therapy in bacterial meningitis is pharmacodynamics, which is concerned with the antimicrobial effect of drug concentrations in a particular site of infection over time. Knowledge of the pharmacodynamic properties of antimicrobials allows for appropriate optimization of bactericidal drug concentrations.[14] Bacterial killing is particularly important in the CSF, in which there is a decreased immune response from relatively lower concentrations of antibody and complement and inefficient phagocytosis.[12]

Antibiotics may exhibit ether time-dependent or concentration-dependent killing. Time-dependent antimicrobial activity, demonstrated by the β-lactam antibiotics and vancomycin, depends on the time that the drug concentration in CSF is above the MBC (T > MBC). An experimental study of cephalosporin-resistant pneumococcal meningitis showed that the T > MBC was the most important single determinant of ceftriaxone efficacy and correlated best with the bacterial kill rate;[28] a direct linear relationship was found between T > MBC and the bacterial killing rate. Aminoglycosides and fluoroquinolones exhibit concentration-dependent killing,[29,30] although fluoroquinolones, particularly trovafloxacin and gatifloxacin, have been shown to have features of time-dependent killing, in which the T > MBC was also considered a factor in bacterial killing.[31,32] The efficacy of concentration-dependent killing depends on attaining high peak CSF concentrations and a prolonged recovery period, or a postantibiotic effect, once the antibiotic concentration falls to below the MIC.

SELECTED ANTIMICROBIAL AGENTS IN THE TREATMENT OF BACTERIAL MENINGITIS

Most clinical trials of antimicrobial agents in patients with bacterial meningitis have compared new agents with standard therapy, although most of these standard agents have not been completely studied themselves, and no placebo-controlled studies exist in humans. Much of what we know is based on studies in experimental animal models, which have been used to develop guidelines for treatment recommendations (**Table 1**) and to determine optimal dosages of agents that achieve adequate CSF concentrations for bactericidal activity (**Table 2**).[33] The most commonly used class of antimicrobial agents in the treatment of bacterial meningitis have been the β-lactams, especially penicillin G and ampicillin, which have proved to be effective against a wide variety of meningeal pathogens. These agents are well tolerated and generally attain CSF concentrations well above the MIC of sensitive pathogens when administered at high doses. The emergence of penicillin resistance in specific meningeal pathogens has led to the use of other β-lactam agents, including third-generation

Table 1

Recommendations for specific antimicrobial therapy in bacterial meningitis based on isolated pathogen and in vitro susceptibility testing

Microorganism	Standard Therapy	Alternative Therapies
Streptococcus pneumoniae		
Penicillin MIC <0.1 µg/mL	Penicillin G or ampicillin	Third-generation cephalosporin;[a] chloramphenicol
Penicillin MIC 0.1–1.0 µg/mL[b]	Third-generation cephalosporin[a]	Cefepime; meropenem
Penicillin MIC ≥2.0 µg/mL; or cefotaxime or ceftriaxone MIC ≥1.0 µg/mL	Vancomycin + a third-generation cephalosporin[a,c]	Fluoroquinolone[d]
Neisseria meningitidis		
Penicillin MIC <0.1 µg/mL	Penicillin G or ampicillin	Third-generation cephalosporin;[a] chloramphenicol
Penicillin MIC 0.1–1.0 µg/mL	Third-generation cephalosporin[a]	Chloramphenicol; fluoroquinolone; meropenem
Listeria monocytogenes	Ampicillin or penicillin G[e]	Trimethoprim-sulfamethoxazole
Streptococcus agalactiae	Ampicillin or penicillin G[e]	Third-generation cephalosporin[a]
Escherichia coli and other Enterobacteriaceae[g]	Third-generation cephalosporin	Aztreonam; fluoroquinolone; meropenem; trimethoprim-sulfamethoxazole; ampicillin
Pseudomonas aeruginosa[g]	Cefepime[e] or ceftazidime[e]	Aztreonam;[e] ciprofloxacin;[e] meropenem[e]
Haemophilus influenzae		
β-lactamase-negative	Ampicillin	Third-generation cephalosporin;[a] cefepime; chloramphenicol; fluoroquinolone
β-lactamase-positive	Third-generation cephalosporin[a]	Cefepime; chloramphenicol, fluoroquinolone
Staphylococcus aureus		
Methicillin-susceptible	Nafcillin or oxacillin	Vancomycin; meropenem; linezolid; daptomycin
Methicillin-resistant	Vancomycin[f]	Trimethoprim-sulfamethoxazole; linezolid; daptomycin
Staphylococcus epidermidis	Vancomycin[f]	Linezolid

a Ceftriaxone or cefotaxime.

b Ceftriaxone/cefotaxime susceptible isolates.

c Consider addition of rifampin if ceftriaxone MIC is > 2 µg/mL.

d Moxifloxacin. No clinical data available; if used, many authorities would combine with vancomycin or a third-generation cephalosporin (eg, cefotaxime or ceftriaxone).

e Addition of an aminoglycoside should be considered.

f Consider addition of rifampin.

g Choice of a specific antimicrobial agent must be guided by in vitro susceptibility testing.

Data from Tunkel AR, Hartman BJ, Kaplan SL, et al. Practice guidelines for the management of bacterial meningitis. Clin Infect Dis 2004;39:1267–84.

Table 2
Recommended dosages of antimicrobial therapy in adult patients with bacterial meningitis with normal renal and hepatic function

Antimicrobial Agent	Total Daily Dose (Dosing Interval in Hours)
Amikacin[a]	15 mg/kg (8)
Ampicillin	12 g (4)
Aztreonam	6–8 g (6–8)
Cefepime	6 g (8)
Cefotaxime	8–12 g (4–6)
Ceftazidime	6 g (8)
Ceftriaxone	4 g (12–24)
Chloramphenicol	4–6 g (6)[b]
Ciprofloxacin	800–1200 mg (8–12)
Gentamicin[a]	5 mg/kg (8)
Meropenem	6 g (8)
Moxifloxacin	400 mg (24)[c]
Nafcillin	9–12 g (4)
Oxacillin	9–12 g (4)
Penicillin G	24 mU (4)
Rifampin	600 mg (24)
Tobramycin[a]	5 mg/kg (8)
Trimethoprim-sulfamethoxazole[d]	10–20 mg/kg (6–12)
Vancomycin[e]	30–60 mg/kg (8–12)

[a] Need to monitor peak and trough serum concentrations.
[b] Higher dose recommended for patients with pneumococcal meningitis.
[c] No data on optimal dosage needed in patients with bacterial meningitis.
[d] Dosage based on trimethoprim component.
[e] Maintain serum trough concentrations of 15–20 µg/mL; one study administered vancomycin as a continuous infusion at a total daily dose of 60 mg/kg (see text for details).[64]

Data from Tunkel AR, Hartman BJ, Kaplan SL, et al. Practice guidelines for the management of bacterial meningitis. Clin Infect Dis 2004;39:1267–84.

cephalosporins and carbapenems. Some organisms also have been difficult to eradicate with standard therapy, necessitating use of alternative agents in selected patients. The following sections review antimicrobial agents that have been studied in experimental animals and patients with bacterial meningitis, with a focus on newer drugs.

Cephalosporins

The cephalosporins, specifically third-generation agents, are integral in the treatment of bacterial meningitis and are the standard of therapy for meningitis caused by pneumococcal and meningococcal strains previously defined as being of intermediate susceptibility to penicillin (MIC 0.1–1 µg/mL).[33] Past clinical trials have clearly demonstrated the superiority of third-generation cephalosporins to chloramphenicol and second-generation cephalosporins (ie, cefuroxime) in the treatment of bacterial meningitis.[34,35] A recent noninferiority trial of 308 patients with confirmed epidemic meningococcal meningitis in Africa supported the use of ceftriaxone as an alternative to intramuscular oily chloramphenicol for short-course therapy.[36] Ceftazidime is a third-generation cephalosporin effective in the therapy of *Pseudomonas aeruginosa* meningitis[37,38] and experimental *Klebsiella pneumoniae* meningitis.[39] A recent study of 25 cases of culture-proven *P aeruginosa* meningitis in Taiwan determined a ceftazidime susceptibility rate of 91.7%.[40]

Cefepime is a fourth-generation cephalosporin with a broad antimicrobial spectrum that was found in early experimental animal models to be effective against a variety of meningeal pathogens, including *S pneumoniae, Streptococcus agalactiae, E coli, K pneumoniae,* and *P aeruginosa.*[41] It also has been used successfully in the treatment of meningitis caused by *Enterobacter aerogenes.*[42] Its efficacy against penicillin-resistant *S pneumoniae* was previously elucidated in two experimental studies using the rabbit model. One of these studies showed that the superior bacterial killing of cefepime compared with ceftriaxone was statistically significant in vivo despite similar antimicrobial activity in vitro. Cefepime monotherapy was also proven to be as effective as the combination of vancomycin plus ceftriaxone against penicillin-resistant *S pneumoniae* isolates with induced fluoroquinolone resistance.[43] Cefepime had similar bacterial killing rates to that of vancomycin and ceftriaxone in vivo, although the fluoroquinolone-resistant strain was killed more slowly by cefepime and ceftriaxone compared with the parent fluoroquinolone-susceptible strain.[44]

A study in hospitalized patients that compared cefepime with ceftriaxone against *S pneumoniae* verified the superior pharmacodynamics of cefepime by determining the pharmacodynamic profiles of ceftriaxone and cefepime in the CSF and serum of hospitalized patients with external ventricular drains.[45] The probability of ceftriaxone achieving 50% and 100% T > MIC in CSF was less than 80%, whereas cefepime had a more than 90% and 82% probability of achieving 50% and 100% T > MIC, respectively, in the CSF against *S pneumoniae.* Although ceftriaxone had a low probability of providing adequate exposure in CSF for *S pneumoniae* strains with MIC values more than 0.03 µg/mL, cefepime had a high probability of ensuring adequate exposure for MIC values up to 0.5 µg/mL. These data are favorable for cefepime, although the model was derived from noninflamed meninges in patients with hydrocephalus. In the setting of pediatric meningitis in Latin America, cefepime was shown to be clinically effective and to have comparable activity to ceftriaxone and cefotaxime,[46] which indicates that cefepime is an important therapeutic option in the empiric treatment of pediatric bacterial meningitis.

Carbapenems

The carbapenems that have been studied for use in bacterial meningitis are imipenem, ertapenem, and meropenem. Imipenem has been shown to be effective in pneumococcal meningitis caused by penicillin- and cephalosporin-resistant strains; however, given its potential for seizure activity (up to 33% in one study),[47] it is not recommended for use in therapy for bacterial meningitis.[33] Ertapenem lacks in vitro activity against *P aeruginosa* and *Enterococcus* species, although it has a broad antimicrobial spectrum and was found to be effective in an experimental study of pneumococcal meningitis in rabbits caused by penicillin-sensitive (MIC 0.03 µg/mL) and penicillin-resistant (MIC 0.5 µg/mL) strains.[48,49] During the entire treatment period, ertapenem achieved CSF concentrations above the MICs of both strains, denoting sufficient penetration into inflamed meninges, and was successful in sterilizing the CSF in animals with infection caused by penicillin-sensitive and penicillin-resistant strains.

Meropenem has been the most studied carbapenem in patients with bacterial meningitis.[33] It is less neurotoxic and has a lower risk of inducing seizures compared with imipenem, likely because of the less basic C-2 side chain of its chemical structure.[50] Four randomized clinical trials in adults and children compared meropenem to cefotaxime and ceftriaxone in the treatment of bacterial meningitis and demonstrated that meropenem was clinically and microbiologically comparable to cefotaxime and ceftriaxone. Meropenem dosages of 40 mg/kg every 8 hours were used, and rapid CSF sterilization was achieved in all patients in all four study groups (18–36 hours in most patients). Clinical cure was seen in 97% to 100% of patients, and no seizure activity was thought to be related to therapy.[51–53] A recent experimental study in guinea pigs also found a comparable efficacy of meropenem compared with ceftazidime in the treatment of *P aeruginosa* meningitis.[54]

Although the clinical data for meropenem in the treatment of bacterial meningitis are favorable, reports of meropenem resistance in cephalosporin-resistant *S pneumoniae* have become a growing concern,[55] and recent experimental studies have further elucidated the activity of meropenem in penicillin- and cephalosporin-resistant pneumococcal meningitis. A study in rabbits evaluated the therapeutic efficacy of meropenem monotherapy compared with the combination of meropenem plus vancomycin caused by a highly penicillin- and cephalosporin-resistant strain of *S pneumoniae*. In that study, intermediate susceptibility to meropenem was found (MIC 0.5 μg/mL in one strain). Despite administration of meropenem at high doses (125 mg/kg) to maintain adequate CSF concentrations, meropenem monotherapy showed only a bacteriostatic effect on the study strain, with regrowth of the isolate at 24 hours. The addition of vancomycin to meropenem showed a statistically significant improvement in bacteriologic response and was comparable to therapy with ceftriaxone and vancomycin, although synergy was not found.[56] Another recent experimental study used two different animals—the rabbit and guinea pig—to evaluate meropenem therapy in meningitis caused by cephalosporin-susceptible and cephalosporin-resistant *S pneumoniae* strains. There was excellent bactericidal activity against the cephalosporin-susceptible strain in both animal species and against the cephalosporin-resistant strain in guinea pigs, but there was therapeutic failure in the rabbits inoculated with the cephalosporin-resistant strain.[57] That result suggested that meropenem may not be useful as monotherapy in the treatment of pneumococcal meningitis caused by highly penicillin- and cephalosporin-resistant strains.

Glycopeptides

Vancomycin has become important in the treatment of bacterial meningitis in the past decade, particularly as a result of the rise of pneumococcal resistance to penicillin. It is recommended that the empiric therapy of bacterial meningitis in all patients 1 month of age and older include vancomycin combined with a third-generation cephalosporin to treat for the possibility of pneumococcal meningitis caused by highly penicillin- and cephalosporin-resistant strains, pending organism identification and in vitro susceptibility testing.[33] Vancomycin has been found to be synergistic when combined with ceftriaxone in cephalosporin-resistant pneumococcal meningitis[58] and when combined with gentamicin against penicillin-resistant pneumococci in vitro and in a rabbit model of meningitis.[59] Important concerns regarding the use of vancomycin are its diminished CSF penetration in the presence of dexamethasone and the emergence of vancomycin tolerance in some *S pneumoniae* isolates.

Past experimental studies of vancomycin use in pneumococcal meningitis have demonstrated the significantly lower CSF concentrations of vancomycin after administration with dexamethasone compared with vancomycin administration alone.[17,18,60] In humans, two published studies demonstrated conflicting results. The first study of 11 adults with pneumococcal meningitis used vancomycin at a dose of 15 mg/kg/d and revealed low to undetectable CSF vancomycin concentrations after concomitant administration of dexamethasone.[61] In the second study, children with bacterial meningitis were given vancomycin at a dose of 60 mg/kg/d with ceftriaxone and dexamethasone, which resulted in acceptable CSF concentrations of vancomycin.[62] The higher dose administered in the second study may have contributed to the favorable results, as was demonstrated by an experimental study of penicillin- and cephalosporin-resistant pneumococci in rabbits, in which regimens of 20 mg/kg/d and 40 mg/kg/d of vancomycin plus dexamethasone were compared.[63] Rates of bacterial clearance from CSF were similar with both dosage regimens, but the coadministration of dexamethasone significantly reduced the CSF penetration of vancomycin and bacterial clearance in animals receiving the 20 mg/kg dose. For animals receiving the 40 mg/kg dose of vancomycin, therapeutic peak CSF concentrations of vancomycin were attained even with use of adjunctive dexamethasone, which suggested that the effects of steroids on antimicrobial penetration may be circumvented by using larger vancomycin doses. A strong positive linear correlation between serum and CSF concentrations of vancomycin was also demonstrated in a recent prospective multicenter observational study of 14 adults with suspected pneumococcal meningitis who received vancomycin (in a continuous infusion of 60 mg/kg/d after a loading dose of 15 mg/kg), combined with cefotaxime and dexamethasone. The mean serum and CSF vancomycin concentrations were 25.2 µg/mL and 7.9 µg/mL, respectively, and follow-up CSF analysis revealed negative bacterial culture results and marked improvement in CSF parameters in all patients. These findings suggest that higher vancomycin dosages may overcome diminished vancomycin CSF penetration associated with dexamethasone administration.[64]

Another concern with the use of vancomycin is the emergence of a genetic trait in pneumococci called tolerance, which is the ability of the bacteria to evade killing through loss of antimicrobial-induced autolysin activity. Tolerance reduces the rate of death on exposure to an antimicrobial agent and allows for a resumption of growth after its removal, effectively changing the antimicrobial activity from bactericidal to bacteriostatic, with attenuated killing at the defined MIC for the given isolate. Once thought to be sporadic, it is currently believed to be present in a large number of pneumococcal serotypes.[65,66] In 1998, a case of vancomycin-tolerant S pneumoniae was reported in a child who developed recrudescent meningitis 8 days after receiving a 10-day course of parenteral vancomycin and cefotaxime.[67] In a recent study, S pneumoniae strains from 215 nasopharyngeal swabs of healthy vaccinated infants and 113 isolates from patients with pneumococcal meningitis were recently tested for vancomycin tolerance.[66] Tolerance to vancomycin was detected in 3.7% of the nasopharyngeal swabs and 10.6% of the invasive isolates. The patients with meningitis caused by the identified tolerant isolates had a worse estimated 30-day survival than patients with meningitis caused by nontolerant isolates (49% versus 86%; $P = .048$).

Two other glycopeptides have been studied for use in bacterial meningitis. Oritavancin, a novel semisynthetic glycopeptide with long half-life and a mechanism of action resembling that of vancomycin, has in vitro activity against vancomycin-resistant microbes and has been studied in experimental animal models of pneumococcal meningitis. One study in animals with penicillin-susceptible S pneumoniae meningitis showed that despite low CSF penetration (1%–5%), oritavancin exhibited similar bacterial killing rates compared with ceftriaxone. It also had a low MIC and MBC against the test pneumococcal isolate (0.015 and 0.03 µg/mL, respectively) and was found to influence the release of a lower amount of proinflammatory bacterial compounds (lipoteichoic and teichoic acids) in vitro than ceftriaxone, although it had comparable effects in vivo.[68] Another study in rabbits examined the treatment of cephalosporin-resistant pneumococci by oritavancin alone and in combination with ceftriaxone. There was a rapid decrease in bacterial concentrations at 2 hours (2 log CFU/mL), and the drug was bactericidal at 6 hours (mean reduction 3.5 log CFU/mL). This activity was improved by addition of ceftriaxone (mean reduction 3.99 log CFU/mL), although not statistically significant, possibly because of the rapid decrease in bacterial concentrations with combination therapy. The bacterial killing rate in most cases was not affected by dexamethasone administration, and there were no therapeutic failures in all study animals.[69] These data are encouraging, although no studies in humans have been performed to define the safety and efficacy of oritavancin in patients with bacterial meningitis.

Teicoplanin, another glycopeptide first discovered in 1978, has been studied for use in bacterial meningitis. When used alone in experimental treatment of pneumococcal meningitis, teicoplanin resulted in effective bacterial killing and bactericidal activity at 24 hours without evidence of therapeutic failures. The addition of dexamethasone did not alter this result, despite a significant reduction in the penetration of teicoplanin into CSF (from 2.31% to 0.71%). Ceftriaxone combined with teicoplanin did not show a significant improvement in bacterial killing despite in vitro synergy.[70] Teicoplanin has been used in the treatment of meningitis caused by methicillin-resistant *Staphylococcus aureus* (MRSA), which has emerged as an important cause of nosocomial CNS infection. It has been reported to be effective in the treatment of staphylococcal meningitis in neonates after intrathecal administration and via intravenous administration in the treatment of six cases of culture-proven MRSA meningitis.[71,72] An experimental study in rabbits with MRSA meningitis compared teicoplanin with vancomycin and showed comparable antimicrobial activity of each, with similar CSF bacterial counts at 28 and 40 hours after inoculation.[73]

Rifampin

Most studies of rifampin in bacterial meningitis investigated its use in combination therapy with other agents, most commonly a cephalosporin and vancomycin, because of the rapid emergence of bacterial resistance that is seen with rifampin monotherapy. One study of a cephalosporin-resistant *S pneumoniae* strain, using the CSF of children treated with a combination of ceftriaxone and rifampin, reported that the addition of rifampin to ceftriaxone enhanced the CSF activity against the isolate.[62] This result was also seen in an earlier experimental study of penicillin- and cephalosporin-resistant pneumococcal meningitis in rabbits, in which prompt bacteriologic cure occurred when rifampin was used with ceftriaxone, with or without the addition of dexamethasone therapy.[17] This study also demonstrated that rifampin concentrations in the CSF were unaffected by dexamethasone administration, an observation further elucidated by a later experimental study,[60] in which rifampin was studied in combination with vancomycin in the treatment of penicillin-resistant pneumococcal meningitis. The interference of dexamethasone on the CSF vancomycin concentrations was less pronounced when rifampin was used simultaneously, likely a result of enhanced dexamethasone metabolism in the presence of rifampin.

Two recent experimental studies in rabbits of penicillin- and cephalosporin-resistant *S pneumoniae* meningitis have compared the use of ceftriaxone and rifampin combination therapy to combination regimens that include vancomycin. In both studies, the addition of rifampin to ceftriaxone was comparable in efficacy to ceftriaxone and vancomycin, one showing it to be equally effective[74] and the other showing it to be superior.[75] The drug combination consisting of vancomycin, rifampin, and ceftriaxone had similar therapeutic efficacy to the combined ceftriaxone and rifampin regimen.[75] Compared to ceftriaxone, rifampin has been found to release less proinflammatory cell wall products from *S pneumoniae* in vitro and a lower amount of reactive oxygen species produced by CSF phagocytes and endothelial cells. This correlated with attenuated neuronal damage and a reduction in mortality in two animal models of pneumococcal meningitis.[76,77]

Fluoroquinolones

The fluoroquinolones have excellent in vitro activity against many of the meningeal pathogens and good penetration into CSF and have been used successfully in patients with gram-negative meningitis.[78–80] Trovafloxacin is one agent that showed great promise in a multicenter, randomized trial in children with bacterial meningitis, in which no significant differences between trovafloxacin and ceftriaxone, with or without vancomycin, were detected in terms of clinical success at 5 to 7 weeks after treatment (79% versus 81%), deaths (2% versus 3%), seizures (22% versus 21%), or severe sequelae (14% versus 14%).[81] Despite these favorable results, however, reports of liver toxicity have largely precluded the use of trovafloxacin. Newer fluoro-quinolones, including gemifloxacin, moxifloxacin, gatifloxacin, and garenoxacin, have been developed and show excellent in vitro activity against gram-positive bacteria. These drugs, along with clinafloxacin, have been studied in experimental cases of pneumococcal meningitis with mostly efficacious results.[58,82–92]

Moxifloxacin is a promising new fluoroquinolone that was recently found in experi-mental rabbit models to have similar antibacterial activity to the combination of ampi-cillin plus gentamicin in the treatment of meningitis caused by *Listeria monocytogenes*.[93] It has also been evaluated in experimental *E coli* meningitis to be at least as effective as ceftriaxone and more effective than meropenem; it was found to have excellent CSF penetration (50%–85%).[30] A recent study in healthy humans evaluated the CSF penetration of moxifloxacin after a single oral dose of 400 mg and found good penetration that would attain CSF concentrations to achieve a satis-factory bactericidal effect against penicillin-resistant *S pneumoniae*.[94] Given the previous experimental data that demonstrated satisfactory penetration of moxifloxa-cin through inflamed meninges, the authors hypothesized that moxifloxacin concen-trations may be even higher in the CSF of patients with meningitis.

Three experimental studies in rabbits demonstrated a synergy between fluoroquino-lones and other antibiotics commonly used in bacterial meningitis. In the first study, the combination of meropenem and levofloxacin was shown to increase the efficacy of levofloxacin against penicillin-resistant pneumococcal strains in vitro, reaching higher efficacy than the standard regimen of ceftriaxone and vancomycin.[95] The second study evaluated cefotaxime and levofloxacin combined and found higher bactericidal activity of combination therapy compared with monotherapy, the efficacy of which was twice that of standard ceftriaxone and vancomycin, and confirmed synergy between the two antimicrobials. The combination almost completely dimin-ished levofloxacin-induced resistance of the test train, with a twofold increase in the MIC.[24] The third study examined the effect of ceftriaxone and levofloxacin combined and found similar synergy with the combination regimen and the reduction of levoflox-acin resistance in the pneumococcal strain. Specifically, it was determined that cef-triaxone prevented the emergence of mutations in the pneumococcal genome that contributed to a high-level resistance (MIC 64 µg/mL) to levofloxacin in the test strain.[23]

Daptomycin

Daptomycin, a cyclic lipopeptide antimicrobial agent, has potent bactericidal activity against multidrug-resistant gram-positive organisms.[96] Its clinical use has largely been in complicated skin and soft tissue infections, and there is little clinical experi-ence with its use in bacterial meningitis. In a rabbit model of meningitis caused by penicillin- and quinolone-resistant pneumococci,[97] there was a 6% penetration of daptomycin into CSF, a concentration sufficient to produce highly bactericidal concentrations (CSF concentration/MIC ratios between 86 and 53). Daptomycin had comparable efficacy and more rapid bacterial killing when compared with cefotaxime and levofloxacin combined but had superior efficacy compared with the combination of ceftriaxone and vancomycin. In a rabbit model of methicillin-sensitive S aureus meningitis, daptomycin was also found to be superior to vancomycin in efficacy in vivo and in time-killing assays in vitro.[98] There was rapid sterilization of the CSF in both models by daptomycin within 4 to 6 hours of initiation of therapy.

Two recent studies have described the nonbacteriolytic activity of daptomycin in the therapy of meningitis, which may be beneficial in preventing the release of proinflammatory mediators from cell wall components after bacterial lysis. The first study compared the measured amount of [3H]choline, a main component of the proinflammatory mediators teichoic acid and lipoteichoic acid, in the CSF of rabbits with penicillin-resistant pneumococcal meningitis after treatment with ceftriaxone and daptomycin.[99] There were drastic increases in [3H]choline concentrations and observed cell wall morphologic alterations via electron microscopy after ceftriaxone administration and only mild elevations in [3H]choline concentrations with no morphologic changes in pneumococcal cell walls after daptomycin administration. The second study examined the effects of ceftriaxone and daptomycin therapy on cortical brain damage in infant rats with pneumococcal meningitis.[100] Only the animals treated with ceftriaxone had cortical brain damage (0.26%–7.26% in 7 of 28 animals) as evidenced by areas of cortical necrosis upon histologic analysis of brain sections of sacrificed animals 40 hours after therapy. None of the 30 animals given daptomycin had evidence of cortical damage on histologic analysis.

Recently, a case report demonstrated the success of daptomycin (combined with rifampin) in the treatment of MRSA meningitis.[101] There was clinical improvement of the patient with eventual discharge from the hospital and no residual neurologic deficits after a treatment course of 42 days. These results supported the potential of daptomycin in patients with bacterial meningitis, although more data are needed.

Linezolid

Linezolid is a novel antimicrobial of the oxazolidinone class with in vitro activity against numerous gram-positive organisms,[102] and it has been used in isolated cases in patients with bacterial meningitis. A recent review of documented CNS infections noted cure or clinical improvement in 90% of cases identified. In these cases, linezolid therapy, dosed at 600 mg twice daily as monotherapy or in a combination regimen, was started after initial therapeutic regimens failed or were associated with adverse effects.[103] Linezolid was reported to be effective in meningitis caused by penicillin-nonsusceptible S pneumoniae, vancomycin-resistant Enterococcus species, methicillin-resistant Staphylococcus epidermidis, MRSA, and heteroresistant vancomycin-intermediate S aureus. To date, no clinical trials have compared linezolid with standard therapy for bacterial meningitis, although an experimental study in rabbits with meningitis caused by penicillin-sensitive and penicillin-resistant pneumococci showed inferior killing rates of linezolid compared with ceftriaxone plus vancomycin despite good CSF penetration (38% ± 4%).[104] There was a more pronounced antibacterial activity of the agent against penicillin-resistant pneumococci than against penicillin-sensitive strains.

Telavancin

A semisynthetic derivative of vancomycin, telavancin, is an investigational lipoglyco-peptide antimicrobial with bactericidal activity against gram-positive bacteria and a favorable spectrum of activity against drug-resistant streptococci, enterococci, and staphylococci. It has an MIC two to eight times lower than vancomycin for these organisms.[105] Clinical experience with the use of telavancin in patients with meningitis has not yet been reported, but an experimental study in rabbits examined its use in meningitis caused by penicillin-resistant pneumococci and methicillin-sensitive S aureus. CSF concentrations of telavancin remained above the MIC for both strains, leading to CSF/MIC ratios from 30 to 63 for the pneumococcal strain and 0.9 to 1.9 for the staphylococcal strain. Penetration was 2% through inflamed meninges and less than 1% through noninflamed meninges. The combination of ceftriaxone and van-comycin proved to be less efficacious than telavancin for the pneumococcal strain. Although telavancin was slightly superior to vancomycin alone against the staphylo-coccal strain, this difference was not statistically significant.[106]

SUMMARY

Bacterial meningitis is a life-threatening disease and is associated with significant long-term sequelae in surviving patients. Success in its treatment relies on knowledge of the fundamental principles of antimicrobial therapy in the unique environment of the CSF, including CSF penetration, activity in purulent CSF, mode of administration of the drug, and pharmacodynamic properties within the CSF. Although promising results have been reported in the prevention of bacterial meningitis through vaccination programs, challenges still remain with the emergence of antimicrobial resistance, particularly in pneumococci, and the changing epidemiology of the disease. In the past decade, new therapies and strategies for disease management have been exam-ined in experimental animal models. Further clinical experience is warranted to deter-mine the impact these strategies may have in the human population.

REFERENCES

1. Tunkel AR. Bacterial meningitis. Philadelphia: Lippincott Williams & Wilkins; 2001.
2. Casado-Flores J, Aristegui J, de Liria CR, et al. Clinical data and factors associ-ated with poor outcome in pneumococcal meningitis. Eur J Pediatr 2006;165: 285–9.
3. van de Beek D, de Gans J, Tunkel AR, et al. Community-acquired bacterial meningitis in adults. N Engl J Med 2006;354:44–53.
4. Makwana N, Riordan FA. Bacterial meningitis: the impact of vaccination. CNS Drugs 2007;21:355–66.
5. Adams WG, Deaver KA, Cochi SL, et al. Decline of childhood Haemophilus influ-enzae type b (Hib) disease in the Hib vaccine era. JAMA 1993;269:221–6.
6. Whitney CG, Farley MM, Hadler J, et al. Decline in invasive pneumococcal disease after the introduction of protein-polysaccharide conjugate vaccine. N Engl J Med 2003;348:137–46.
7. Swartz M. Bacterial meningitis: a view of the past 90 years. N Engl J Med 2004; 351:1826–8.
8. Tzanakaki G, Mastrantonio P. Aetiology of bacterial meningitis and resistance to antibiotics of causative pathogens in Europe and in the Mediterranean region. Int J Antimicrob Agents 2007;29:621–9.

9. Nigrovic LE, Kupperman N, Malley R. Children with bacterial meningitis presenting to the emergency department during the pneumococcal conjugate vaccine era. Acad Emerg Med 2008;15:522–8.
10. Centers for Disease Control and Prevention (CDC). Emergence of antimicrobial-resistant serotype 19A *Streptococcus pneumoniae:* Massachusetts, 2001–2006. MMWR Morb Mortal Wkly Rep 2007;56:1077–80.
11. Sinner SW, Tunkel AR. Antimicrobial agents in the treatment of bacterial meningitis. Infect Dis Clin North Am 2004;18:581–602.
12. Tunkel AR, Scheld WM. Applications of therapy in animal models to bacterial infection in human disease. Infect Dis Clin North Am 1989;3:441–59.
13. Andes DR, Craig WA. Pharmacokinetics and pharmacodynamics of antibiotics in meningitis. Infect Dis Clin North Am 1999;13:595–618.
14. Lutsar I, McCracken GH Jr, Friedland IR. Antibiotic pharmacodynamics in cerebrospinal fluid. Clin Infect Dis 1998;27:1117–29.
15. Spector R. Advance in understanding the pharmacology of agents used to treat bacterial meningitis. Pharmacology 1990;41:113–8.
16. Quagliarello VJ, Long WJ, Scheld WM. Morphologic alterations of the blood brain barrier with experimental meningitis in the rat. J Clin Invest 1986;77: 1084–95.
17. Paris MM, Hickey SM, Uscher MI, et al. Effect of dexamethasone on therapy of experimental penicillin- and cephalosporin-resistant pneumococcal meningitis. Antimicrob Agents Chemother 1994;38:1320–4.
18. Cabellos C, Martinez-Lacasa J, Martos A, et al. Influence of dexamethasone on efficacy of ceftriaxone and vancomycin therapy in experimental pneumococcal meningitis. Antimicrob Agents Chemother 1995;39:2158–60.
19. Scheld WM, Brodeur JP. Effect of methylprednisolone on entry of ampicillin and gentamicin into cerebrospinal fluid in experimental pneumococcal and *Escherichia coli* meningitis. Antimicrob Agents Chemother 1983;23:108–12.
20. Chowdhury MH, Tunkel AR. Antibacterial agents in infections of the central nervous system. Infect Dis Clin North Am 2000;14:391–408.
21. Dragan R, Velghe L, Rodda JL, et al. Penetration of meropenem into cerebrospinal fluid of patients with inflamed meninges. J Antimicrob Chemother 1994; 34:175–9.
22. Schmidt T, Floula J, Täuber MG. Clarithromycin lacks bactericidal activity in cerebrospinal fluid in experimental pneumococcal meningitis. J Antimicrob Chemother 1993;32:627–32.
23. Flatz L, Cottagnoud M, Kuhn F, et al. Ceftriaxone acts synergistically with levofloxacin in experimental meningitis and reduces levofloxacin-induced resistance in penicillin-resistant pneumococci. J Antimicrob Chemother 2004;53:305–10.
24. Kuhn F, Cottagnoud M, Acosta F, et al. Cefotaxime acts synergistically with levofloxacin in experimental meningitis due to penicillin-resistant pneumococci and prevents selection of levofloxacin-resistant mutants in vitro. Antimicrob Agents Chemother 2003;47:2487–91.
25. Steinberg E, Overturf GD, Wilkins J, et al. Failure of cefamandole in treatment of meningitis due to *Haemophilus influenzae* type b. J Infect Dis 1978;137:S180–6.
26. Syriopoulou VP, Scheifele DW, Sack CM, et al. Effect of inoculum size on the susceptibility of *Haemophilus influenzae* b to beta-lactam antibiotics. Antimicrob Agents Chemother 1979;16:510–3.
27. Kasiakou SK, Sermaides GJ, Michalopoulos A, et al. Continuous versus intermittent intravenous administration of antibiotics: a meta-analysis of randomized controlled trials. Lancet Infect Dis 2005;5:581–9.

28. Lutsar I, Ahmed A, Friedland IR, et al. Pharmacodynamics and bactericidal activity of ceftriaxone therapy in experimental cephalosporin-resistant pneumococcal meningitis. Antimicrob Agents Chemother 1997;41:2414–7.

29. Ahmed A, Paris MM, Trujillo M, et al. Once-daily gentamicin therapy for experimental *Escherichia coli* meningitis. Antimicrob Agents Chemother 1997;41:49–53.

30. Rodriguez-Cerrato V, McCoid CC, Michelow IC, et al. Pharmacodynamics and bactericidal activity of moxifloxacin in experimental *Escherichia coli* meningitis. Antimicrob Agents Chemother 2001;45:3092–7.

31. Kim YS, Liu Q, Chow LL, et al. Trovafloxacin in treatment of rabbits with experimental meningitis caused by high-level penicillin-resistant *Streptococcus pneumoniae*. Antimicrob Agents Chemother 1997;41:1186–9.

32. McCracken G. Pharmacodynamics of gatifloxacin in experimental models of pneumococcal meningitis. Clin Infect Dis 2000;31(Suppl 2):S45–50.

33. Tunkel AR, Hartman BJ, Kaplan SL, et al. Practice guidelines for the management of bacterial meningitis. Clin Infect Dis 2004;39:1267–84.

34. Peltola H, Anttila M, Renkonen OV, et al. Randomised comparison of chloramphenicol, ampicillin, cefotaxime, and ceftriaxone for childhood bacterial meningitis. Lancet 1989;1:1281–7.

35. Lebel MH, Hoyt MJ, McCracken GH Jr. Comparative efficacy of ceftriaxone and cefuroxime for treatment of bacterial meningitis. J Pediatr 1989;114:1049–54.

36. Nathan N, Borel T, Djibo A, et al. Ceftriaxone as effective as long-acting chloramphenicol in short-course treatment of meningococcal meningitis during epidemics: a randomized non-inferiority study. Lancet 2005;366:308–13.

37. Norby SR. Role of cephalosporins in the treatment of bacterial meningitis in adults: overview with special emphasis on ceftazidime. Am J Med 1985;79: 56–61.

38. Rodriguez WJ, Khamn WN, Cocchetto DM, et al. Treatment of *Pseudomonas* meningitis with ceftazidime with or without concurrent therapy. Pediatr Infect Dis J 1990;9:83–7.

39. Mizen L, Woodnutt G, Kernutt I, et al. Simulation of human serum pharmacokinetics of ticarcillin-clavulanic acid and ceftazidime in rabbits, and efficacy against experimental *Klebsiella pneumoniae* meningitis. Antimicrob Agents Chemother 1989;33:693–9.

40. Huang CR, Lu CH, Chuang YC, et al. Adult *Pseudomonas aeruginosa* meningitis: high incidence of underlying medical and/or postneurosurgical conditions and high mortality rate. Jpn J Infect Dis 2007;60:397–9.

41. Tsai YH, Bies M, Leitner F, et al. Therapeutic studies of cefepime (BMY 28142) in murine meningitis and pharmacokinetics in neonatal rats. Antimicrob Agents Chemother 1990;34:733–8.

42. Rousseau JM, Soullie B, Villevieille T, et al. Efficiency of cefepime in postoperative meningitis attributable to *Enterobacter aerogenes* [letter]. J Trauma 2001;50:971.

43. Gerber CM, Cottagnoud M, Neftel K, et al. Evaluation of cefepime alone and in combination with vancomycin against penicillin-resistant pneumococci in the rabbit meningitis model and in vitro. J Antimicrob Chemother 2000;45:63–8.

44. Cottagnoud P, Acosta F, Cottagnoud M, et al. Cefepime is efficacious against penicillin- and quinolone-resistant pneumococci in experimental meningitis. J Antimicrob Chemother 2002;49:327–30.

45. Lodise TP Jr, Nau R, Kinzig M, et al. Comparison of the probability of target attainment between ceftriaxone and cefepime in the cerebrospinal fluid and serum against *Streptococcus pneumoniae*. Diagn Microbiol Infect Dis 2007; 58:445–52.

46. Saez-Llorens X, O'Ryan M. Cefepime in the empiric treatment of meningitis in children. Pediatr Infect Dis J 2001;20:356–61.
47. Wong VK, Wright HT Jr, Ross LA, et al. Imipenem/cilastatin treatment of bacterial meningitis in children. Pediatr Infect Dis J 1991;10:122–5.
48. Zhanel GG, Wiebe R, Dilay L, et al. Comparative review of the carbapenems. Drugs 2007;67:1027–52.
49. Cottagnoud P, Pfister M, Cottagnoud M, et al. Activities of ertapenem, a new long acting carbapenem, against penicillin-sensitive or -resistant pneumococci in experimental meningitis. Antimicrob Agents Chemother 2003;47:1943–7.
50. Norrby SR. Neurotoxicity of carbapenem antibiotics: consequences for their use in bacterial meningitis. J Antimicrob Chemother 2000;45:5–7.
51. Schmutzhard E, Williams KJ, Vukmirovits G, et al. A randomized comparison of meropenem with cefotaxime and ceftriaxone for the treatment of bacterial meningitis in adults: meropenem meningitis study group. J Antimicrob Chemother 1995;36(Suppl A):85–97.
52. Klugman KP, Dagan R. Randomized comparison of meropenem with cefotaxime for treatment of bacterial meningitis. Antimicrob Agents Chemother 1995;39:1140–6.
53. Odio CM, Puig JR, Feris JM, et al. Prospective, randomized, investigator-blinded study of the efficacy and safety of meropenem vs. cefotaxime therapy in bacterial meningitis in children. Pediatr Infect Dis J 1999;18:581–90.
54. Maiques JM, Domenech A, Cabellos C, et al. Evaluation of antimicrobial regimens in a guinea-pig model of meningitis caused by Pseudomonas aeruginosa. Microbes Infect 2007;9:435–41.
55. Buckingham SC, Davis Y, English BK. Pneumococcal susceptibility to meropenem in a mid-south children's hospital. South Med J 2002;95:1293–6.
56. Kim SW, Jim JH, Kang SJ, et al. Therapeutic efficacy of meropenem for treatment of experimental penicillin-resistant pneumococcal meningitis. J Korean Med Sci 2004;19:21–6.
57. Force E, Taberner F, Cabellos C, et al. Experimental study of meropenem in the therapy of cephalosporin-susceptible and -resistant pneumococcal meningitis. Eur J Clin Microbiol Infect Dis 2008;27:685–90.
58. Friedland IR, Paris M, Ehrett S, et al. Evaluation of antimicrobial regimens for treatment of experimental penicillin- and cephalosporin-resistant pneumococcal meningitis. Antimicrob Agents Chemother 1999;43:2372–5.
59. Cottagnoud P, Cottagnoud M, Täuber MG. Vancomycin acts synergistically with gentamicin against penicillin-resistant pneumococci by increasing the intracellular penetration of gentamicin. Antimicrob Agents Chemother 2003;47:144–7.
60. Martinez-Lacasa J, Cabellos C, Martos A, et al. Experimental study of the efficacy of vancomycin, rifampicin and dexamethasone in the therapy of pneumococcal meningitis. J Antimicrob Chemother 2002;49:507–13.
61. Viladrich PF, Gudiol F, Linares J, et al. Evaluation of vancomycin for therapy of adult pneumococcal meningitis. Antimicrob Agents Chemother 1991;35:2467–72.
62. Klugman KP, Friedland IR, Bradley JS. Bactericidal activity against cephalosporin-resistant Streptococcus pneumoniae in cerebrospinal fluid of children with acute bacterial meningitis. Antimicrob Agents Chemother 1995;39:1988–92.
63. Ahmed A, Jafri H, Lutsar I, et al. Pharmacodynamics of vancomycin for the treatment of experimental penicillin- and cephalosporin-resistant pneumococcal meningitis. Antimicrob Agents Chemother 1999;43:876–81.

64. Ricard JD, Wolff M, Lacherade JC, et al. Levels of vancomycin in cerebrospinal fluid of adult patients receiving adjunctive corticosteroids to treat pneumococcal meningitis: a prospective multicenter observational study. Clin Infect Dis 2007; 44:250–5.
65. Novak R, Henriques B, Charpentier E, et al. Emergence of vancomycin tolerance in Streptococcus pneumoniae. Nature 1999;399:590–3.
66. Rodriguez CA, Atkinson R, Bitar W, et al. Tolerance to vancomycin in pneumococci: detection with a molecular marker and assessment of clinical impact. J Infect Dis 2004;190:1481–7.
67. McCullers JA, English BK. Isolation and characterization of vancomycin-tolerant Streptococcus pneumoniae from the cerebrospinal fluid of a patient who developed recrudescent meningitis. J Infect Dis 2000;181:369–73.
68. Gerber J, Smirnov A, Wellmer A, et al. Activity of LY333328 in experimental meningitis caused by a Streptococcus pneumoniae strain susceptible to penicillin. Antimicrob Agents Chemother 2001;45:2169–72.
69. Cabellos C, Fernandez A, Maiques JM. Experimental study of LY333328 (oritavancin), alone and in combination, in therapy of cephalosporin-resistant pneumococcal meningitis. Antimicrob Agents Chemother 2003;47:1907–11.
70. Cabellos AF, Tubau F, Maiques JM, et al. Experimental study of teicoplanin, alone and in combination, in the therapy of cephalosporin-resistant pneumococcal meningitis. J Antimicrob Chemother 2005;55:78–83.
71. Kralinsky K, Lako J, Dluhollucky S, et al. Nosocomial staphylococcal meningitis in neonates successfully treated with intraventricular teicoplanin. Chemotherapy 1999;45:313–4.
72. Arda B, Yamazhan T, Sipahi OR, et al. Meningitis due to methicillin-resistant Staphylococcus aureus (MRSA): Review of 10 cases. Int J Antimicrob Agents 2005;25:414–8.
73. Sipahi OR, Arda B, Yurtseven T, et al. Vancomycin versus teicoplanin in the therapy of experimental methicillin-resistant Staphylococcus aureus (MRSA) meningitis. Int J Antimicrob Agents 2005;26:412–5.
74. Suntur BM, Yurtseven T, Sipahi OR, et al. Rifampicin + ceftriaxone versus vancomycin + ceftriaxone in the treatment of penicillin- and cephalosporin-resistant pneumococcal meningitis in an experimental rabbit model. Int J Antimicrob Agents 2005;26:258–60.
75. Lee H, Song JH, Kim SW, et al. Evaluation of a triple drug combination for treatment of experimental multidrug-resistant pneumococcal meningitis. Int J Antimicrob Agents 2004;23:307–10.
76. Nau R, Wellmer A, Soto A, et al. Rifampin reduces early mortality in experimental Streptococcus pneumoniae meningitis. J Infect Dis 1999;179:1557–60.
77. Bottcher T, Gerber J, Wellmer A, et al. Rifampin reduces production of reactive oxygen species of cerebrospinal fluid phagocytes and hippocampal neuronal apoptosis in experimental Streptococcus pneumoniae meningitis. J Infect Dis 2000;181:2095–8.
78. Schonwald S, Geus I, Lisic M, et al. Ciprofloxacin in the treatment of gram-negative bacillary meningitis. Am J Med 1989;87:248S–9S.
79. Wong-Beringer A, Beringer P, Lovett MA. Successful treatment of multidrug-resistant Pseudomonas aeruginosa meningitis with high dose ciprofloxacin. Clin Infect Dis 1997;25:936–7.
80. Krcmery V Jr, Filka J, Uher J, et al. Ciprofloxacin in treatment of nosocomial meningitis in neonates and in infants: report of 12 cases and review. Diagn Microbiol Infect Dis 1999;35:75–80.

81. Saez-Llorens X, McCoig C, Feris JM, et al. Quinolone treatment for pediatric bacterial meningitis: a comparative study of trovafloxacin and ceftriaxone with or without vancomycin. Pediatr Infect Dis J 2002;21:14–22.

82. Shapiro MA, Donovan KD, Gage JW. Comparative therapeutic efficacy of clinafloxacin in a pneumococcal meningitis mouse model. J Antimicrob Chemother 2000;45:489–92.

83. Smirnov A, Wellmer A, Gerber J, et al. Gemifloxacin is effective in experimental pneumococcal meningitis. Antimicrob Agents Chemother 2000;44:767–70.

84. Cottagnoud P, Acosta F, Cottagnoud M, et al. Gemifloxacin is efficacious against penicillin-resistant and quinolone resistant pneumococci in experimental meningitis. Antimicrob Agents Chemother 2002;46:1607–9.

85. Schmidt H, Dalhoff A, Steurtz K, et al. Moxifloxacin in the therapy of experimental pneumococcal meningitis. Antimicrob Agents Chemother 1998;42:1397–401.

86. Ostergaard C, Sorensen TK, Knudsen JD, et al. Evaluation of moxifloxacin, a new 8-methoxyquinolone, for treatment of meningitis caused by a penicillin-resistant pneumococcus in rabbits. Antimicrob Agents Chemother 1998;42:1706–12.

87. Tarasi A, Capone A, Tarasi D, et al. Comparative in-vitro activity of moxifloxacin, penicillin, ceftriaxone and ciprofloxacin against pneumococci isolated from meningitis. J Antimicrob Chemother 1999;43:833–5.

88. Lutsar I, Friedland IR, Jafri HS, et al. Efficacy of gatifloxacin in experimental Escherichia coli meningitis. Antimicrob Agents Chemother 1999;43:1805–7.

89. Perrig M, Acosta F, Cottagnoud M, et al. Efficacy of gatifloxacin alone and in combination with cefepime against penicillin-resistant Streptococcus pneumoniae in a rabbit meningitis model and in vitro. J Antimicrob Chemother 2001;47:701–4.

90. Rodriguez-Cerrato V, Ghaffar F, Saavedra J, et al. BMS-284756 in experimental cephalosporin-resistant pneumococcal meningitis. Antimicrob Agents Chemother 2001;45:3098–103.

91. Cottagnoud P, Acosta F, Cottagnoud M, et al. Efficacies of BMS 284756 against penicillin-sensitive, penicillin-resistant and quinolone-resistant pneumococci in experimental meningitis. Antimicrob Agents Chemother 2002;46:184–7.

92. Rodriguez-Cerrato V, McCoig CC, Saavedra J, et al. Garenoxacin (BMS-284756) and moxifloxacin in experimental meningitis caused by vancomycin-tolerant pneumococci. Antimicrob Agents Chemother 2003;47:211–5.

93. Sipahi OR, Turhan T, Pullukcu H, et al. Moxifloxacin versus ampicillin + gentamicin in the therapy of experimental Listeria monocytogenes meningitis. J Antimicrob Chemother 2008;61:670–3.

94. Kanellakopoulou K, Pagoulatou A, Stroumpoulis K, et al. Pharmacokinetics of moxifloxacin in non-inflamed cerebrospinal fluid in humans: implication for a bactericidal effect. J Antimicrob Chemother 2008;61:1328–31.

95. Cottagnoud P, Cottagnoud M, Acosta F, et al. Meropenem prevents levofloxacin-induced resistance in penicillin-resistant pneumococci and acts synergistically with levofloxacin in experimental meningitis. Eur J Clin Microbiol Infect Dis 2003;22:656–62.

96. Steenbergen J, Alder J, Thorne GM, et al. Daptomycin: a lipopeptide for the treatment of serious gram-positive infections. J Antimicrob Chemother 2005;55:283–8.

97. Cottagnoud P, Pfister M, Acosta F, et al. Daptomycin is highly efficacious against penicillin-resistant and penicillin- and quinolone-resistant pneumococci in experimental meningitis. Antimicrob Agents Chemother 2004;48:3928–33.

98. Gerber P, Stucki A, Acosta F, et al. Daptomycin is more efficacious than vancomycin against a methicillin-susceptible *Staphylococcus aureus* in experimental meningitis. J Antimicrob Chemother 2006;57:720–3.

99. Stucki A, Cottagnoud M, Winkelmann V, et al. Daptomycin produces an enhanced bactericidal activity compared to ceftriaxone, measured by [^{3}H]choline release in the cerebrospinal fluid, in experimental meningitis due to a penicillin-resistant pneumococcal strain without lysing its cell wall. Antimicrob Agents Chemother 2007;51:2249–52.

100. Grandgirard D, Schurch C, Cottagnoud P, et al. Prevention of brain injury by the nonbacteriolytic antibiotic daptomycin in experimental pneumococcal meningitis. Antimicrob Agents Chemother 2007;51:2173–8.

101. Lee DH, Palermo B, Chowdhury M. Successful treatment of methicillin-resistant *Staphylococcus aureus* meningitis with daptomycin. Clin Infect Dis 2008;47: 588–90.

102. Jones RN, Ross JE, Castanheira M, et al. United States resistance surveillance results for linezolid (LEADER program for 2007). Diagn Microbiol Infect Dis 2008;62:416–26.

103. Ntziora F, Falagas ME. Linezolid for the treatment of patients with central nervous system infection. Ann Pharmacother 2007;41:296–308.

104. Cottagnoud P, Gerber CM, Acosta F, et al. Linezolid against penicillin-sensitive and -resistant pneumococci in the rabbit meningitis model. J Antimicrob Chemother 2000;46:981–5.

105. Attwood RJ, LaPlante KL. Telavancin: a novel lipoglycopeptide antimicrobial agent. Am J Health Syst Pharm 2007;64:2335–48.

106. Stucki A, Gerber P, Acosta F, et al. Efficacy of telavancin against penicillin-resistant pneumococci and *Staphylococcus aureus* in a rabbit meningitis model and determination of kinetic parameters. Antimicrob Agents Chemother 2006;50: 770–3.

Topical Antibacterial Agents

Peter A. Lio, MD[a],*, Elaine T. Kaye, MD[b]

KEYWORDS

- Antiseptics • Mupirocin • Neomycin • Gentamicin
- Bacitracin • Polymyxin

The skin presents a first line of defense against a wide range of bacterial invaders. When the integrity of the skin is compromised accidentally or intentionally, its natural defenses weaken and a role for antibacterials emerges. The topical route of application offers several advantages over systemic administration, including the avoidance of systemic toxicity and side effects, the decreased induction of bacterial resistance, and the high concentration of antibacterial agent at the site of infection. However, a treatment that must be physically applied to the skin is limited by patient compliance, local side effects such as allergic contact dermatitis, and the depth of penetration of the agent. Despite their shortcomings, topical antibacterial agents are highly versatile and can be used successfully for both prophylaxis and treatment of bacterial infections.

Outside of the hospital setting, *Staphylococcus aureus* and group A streptococci are classically considered the pathogens most often involved in infections of the skin. Recent data from hospitalized patients demonstrate that *S aureus*, *Enterococcus* spp, coagulase-negative staphylococci, *Escherichia coli* and *Pseudomonas aeruginosa* are the most prevalent pathogens involved in skin and soft tissue infections.[1]

These well-known offenders, as well as the panoply of more exotic pathogens that have been reported to cause skin infections, must be kept in mind while exploring the topical antibacterial agents at one's disposal.

PROFILES OF SELECTED ANTIBACTERIAL AGENTS
Antiseptics

Antiseptics, also known as disinfectants, are chemical agents primarily used to decrease the risk of infection in intact skin or in minor wounds. Alcohol and iodophors have rapid action against bacteria but little persistent activity, whereas chlorhexidine

---

[a] Department of Dermatology, Northwestern University Feinberg School of Medicine, 676 N. St. Clair, Suite 1600, Chicago, IL 60611, USA
[b] Department of Dermatology, Harvard Medical School, Children's Hospital Medical Center, 65 Walnut Street, Wellesley Hills, Boston, MA 02481, USA
* Corresponding author.
E-mail address: p-lio@northwestern.edu (P. A. Lio).

Infect Dis Clin N Am 23 (2009) 945–963
doi:10.1016/j.idc.2009.06.006

id.theclinics.com

and triclosan are slower to act but persist on the stratum corneum for continued anti-microbial effects.[2,3] Most antiseptics are not suitable for open wounds as they may impede wound healing by direct cytotoxic effects to keratinocytes and fibroblasts.[4]

Hydrogen peroxide

Hydrogen peroxide is a common antiseptic agent used on intact skin and minor wounds. It is thought to kill bacteria in two distinct modes: rapidly by way of DNA damage from highly reactive hydroxyl radicals, and more slowly in a manner that may involve the inactivation of housekeeping enzymes.[5,6] It has limited bactericidal activity, however. In one study of mixed microorganism disinfection of a glass, it was found to be entirely ineffective.[7] A prospective study in human appendectomy wounds found that there was no statistical difference in the infection rate between a control group and a group receiving hydrogen peroxide.[8]

Hydrogen peroxide may be detrimental to wound healing, however, as it has been shown to be directly cytotoxic to keratinocytes, and even at very low concentrations inhibits keratinocyte migration and proliferation.[9]

Chlorhexidine

Chlorhexidine's role continues to expand as an effective and versatile agent for both infection control and prevention.[10] Chlorhexidine gluconate is active against a wide range of gram-positive and gram-negative bacteria, yeast, and molds.[11] Chlorhexidine acts by disrupting cytoplasmic membranes and remains active for hours after application.[3,12,13] It has a major role in antisepsis for both general skin cleansing and preoperative bathing and surgical site preparation. Chlorhexidine is consistently superior to povidone-iodine and a number of other antiseptics in reducing colonizing flora immediately and several days after application.[2,14,15] It is useful in decolonization of methicillin-resistant *Staphylococcus aureus* (MRSA) carriers and has been shown to reduce MRSA infection in ICU patients treated with a combination of chlorhexidine bath along with intranasal mupirocin.[16,17] Daily chlorhexidine baths alone reduced contamination and acquisition of vancomycin-resistant enterococcus.[10,18] In addition, chlorhexidine is widely used for skin preparation before catheter insertion. More recent developments include chlorhexidine-impregnated dressings or sponges for maintenance of indwelling catheters and impregnated or coated catheters and catheter cuffs.[19,20] Finally, chlorhexidine is playing an emerging role in decontamination of the oropharynx as it impacts on nosocomial pneumonia. A meta-analysis found that chlorhexidine decontamination was responsible for a 30% decrease in the incidence of ventilator-associated pneumonia.[10,21]

Triclosan

Triclosan is a broad-spectrum cationic antimicrobial agent that is widely used in consumer products such as soaps, detergents, toothpastes, and cutting boards. Its mechanism of action is bacterial membrane disruption through blockade of lipid synthesis. This was elucidated recently when triclosan resistance was found in *E coli* strains. These strains were found to have a mutation in the *fabI* gene, which encodes an enzyme involved in fatty acid biosynthesis.[22] The emergence of resistance, although not yet clinically relevant, has sparked concern about the widespread use of this agent promoting resistance.

Iodophors

The iodophors are complexes of iodine and organic carrier compounds that have a broad spectrum of activity against bacteria and fungi. Its mechanism is thought to be by way of destroying microbial protein and DNA.[23] They were formulated to be less irritating and allergenic, but are also less active than pure iodine solutions.[24] Iodo-phors require at least 2 minutes of contact to release free iodine that exerts the anti-bacterial activity. In vitro data shows a large number of gram-positive isolates after exposure for 15 seconds but essentially none after 120 seconds of exposure.[25]

Iodophors are used most commonly for preoperative skin preparation. Povidone-iodine is a complex of the bactericidal iodine with the polymer polyvinylpyrrolidone (povidone). It is available in various commercial forms, including cleansers, surgical scrubs, and ointments. It is effective against MRSA and *Enterococcus* spp; clinically significant resistance to povidone-iodine has not been documented.[26]

The rate of adverse reactions with povidone-iodine is low although there are reports of contact dermatitis as well as metabolic acidosis with prolonged use.[27] In addition, iodine has been considered cytotoxic and deleterious to wound healing. One review concluded that in the majority of in vivo studies reviewed, povidone-iodine seemed to impair wound healing.[28]

Benzoyl peroxide and other antiacne agents

A powerful oxidizing agent, benzoyl peroxide has broad-spectrum bactericidal effects.[29] It is available in gels, creams, lotions, and washes and in various concentra-tions from 2.5% to 20%. Most commonly, benzoyl peroxide is used as a treatment for acne vulgaris; however, in vitro tests confirm that it is effective against a wide range of organisms including *Staphylococcus capitis, Staphylococcus epidermidis, Propioni-bacterium avidum, Propionibacterium granulosum, and Pityrosporum ovale*, in addi-tion to *P acnes*.[29]

Increasingly, benzoyl peroxide is being formulated in combination with antibiotics, such as clindamycin and erythromycin. These topical combinations are more effective clinically and induce less resistance of *P acnes*.[30] Topical erythromycin alone is used to treat erythrasma, pitted keratolysis, and trichomycosis axillaris caused by corynebacterium.[31]

Topical azelaic acid is a dicarboxylic acid that is used in both acne vulgaris and rosacea. It works by killing *P acnes* as well as decreasing keratin production.

Hypochlorite

Sodium hypochlorite (NaOCl) has historical significance as well as an emerging prom-inence because of its bleaching and disinfecting properties.[32] It was discovered in 1788 and used in 1820 to help embalm the decomposing body of Louis XVIII. Later, it was reformulated as Dakin's solution and used widely in World War II to treat both burns and wounds. Despite hypochlorite's broad spectrum activity against both gram-positive and gram-negative organisms, concerns have been raised about its potential for cytotoxicity.

More recently, NaOCl (bleach) has been used empirically in pediatric patients with impetiginized atopic dermatitis, most commonly in the proportion of one-quarter to one-half cup per full bath, for 15 minutes, twice weekly.[33,34] A series of in vitro exper-iments demonstrated that maximal killing of isolates of community-associated MRSA optimally requires a 5-minute exposure to hypochlorite at a concentration of 2.5µl/mL.[35] This is equivalent to one-half cup of bleach in a quarter of a bathtubful of water. However, the clinical safety and efficacy of this approach is not well documented, though studies are in progress.

Other antiseptic agents

A number of other antiseptics find service in more limited capacities. Benzalkonium chloride is a quaternary ammonium compound traditionally used for preparation of the urethral area for catheterization. It is thought to work by binding and disorganizing the bacterial membrane.[36]

Hexachlorophene is a chlorinated bisphenol compound with bacteriostatic activity against gram-positive bacteria. Its residue remains active for several days on skin. Neurotoxicity has resulted from excessive absorption and studies have also suggested a possible teratogenic effect.[37]

A number of botanic products such as thyme oil (thymol)[38] and clove oil (eugenol)[39] have been shown to have antibacterial properties. Undoubtedly, the list will continue to grow as new compounds are discovered and tested.

Antibiotic Agents

Mupirocin

Mupirocin, known formerly as pseudomonic acid A, is the major fermentation product of *Pseudomonas fluorescens*. It works by the reversible inhibition of bacterial isoleucyl-tRNA synthetase, thereby preventing protein and, subsequently, cell wall synthesis.[29] Mupirocin is highly effective against aerobic gram-positive cocci, especially *S aureus*, for which it is bactericidal at the concentrations present with the commonly used 2% ointment.[40] It is not effective against enterococci and generally has poor activity against gram-negative bacteria.[41]

Mupirocin is a versatile agent used in treating primary skin infections, such as impetigo and secondarily infected lesions. It is also useful for eradication of nasal staphylococcus carriage. It rarely causes local adverse effects, such as pruritus or contact dermatitis. Systemic absorption of mupirocin or its major metabolite, monic acid, has not been detected with short courses of administration.[40]

Despite mupirocin's unique mechanism of action, resistant strains have emerged.[42] In the context of widespread mupirocin use, rates have ranged from 11% to as high as 65%. In the absence of widespread use, one study still found 13% mupirocin resistance in MRSA isolates from SICU subjects, with 9% demonstrating high levels of resistance.[43] Such reports of mupirocin-resistant MRSA[44] argues for more judicious use of this important topical antibiotic.

Retapamulin

Retapamulin is one of a new class of antibiotics called pleuromutilins, which selectively inhibit the elongation phase of bacterial protein synthesis at a unique site on the ribosome.[45] Retapamulin is licensed in the United States for the topical treatment of impetigo caused by *S aureus* (MSSA) and *S pyogenes*. Retapamulin shows in vitro activity against *S aureus* and *S pyogenes*, including isolates resistant to β-lactams, macrolides, quinolones, and mupirocin. In 664 isolates of *S aureus*, including many with high levels of resistance to mupirocin and fusidic acid. and 448 (73%) MRSA isolates, retapamulin demonstrated excellent in vitro activity.[46] More clinical studies of retapamulin in treatment of resistant *S aureus* are needed.

Dapsone

A sulfone synthesized initially in 1908, dapsone was initially put to use as an antileprosy medication.[47] Known for its powerful antiinflammatory effects in addition to its antimicrobial abilities, it was frequently used for severe inflammatory forms of acne before the advent of systemic retinoids but was limited by systemic toxicity. Recently, a 5% topical gel formulation has been approved for the treatment of mild-to-moderate acne.[48] Early studies suggest that the topical formulation is safe and that monitoring for hemolytic anemia is not necessary, even among these with known glucose 6-phosphate dehydrogenase deficiency. Although it is in the sulfa family, it appears that dapsone may not be very effective against the bacteria that are commonly treated with topical agents. In one study, the minimum inhibitory concentration (MIC) for dapsone was measured for *S pyogenes*, *S aureus*, and *E coli*, and found to have essentially no antibacterial effects against these pathogens.[49] Despite these negative findings, it is possible that other uses for topical dapsone will be uncovered as it becomes more widely available.

Neomycin and gentamicin

Neomycin is an aminoglycoside produced by *Streptomyces fradiae*. It is bactericidal by binding the 30s subunit of the bacterial ribosome to inhibit protein synthesis.[29] Neomycin is highly active against most gram-negative bacteria but is less active against *P aeruginosa* and anaerobic species such as *Bacteroides*. It is active against staphylococci but is not effective against other gram-positive bacteria such as streptococci.[41] Resistance has been reported in staphylococci and gram-negative bacilli including *E coli*, *Klebsiella*, and *Proteus*.

Neomycin is usually formulated as 20% neomycin sulfate in petrolatum, and is widely used by itself and in combination with other antibiotics, such as bacitracin and polymyxin B. One of the major drawbacks of neomycin is the perceived high prevalence of allergic contact dermatitis, estimated at 1%–6%, but perhaps higher still in patients who have a compromised skin barrier.[50,51] A recent review, however, highlights the fact that data from thousands of subjects show the actual incidence of allergic contact dermatitis to neomycin to be 1% or less in the general population.[51] Neomycin can be systemically absorbed if applied to large body surfaces in which skin is damaged, causing systemic toxicity such as ototoxicity and nephrotoxicity.[52]

Topical gentamicin is another aminoglycoside with the same mechanism of action as neomycin. It is highly active against gram-negative organisms such as *Pseudomonas* and some gram-positive bacteria, including some staphylococcal strains. It has been used to treat wounds, anogenital infections, and pseudomonas folliculitis. It should be applied with caution because of its history of causing ear and kidney toxicity when used on burn wounds, where it is rapidly absorbed.[31]

Polymyxin

Polymyxins are cationic decapeptides that are products of *Bacillus polymyxa*. Polymyxin acts as a surfactant that disrupts bacterial membranes. Polymyxins have bactericidal activity against some gram-negative organisms including *P aeruginosa*, *E coli*, *Enterobacter* sp and *Klebsiella* sp, but do not have activity against *Proteus*, most *Serratia*, or gram-positive bacteria.[41] Polymyxins only rarely cause allergic contact dermatitis, and are most often used in combination with bacitracin, zinc, and neomycin in a petrolatum base.

Bacitracin

Bacitracin is a polypeptide produced by *Bacillus subtilis*, named for Margaret Tracy, the 7-year-old girl from whose wound the strain was originally isolated.[32] Initially developed for systemic administration, nephrotoxicity limited its use.[29] Bacitracin A is the form most commonly used, often formulated as 20% bacitracin zinc in petrolatum. It exerts its antibacterial activity by complexing with C55-prenol pyrophosphate, a constituent of the bacterial cell wall, thus blocking cell wall formation.[29]

Bacitracin is primarily active against gram-positive organisms, including staphylococci, streptococci, clostridia, and corynebacteria. It is used for treatment of local infection and is a popular topical antibiotic for wound prophylaxis because of its low cost and low toxicity. Historically, bacitracin rarely caused sensitization[41] but, in recent years, it has become a frequent cause of allergic contact dermatitis.[53,54]

INTACT SKIN

Topical antibacterial agents can be used as prophylaxis against infection in a variety of inpatient and outpatient settings. In this capacity, antiseptics—chemicals used to disinfect, and antibiotics—biologically derived substances, serve this role.

Resident Skin Flora

The skin normally provides host to a number of bacteria, fungi, and even mites (ie, *Demodex* spp). Coagulase-negative staphylococci represent the dominant bacterial resident in the stratum corneum and on the skin surface, with a reservoir in the sebaceous glands. A number of agents successfully eradicate surface bacteria but are short-acting and are unable to clear bacteria that reside more deeply in the stratum corneum. A comparison of antiseptic agents and antimicrobial agents was performed on various sites in 14 healthy subjects.[55] The study results are summarized in **Table 1**.

Another study of 50 healthy subjects demonstrated that treatment with triple-antibiotic ointment (TAO) containing bacitracin, polysporin, and neomycin eradicated coagulase-negative staphylococci from 96% of skin surface sites versus mupirocin ointment, which eradicated the bacteria at 40% of the skin surface sites.[55] This study also showed that without neomycin, TAO was essentially equivalent to placebo.

Hand Hygiene

Alcohols are antiseptics that exhibit significant pan-antimicrobial and bactericidal activity,[56] predominantly by way of protein denaturation.[57] In concentrations ranging from 60% to 95%, alcohol-based hand washes (usually ethyl or isopropyl alcohol with emollients often added) safely, quickly, and effectively reduce microorganisms on the skin surface. As a point of reference, a 62% gel preparation of ethyl alcohol exhibited a 99.99% reduction in bacteria from baseline levels after one application.[58] A number of studies in both clinical and nonclinical settings demonstrate significant

Table 1
Eradication of coagulase-negative staphylococci by topical antibacterial agents

Agent	Sterilization of Skin Surface	Sterilization of Stratum Corneum	Prevention of Repopulation After 16 h
10% povidone-iodine	Yes	No	—
2% aqueous iodine	Yes	Yes	—
2% tincture of iodine	Yes	Yes	No
70% ethanol	Yes	No	—
0.5% chlorhexidine-ethanol	Yes	No	—
Iodophor	Yes	Yes	No
Silver sulfadiazine	No	—	—
Mupirocin	Yes	Yes	No
TAO	Yes	Yes	Yes
Control	No	No	No

10% povidone-iodine, 2% aqueous iodine, 2% tincture of iodine, 70% ethanol, and 0.5% chlorhexidine-ethanol were applied for 15 seconds with a gauze sponge. Iodophor, silver sulfadiazine, mupirocin, and TAO were applied and covered for 6 hours with gauze. (*Based on data from* Hendley JO, Ashe KM. Effect of topical antimicrobial treatment on aerobic bacteria in the stratum corneum of human skin. Antimicrob Agents Chemother 1991;35(4):627–31).

decrease in bacterial counts on hands and in infection rates, significantly better than hand washing with antiseptic soap.[59–61]

A major limitation of alcohol is the transient effect of antibacterial action. Compounding alcohol with a preservative or another antibacterial agent can overcome this normally transient reduction of bacterial counts. In one study, 70% ethyl alcohol with 0.5% chlorhexidine gluconate was compared with 4% aqueous chlorhexidine, triclosan, 7.5% povidone-iodine or vehicle control for surgical scrubbing. Although all preparations reduced flora when compared with control on day 1, the combination of alcohol and chlorhexidine outperformed other preparations when evaluated on day 5.[2]

The powerful antimicrobial effect with relatively few drawbacks has led to rapid adoption of alcohol-based hand washes by numerous medical institutions and discussions of replacing traditional surgical scrubs with alcohol-based agents.[62]

Staphylococcal Colonization

Nasal colonization of S aureus predisposes the carrier to S aureus infections. Both logic and some clinical studies support the assertion that eradication of carriage results in significantly decreased rates of infection.[63,64] A number of techniques for eliminating the bacteria have been attempted, including systemic antibacterial agents, antiseptics, and topical antibacterials. Topical antibiotics such as bacitracin, tetracycline, and vancomycin applied to the nares have resulted in only temporary eradication of S aureus.[65]

Mupirocin demonstrates superior efficacy against a host of antibiotic-resistant strains and significant duration of clearing. A recent review of the evidence for mupirocin in treating S aureus colonization[63] highlighted some of the following results:

In one series, 5 days of intranasal mupirocin twice daily resulted in 13% positive culture results in the experimental group versus 93% in the placebo control group at 48 to 72 hours, 18% versus 88% at 4 weeks, and 53% versus 76% at 1 year.

A comparison between intranasal mupirocin and bacitracin in health care workers demonstrated 20% carriage for mupirocin recipients versus 77% carriage for the bacitracin group at 30 days follow-up.

Intranasal neomycin was compared with mupirocin (both thrice daily for 7 days) in a small study that showed 42% of the mupirocin group and 75% of the neomycin group had positive cultures at 3 months posttreatment.

While the data are convincing in terms of reducing carriage, subsequent differential infection rates are a more meaningful measure. Benefits of decolonization have been demonstrated in patients who are undergoing surgery as well as those receiving peritoneal dialysis and hemodialysis. In one large study of 4030 subjects who received intranasal mupirocin twice daily for 5 days preoperatively, 4% of nasal carriers of S aureus in the treated group developed surgical site infection versus 7.7% of placebo-treated carriers.[66] A study of 267 nasal carriers of S aureus on peritoneal dialysis showed that the group treated with mupirocin twice daily for 5 days per month had 14 exit-site infections versus 44 in the placebo group.[67] Other types of infections such as peritonitis were not significantly reduced. Of note, the study revealed that treating large numbers of nonnasal carriers did not affect their infection rate.

Unlike the surgical and dialysis populations, however, nonsurgical subjects did not seem to benefit from mupirocin prophylaxis. 1602 nonsurgical subjects were found to be nasal S aureus carriers at the time of admission and treated with mupirocin or placebo ointment twice daily for 5 days. Nosocomial S aureus infections did not differ between the two groups.[68] While mupirocin resistance and dosing regimen may be factors that affected the results, the study suggests that nonsurgical patients do not benefit from such screening and intervention.[69] Future studies may better define subsets of individuals with identifiable risk factors that may be appropriate candidates for decolonization.

MRSA

Although there was an overall decrease in *Staphylococcal* nasal colonization in the United States between 2001 and 2004, the prevalence of nasal colonization with MRSA has increased.[70] Individuals who have newly acquired MRSA as well as individuals who have harbored MRSA for greater than 1 year are at high risk for MRSA morbidity.[71]

Traditionally mupirocin has shown efficacy against MRSA. One study used mupirocin intranasally thrice weekly as a prophylatic regimen on a ward with endemic MRSA. This was effective at decreasing serious MRSA infection and resistance to mupirocin was not seen.[72] Mupirocin resistance has emerged, however, and there is speculation that this may be due to low concentrations of mupirocin in the pharynx during intranasal administration.[73] In one provocative study, mupirocin resistance was overcome by the use of intranasal TAO containing bacitracin, polymyxin B, and gramicidin.[74] With reports of high rates of mupirocin resistance (see above), including high-level resistance, infection control strategies for MRSA should not rely too heavily on mupirocin alone, especially as testing for mupirocin resistance is not routine at most institutions.[43]

MRSA decolonization as a strategy for infection control is controversial, primarily because there is no clear antibacterial regimen that succeeds in long-term eradication in hospitalized patients. Previous studies of mupirocin have focused on detection and treatment of MRSA carriage in the nose; however, there is ample evidence that MRSA colonizes multiple sites which, in addition to the nose, include the throat, axilla, groin, and rectal area.[75] Therefore, it follows that effective decolonization would need to address these broad anatomic sites.

Studies using multiple modes of treatment, including directed nasal mupirocin application and generalized antiseptic washes and systemic agents, hold promise in successful decolonization. In one randomized study, hospitalized subjects who had MRSA received a 7-day course of chlorhexidine washes, intranasal mupirocin, rifampin and doxycycline.[76] 92% of these subjects were cleared of MRSA from all sites and 74% remained clear at 3 months. A previous study used a similar combined regimen of topical and oral antimicrobial agents and achieved 90% in the subjects followed up at 3 months.[77]

Although these studies imply that there may be effective regimens, likely including topical antibacterial agents, for long-term *S aureus* eradication there are still many important questions. The optimal dosing regimen remains unclear and its ability to alter infection rates needs to be better elucidated. It may even be argued that widespread MRSA decolonization may be detrimental as it might select for more virulent strains.

Newer agents such as lysostaphin, an endopeptidase, show promising success in animal models.[78] A recent study examined the MIC at which 50% of the isolates tested were inhibited for MRSA. They found that the lysostaphin had an MIC^{50} that was an impressive four times lower than that of mupriocin.[79]

Less conventional antibacterial agents such as tea tree oil (*Melaleuca alternifolia*) have been studied as well. In one small study, tea tree oil was applied in a 4% nasal ointment with a 5% tea tree oil–based body wash and compared with mupirocin nasal ointment with triclosan body wash for MRSA eradiacation. The tea tree oil regimen was found to be more efficacious, although not significantly so.[80] Newer studies suggest that habituation may occur with tea tree oil and caution that this may decrease efficacy of other topical antibiotics.[81,82] The increasing importance of MRSA infections calls for more work in this area.

SUPERFICIAL WOUNDS

An Australian study of 177 superficial wounds in schoolchildren found infection rates of 8.5% and 12.5% by microbiologic and clinical criteria, respectively.[83] A landmark study on the natural history of superficial wound infection demonstrated a 47% streptococcal colonization rate of minor skin trauma (largely mosquito bites and abrasions) in a control group.[84] This same study showed that TAO containing bacitracin, polysporin, and neomycin decreased this rate to 15% when applied thrice daily.

Topical antibacterial agents also appear to have effects on wound healing in a manner seemingly unrelated to their antimicrobial properties. TAO has been shown to increase the reepithelialization rate of experimentally induced wounds by up to 25%[85] and minimize scarring and dyspigmentation compared with other agents and placebo.[86]

OPERATIVE WOUNDS
Preoperative Prophylaxis

Preoperative disinfection of the skin is widely accepted as the standard of care for decreasing postoperative wound infection.[87] Chlorhexidine and iodophors are generally accepted as among the most effective and widely used agents.[88] One prospective study found that preoperative showering with 4% chlorhexidine gluconate was more effective than povidone-iodine soap in reducing positive intraoperative wound cultures (4% versus 9%, respectively).[89] A more recent study suggested that a 2% chlorhexidine gluconate preparation with 70% isopropyl alcohol was more effective than either of the two constituents alone at reducing microbial counts at different time points.[12]

Postoperative Wound Care

Despite their excellent preoperative performance, disinfectants such as chlorhexidine, NaOCl, and povidone-iodine are generally not helpful in preventing infections in postoperative wounds; moreover, many experimental studies have demonstrated significant cytotoxicity from these agents.[4,90–92] Better suited for this task are the topical antibiotics such as bacitracin, mupirocin, and silver sulfadiazine (SSD), which appear to decrease infection rates and enhance wound healing.[85,93–95] In one large study of 6,000 surgical cases, neomycin-bacitracin-polymyxin spray was found to decrease infection rates.[96] Another trial of the neomycin-bacitracin-polymyxin spray versus no treatment of 851 surgical wounds demonstrated significant reduction in infection in the experimental group.[97]

In a mouse surgical wound model, mupirocin cream showed equal efficacy to the oral penicillin flucloxacillin and greater efficacy than oral erythromycin in reducing bacterial counts. It was also similar in efficacy to oral cephalexin against S pyogenes but superior against S aureus.[98]

Honey has been studied in a number of clinical settings, including as an agent for wound healing. The hyperosmolarity of honey impedes bacterial growth, whereas factors in honey called inhibines, which include hydrogen peroxide, flavonoids, and phenolic acids, appear to elicit antibacterial effects directly.[99] A systematic review of the data on honey concluded that, with some reservation due to study quality and small numbers, wound healing and infection rates were consistently better in those subjects treated with topical honey compared with several other active agents.[100]

BURNS

The moist, necrotic tissue in a burn patient is an ideal environment for bacterial growth. The large areas of ischemic tissue around the wounds may limit the availability and, thus, the usefulness of systemic antibiotics. Before 1965, the rate of burn wound sepsis was reported to be as high as 60%; this quickly fell to 28% after the widespread use of topical silver nitrate.[101] A 2008 review of wound management in the *New England Journal of Medicine* concluded that the optimal therapy for highly contaminated or infected burns with significant exudate is the application of topical antimicrobial agents and absorbent gauze dressings.[102]

Numerous topical agents and regimens have been proposed and tested, but SSD has long been recognized as the mainstay of topical burn therapy. With broad antimicrobial properties and a relatively small side-effect profile, it continues to be the standard by which other treatments are measured, especially for second- and third-degree burns.[102] Because SSD can cause cytotoxicity and thereby delay healing, newer synthetic dressings that release the silver slowly and reduce cytotoxicity are being developed.

A recent study demonstrates that the addition of 0.2% chlorhexidine digluconate to SSD results in superior antimicrobial effects against all bacteria studied in an in vitro model.[101] SSD has several documented side effects, however rare, including neutropenia, erythema multiforme, crystalluria, and methemoglobinemia.[103] These, in part, continue to drive the search for other agents.

Several studies have demonstrated the efficacy of mupirocin ointment for burn wounds, particularly those that are infected with MRSA. One such study of 45 children with burn wounds who developed MRSA infections despite treatment with SSD with chlorhexidine or povidone-iodine showed complete eradication of MRSA within 4 days of initiating mupirocin therapy.[104]

A large study compared 1053 burn subjects treated with povidone-iodine plus neomycin-framycetin-bacitracin ointment (PVP+N) with 1089 subjects treated with SSD and found that healing times and infection rates were statistically favorable for the PVP+N group.[105]

Honey has been studied as an alternative to SSD in burns. A 1998 study of 50 subjects, 25 of them treated with honey and 25 with SSD-impregnated gauze, showed that 100% of the honey-treated subjects showed evidence of wound healing by day 21 versus only 84% by day 21 in the SSD-treated group, although this was not statistically significant.[106] The study also found similar infection eradication rates in both groups. A systematic review of six studies with honey in burn wound treatment found that wound healing infection rates were consistently better in those subjects treated with topical honey compared with other active agents.[100] Recently, there has been some promising new data on honey. Using a standardized medical-grade honey, it was demonstrated that the bacteria on the arms of 42 healthy adults was reduced by 100-fold versus the placebo group, including multiple antibiotic-resistant strains.[107] The investigators suggest that with a more standardized honey preparation, future studies may show more consistent results and open the door for new possibilities for honey as a topical therapy.

The adverse effects associated with SSD are thought to be associated with the sulfa moiety; several attempts have been made to use silver alone. Silver is thought to exhibit its antibacterial properties by interacting with thiol groups in bacterial proteins, which leads to inactivation and by direct DNA condensation and loss of replication abilities.[108] Earlier studies demonstrated that coating nylon fibers with silver resulted in sustained broad bactericidal effects similar to those of SSD without the potential adverse effects of the sulfa moiety.[109] A modern version of this principle, in the form of a dressing of nanocrystalline silver (Acticoat, Smith & Nephew, London, England) was found nearly equivalent to SSD in terms of antimicrobial effects in an in vitro model.[101]

Despite great advances, burn management continues to be a highly challenging area. The authors follow the developments of some of these newer agents with great interest.

IMPETIGO

Impetigo is a superficial skin infection that can be divided into primary—arising in previously intact skin; and secondary—arising in skin that has had barrier damage, such as dermatitis. Whether primary or secondary, the skin manifestation is classically a superficial erosion and honey-colored crust. S aureus and S pyogenes are most often the causative agents. A Cochrane systematic review of impetigo[45] and a recent large systematic review[110] highlighted the following points:

- The peak incidence occurs between the ages of 2 and 6 years.
- Topical antibiotics are more effective than placebo.
- There is evidence that topical antibiotics are more effective than some systemic antibiotics for the treatment of impetigo.
- Topical antibiotics are the preferable first-line treatment.

One study compared oral erythromycin to topical mupirocin in 75 subjects who had impetigo. The mupirocin performed similarly on clinical grounds and superiorly on microbiological data.[111] Another more recent study in 159 subjects who had secondarily impetiginized eczema demonstrated that mupirocin cream applied thrice daily was bacteriologically superior to oral cephalexin.[112] Finally, experiments in a hamster impetigo model infected with S aureus demonstrated that mupirocin cream was significantly more effective than mupirocin ointment, not significantly different from neomycin-bacitracin cream, but significantly superior to oral erythromycin and cephalexin.[98]

More recently, retapamulin has been approved for use in impetigo caused by MSSA and S pyogenes, as described above.[45]

ULCERS

Preventing bacterial colonization and infection of deeper wounds likely depends on a number of factors, including debridement, active cleansing, and dressing choice. It is therefore difficult to evaluate the role of topical antibacterial agents when divorced from these other factors. Nonetheless, a systematic review of topical antimicrobials in chronic wounds in 2001[113] distilled some of the following points from a total of 17 relevant, although highly disparate, trials:

- Dimethyl sulphoxide (an agent thought to have antiinflammatory and antimicrobial properties) showed a higher rate of complete healing and greater reduction in ulcer area compared with placebo in venous leg ulcer treatment.
- SSD proved to be significantly more effective than a tripeptide-copper complex or placebo in terms of reducing ulcer area.

- 10% and 20% benzoyl peroxide applied to wound dressings proved to be significantly more effective than saline in reducing ulcer area.
- Hexachlorophane lotion compared with placebo for prevention of pressure ulcers revealed no statistically significant difference in the time to develop new lesions or the incidence of new lesions.

Daily application of gentian violet 0.1% solution and ointment (an antiseptic) was shown to eradicate 18 cases of MRSA-infected ulcers that had failed previous treatment with povidone-iodine and systemic antibiotics.[114] The mechanism of gentian violet is not fully understood, but early studies demonstrated nonspecific protein and cell wall synthesis inhibition, as well as accumulation of cytidine diphosphoribitol and peptidoglycan precursors.[115]

Honey has also been used successfully for clearance of MRSA infection and improved healing in ulcers.[100,116]

Disinfectants are often considered too harsh for use in wounds. In vitro studies have demonstrated that antiseptics such as povidone-iodine and chlorhexidine show cytotoxic properties and may therefore delay healing of ulcers.[117]

INTRAVASCULAR CATHETERS

There is a 10%–20% mortality attributed to catheter-related bloodstream infection.[118] Appropriate antiseptic care of intravascular catheters should ideally decrease the incidence of infection and, thus, the risk of sepsis. Impregnation of central venous catheter cuffs with antibacterials is beyond the scope of this article.

A large meta-analysis involving a total of 4143 catheters concluded that chlorhexidine gluconate reduced the risk for catheter-related bloodstream infection by 49% compared with povidone-iodine.[118] The investigators hypothesized that chlorhexidine was more effective due to the fact that blood and serum can lessen the microbicidal effect of povidone-iodine but not chlorhexidine, and that chlorhexidine has both a more potent and a longer residual antimicrobial effect compared with povidone-iodine. A follow-up analysis by the same group calculated that the slightly higher cost of chlorhexidine compared with the decreased morbidity and mortality from its use in this clinical context resulted in a $113 savings per catheter used.[119]

Other topical antibiotics have been used for intravascular catheter care. A study of 709 consecutive subjects with venous catheters treated with neomycin-bacitracin-polymyxin spray or control demonstrated decreased colonization by more virulent potential pathogens such as E coli, Klebsiella, and Staphylococcus when the antibiotic spray was used.[120]

Despite decreasing colonization successfully, a prospective study of 827 catheters treated with neomycin-bacitracin-polymyxin ointment at the insertion of a catheter and every 48 hours thereafter failed to show a difference from placebo in the rate of local infection or catheter-associated sepsis.[121]

SUMMARY

Topical antibacterial agents have an important role in antimicrobial therapy. Antiseptics and antibiotic preparations offer important alternatives and supplements to systemic agents in a variety of clinical scenarios. These agents are highly versatile. Uses include prophylaxis of infection for traumatic and surgical wounds, S aureus decolonization, treatment of burns, and treatment of primary and secondary pyodermas. Although topical antibacterials are widely used in clinical practice, ongoing trials continue to elucidate their relative efficacies.

REFERENCES

1. Jones ME, Karlowsky JA, Draghi DC, et al. Epidemiology and antibiotic susceptibility of bacteria causing skin and soft tissue infections in the USA and Europe: a guide to appropriate antimicrobial therapy. Int J Antimicrob Agents 2003;22(4): 406–19.

2. Larson EL, Butz AM, Gullette DL, et al. Alcohol for surgical scrubbing? Infect Control Hosp Epidemiol 1990;11(3):139–43.

3. Fuursted K, Hjort A, Knudsen L. Evaluation of bactericidal activity and lag of regrowth (postantibiotic effect) of five antiseptics on nine bacterial pathogens. J Antimicrob Chemother 1997;40(2):221–6.

4. Tatnall FM, Leigh IM, Gibson JR. Comparative study of antiseptic toxicity on basal keratinocytes, transformed human keratinocytes and fibroblasts. Skin Pharmacol 1990;3(3):157–63.

5. Pericone CD, Park S, Imlay JA, et al. Factors contributing to hydrogen peroxide resistance in *Streptococcus pneumoniae* include pyruvate oxidase (spxb) and avoidance of the toxic effects of the Fenton reaction. J Bacteriol 2003;185(23): 6815–25.

6. Repine JE, Fox RB, Berger EM. Hydrogen peroxide kills *Staphylococcus aureus* by reacting with staphylococcal iron to form hydroxyl radical. J Biol Chem 1981; 256(14):7094–6.

7. Best M, Springthorpe VS, Sattar SA. Feasibility of a combined carrier test for disinfectants: studies with a mixture of five types of microorganisms. Am J Infect Control 1994;22(3):152–62.

8. Lau WY, Wong SH. Randomized, prospective trial of topical hydrogen peroxide in appendectomy wound infection. High risk factors. Am J Surg 1981;142(3): 393–7.

9. O'Toole EA, Goel M, Woodley DT. Hydrogen peroxide inhibits human keratinocyte migration. Dermatol Surg 1996;22(6):525–9.

10. Milstone AM, Passaretti CL, Perl TM. Chlorhexidine: expanding the armamentarium for infection control and prevention. Clin Infect Dis 2008;46(2):274–81.

11. Nicoletti G, Boghossian V, Gurevitch F, et al. The antimicrobial activity in vitro of chlorhexidine, a mixture of isothiazolinones ('kathon' cg) and cetyl trimethyl ammonium bromide (ctab). J Hosp Infect 1993;23(2):87–111.

12. Hibbard JS, Mulberry GK, Brady AR. A clinical study comparing the skin antisepsis and safety of chloraprep, 70% isopropyl alcohol, and 2% aqueous chlorhexidine. J Infus Nurs 2002;25(4):244–9.

13. Tattawasart U, Hann AC, Maillard JY, et al. Cytological changes in chlorhexidine-resistant isolates of *Pseudomonas stutzeri*. J Antimicrob Chemother 2000;45(2): 145–52.

14. Kaul AF, Jewett JF. Agents and techniques for disinfection of the skin. Surg Gynecol Obstet 1981;152(5):677–85.

15. Mermel L. Choice of disinfectants in obtaining blood cultures. Pediatr Infect Dis J 1994;13(5):425–6.

16. Sandri AM, Dalarosa MG, Ruschel de Alcantara L, et al. Reduction in incidence of nosocomial methicillin-resistant staphylococcus aureus (MRSA) infection in an intensive care unit: role of treatment with mupirocin ointment and chlorhexidine baths for nasal carriers of MRSA. Infect Control Hosp Epidemiol 2006;27(2): 185–7.

17. Wendt C, Schinke S, Wurttemberger M, et al. Value of whole-body washing with chlorhexidine for the eradication of methicillin-resistant *Staphylococcus*

aureus: a randomized, placebo-controlled, double-blind clinical trial. Infect Control Hosp Epidemiol 2007;28(9):1036–43.

18. Vernon MO, Hayden MK, Trick WE, et al. Chlorhexidine gluconate to cleanse patients in a medical intensive care unit: the effectiveness of source control to reduce the bioburden of vancomycin-resistant enterococci. Arch Intern Med 2006;166(3):306–12.

19. Levy I, Katz J, Solter E, et al. Chlorhexidine-impregnated dressing for prevention of colonization of central venous catheters in infants and children: a randomized controlled study. Pediatr Infect Dis J 2005;24(8):676–9.

20. Rupp ME, Lisco SJ, Lipsett PA, et al. Effect of a second-generation venous catheter impregnated with chlorhexidine and silver sulfadiazine on central catheter-related infections: a randomized, controlled trial. Ann Intern Med 2005;143(8):570–80.

21. Chlebicki MP, Safdar N. Topical chlorhexidine for prevention of ventilator-associated pneumonia: a meta-analysis. Crit Care Med 2007;35(2):595–602.

22. Heath RJ, Rubin JR, Holland DR, et al. Mechanism of triclosan inhibition of bacterial fatty acid synthesis. J Biol Chem 1999;274(16):11110–4.

23. Noronha C, Almeida A. Local burn treatments—topical antimicrobial agents. Ann Burn Fire Disasters 2000;8(4):216–9.

24. Ward RS, Saffle JR. Topical agents in burn and wound care. Phys Ther 1995;75(6):526–38.

25. Gocke DJ, Ponticas S, Pollack W. In vitro studies of the killing of clinical isolates by povidone-iodine solutions. J Hosp Infect 1985;6(Suppl A):59–66.

26. Fleischer W, Reimer K. Povidone-iodine in antisepsis–state of the art. Dermatology 1997;195(Suppl 2):3–9.

27. Niedner R. Cytotoxicity and sensitization of povidone-iodine and other frequently used anti-infective agents. Dermatology 1997;195(Suppl 2):89–92.

28. Kramer SA. Effect of povidone-iodine on wound healing: a review. J Vasc Nurs 1999;17(1):17–23.

29. Hsu S, Quan L. Topical antibacterial agents. In: Wolverton SE, editor. Comprehenisve dermatologic drug therapy. Phildelphia: WB Saunders; 2001. p. 472–96.

30. Harkaway KS, McGinley KJ, Foglia AN, et al. Antibiotic resistance patterns in coagulase-negative staphylococci after treatment with topical erythromycin, benzoyl peroxide, and combination therapy. Br J Dermatol 1992;126(6):586–90.

31. Gelmetti C. Local antibiotics in dermatology. Dermatol Ther 2008;21(3):187–95.

32. Barillo DJ. Topical antimicrobials in burn wound care: a recent history. Wounds 2008;20:192–8.

33. Jacin B. Bleach baths fights *S. aureus* infections in eczema patients. Pediatr News 2007;41(7):58.

34. Kaplan SL. Commentary: prevention of recurrent staphylococcal infections. Pediatr Infect Dis J 2008;27(10):935–7.

35. Fisher RG, Chain RL, Hair PS, et al. Hypochlorite killing of community-associated methicillin-resistant *Staphylococcus aureus*. Pediatr Infect Dis J 2008;27(10):934–5.

36. Nagai K, Murata T, Ohta S, et al. Two different mechanisms are involved in the extremely high-level benzalkonium chloride resistance of a *Pseudomonas fluorescens* strain. Microbiol Immunol 2003;47(10):709–15.

37. Halling H. Suspected link between exposure to hexachlorophene and malformed infants. Ann N Y Acad Sci 1979;320:426–35.

38. Thuille N, Fille M, Nagl M. Bactericidal activity of herbal extracts. Int J Hyg Environ Health 2003;206(3):217–21.

39. Kalemba D, Kunicka A. Antibacterial and antifungal properties of essential oils. Curr Med Chem 2003;10(10):813–29.
40. Pappa KA. The clinical development of mupirocin. J Am Acad Dermatol 1990; 22(5 Pt 1):873–9.
41. Spann CT, Tutrone WD, Weinberg JM, et al. Topical antibacterial agents for wound care: a primer. Dermatol Surg 2003;29(6):620–6.
42. Antonio M, McFerran N, Pallen MJ. Mutations affecting the Rossman fold of iso-leucyl-tRNA synthetase are correlated with low-level mupirocin resistance in Staphylococcus aureus. Antimicrob Agents Chemother 2002;46(2):438–42.
43. Jones JC, Rogers TJ, Brookmeyer P, et al. Mupirocin resistance in patients colo-nized with methicillin-resistant Staphylococcus aureus in a surgical intensive care unit. Clin Infect Dis 2007;45(5):541–7.
44. Walker ES, Vasquez JE, Dula R, et al. Mupirocin-resistant, methicillin-resistant Staphylococcus aureus: does mupirocin remain effective? Infect Control Hosp Epidemiol 2003;24(5):342–6.
45. Koning S, van der Wouden JC, Chosidow O, et al. Efficacy and safety of retapa-mulin ointment as treatment of impetigo: randomized double-blind multicentre placebo-controlled trial. Br J Dermatol 2008;158(5):1077–82.
46. Woodford N, Afzal-Shah M, Warner M, et al. In vitro activity of retapamulin against Staphylococcus aureus isolates resistant to fusidic acid and mupirocin. J Antimicrob Chemother 2008;62(4):766–8.
47. Wolf R, Matz H, Orion E, et al. Dapsone. Dermatol Online J 2002;8(1).
48. Draelos ZD, Carter E, Maloney JM, et al. Two randomized studies demonstrate the efficacy and safety of dapsone gel, 5% for the treatment of acne vulgaris. J Am Acad Dermatol 2007;56(3):439.e1–10.
49. Wolf R, Orni-Wasserlauf R. A century of the synthesis of dapsone: its anti-infec-tive capacity now and then. Int J Dermatol 2000;39(10):779–83.
50. Gette MT, Marks JG Jr, Maloney ME. Frequency of postoperative allergic contact dermatitis to topical antibiotics. Arch Dermatol 1992;128(3):365–7.
51. Leyden JJ. The role of topical antibiotics in dermatologic practice. Medscape. Available at: http://www.medscape.com/viewprogram/2501. Accessed November 30, 2008.
52. Winkelman W, Gratton D. Topical antibacterials. Clin Dermatol 1989;7(3):156–62.
53. Kuznar W. Allergen of the year: reactions to common antibiotic bacitracin may be on the rise. Dermatology times 2003, June 1. Available at: http://www.modernmedicine.com/modernmedicine/article/articledetail.Jsp?Ts=1228065479155&id=60907. Ac-cessed November 30, 2008.
54. Jacob SE, James WD. From road rash to top allergen in a flash: bacitracin. Der-matol Surg 2004;30(4 Pt 1):521–4.
55. Hendley JO, Ashe KM. Eradication of resident bacteria of normal human skin by antimicrobial ointment. Antimicrob Agents Chemother 2003;47(6): 1988–90.
56. Hammond B, Ali Y, Fendler E, et al. Effect of hand sanitizer use on elementary school absenteeism. Am J Infect Control 2000;28(5):340–6.
57. Boyce JM. Using alcohol for hand antisepsis: dispelling old myths. Infect Control Hosp Epidemiol 2000;21(7):438–41.
58. Paulson DS, Fendler EJ, Dolan MJ, et al. A close look at alcohol gel as an anti-microbial sanitizing agent. Am J Infect Control 1999;27(4):332–8.
59. Girou E, Loyeau S, Legrand P, et al. Efficacy of handrubbing with alcohol-based solution versus standard handwashing with antiseptic soap: randomised clinical trial. BMJ 2002;325(7360):362.

60. Hilburn J, Hammond BS, Fendler EJ, et al. Use of alcohol hand sanitizer as an infection control strategy in an acute care facility. Am J Infect Control 2003; 31(2):109–16.
61. White C, Kolble R, Carlson R, et al. The effect of hand hygiene on illness rate among students in university residence halls. Am J Infect Control 2003;31(6):364–70.
62. Gruendemann BJ, Bjerke NB. Is it time for brushless scrubbing with an alcohol-based agent? AORN J 2001;74(6):859–73.
63. Laupland KB, Conly JM. Treatment of Staphylococcus aureus colonization and prophylaxis for infection with topical intranasal mupirocin: an evidence-based review. Clin Infect Dis 2003;37(7):933–8.
64. von Eiff C, Becker K, Machka K, et al. Nasal carriage as a source of Staphylococcus aureus bacteremia. Study group. N Engl J Med 2001;344(1):11–6.
65. Bradley SF. Effectiveness of mupirocin in the control of methicillin-resistant Staphylococcus aureus. Infect Med 1993;10:23–31.
66. Perl TM, Cullen JJ, Wenzel RP, et al. Intranasal mupirocin to prevent postoperative Staphylococcus aureus infections. N Engl J Med 2002;346(24):1871–7.
67. Mupirocin Study Group. Nasal mupirocin prevents Staphylococcus aureus exit-site infection during peritoneal dialysis. Mupirocin Study Group. J Am Soc Nephrol 1996;7(11):2403–8.
68. Wertheim HF, Vos MC, Ott A, et al. Mupirocin prophylaxis against nosocomial Staphylococcus aureus infections in nonsurgical patients: a randomized study. Ann Intern Med 2004;140(6):419–25.
69. Chambers HF 3rd, Winston LG. Mupirocin prophylaxis misses by a nose. Ann Intern Med 2004;140(6):484–5.
70. Gorwitz RJ, Kruszon-Moran D, McAllister SK, et al. Changes in the prevalence of nasal colonization with Staphylococcus aureus in the United States, 2001–2004. J Infect Dis 2008;197(9):1226–34.
71. Datta R, Huang SS. Risk of infection and death due to methicillin-resistant Staphylococcus aureus in long-term carriers. Clin Infect Dis 2008;47(2):176–81.
72. Mayall B, Martin R, Keenan AM, et al. Blanket use of intranasal mupirocin for outbreak control and long-term prophylaxis of endemic methicillin-resistant Staphylococcus aureus in an open ward. J Hosp Infect 1996;32(4):257–66.
73. Watanabe H, Masaki H, Asoh N, et al. Low concentrations of mupirocin in the pharynx following intranasal application may contribute to mupirocin resistance in methicillin-resistant Staphylococcus aureus. J Clin Microbiol 2001;39(10):3775–7.
74. Fung S, O'Grady S, Kennedy C, et al. The utility of polysporin ointment in the eradication of methicillin-resistant Staphylococcus aureus colonization: a pilot study. Infect Control Hosp Epidemiol 2000;21(10):653–5.
75. Jeyaratnam D, Gottlieb A, Ajoku U, et al. Validation of the IDI-MRSA system for use on pooled nose, axilla, and groin swabs and single swabs from other screening sites. Diagn Microbiol Infect Dis 2008;61(1):1–5.
76. Simor AE, Phillips E, McGeer A, et al. Randomized controlled trial of chlorhexidine gluconate for washing, intranasal mupirocin, and rifampin and doxycycline versus no treatment for the eradication of methicillin-resistant Staphylococcus aureus colonization. Clin Infect Dis 2007;44(2):178–85.
77. Fung SK, Louie M, Simor AE. Combined topical and oral antimicrobial therapy for the eradication of methicillin-resistant Staphylococcus aureus (MRSA) colonization in hospitalized patients. Can J Infect Dis 2002;13(5):287–92.
78. Kokai-Kun JF, Walsh SM, Chanturiya T, et al. Lysostaphin cream eradicates Staphylococcus aureus nasal colonization in a cotton rat model. Antimicrob Agents Chemother 2003;47(5):1589–97.

79. LaPlante KL. In vitro activity of lysostaphin, mupirocin, and tea tree oil against clinical methicillin-resistant *Staphylococcus aureus*. Diagn Microbiol Infect Dis 2007;57(4):413–8.

80. Caelli M, Porteous J, Carson CF, et al. Tea tree oil as an alternative topical decolonization agent for methicillin-resistant *Staphylococcus aureus*. J Hosp Infect 2000;46(3):236–7.

81. McMahon MA, Blair IS, Moore JE, et al. Habituation to sub-lethal concentrations of tea tree oil (*Melaleuca alternifolia*) is associated with reduced susceptibility to antibiotics in human pathogens. J Antimicrob Chemother 2007;59(1):125–7.

82. McMahon MA, Tunney MM, Moore JE, et al. Changes in antibiotic susceptibility in staphylococci habituated to sub-lethal concentrations of tea tree oil (*Melaleuca alternifolia*). Lett Appl Microbiol 2008;47(4):263–8.

83. Langford JH, Artemi P, Benrimoj SI. Topical antimicrobial prophylaxis in minor wounds. Ann Pharmacother 1997;31(5):559–63.

84. Maddox JS, Ware JC, Dillon HC Jr. The natural history of streptococcal skin infection: prevention with topical antibiotics. J Am Acad Dermatol 1985; 13(2 Pt 1):207–12.

85. Geronemus RG, Mertz PM, Eaglstein WH. Wound healing. The effects of topical antimicrobial agents. Arch Dermatol 1979;115(11):1311–4.

86. Berger RS, Pappert AS, Van Zile PS, et al. A newly formulated topical triple-antibiotic ointment minimizes scarring. Cutis 2000;65(6):401–4.

87. Proposed recommended practices for surgical skin preparation. Association of operating room nurses. AORN J 1996;63(1):221–7.

88. Gilmore OJ, Martin TD, Fletcher BN. Prevention of wound infection after appendicectomy. Lancet 1973;1(7797):220–2.

89. Garibaldi RA. Prevention of intraoperative wound contamination with chlorhexidine shower and scrub. J Hosp Infect 1988;11(Suppl B):5–9.

90. de Jong TE, Vierhout RJ, van Vroonhoven TJ. Povidone-iodine irrigation of the subcutaneous tissue to prevent surgical wound infections. Surg Gynecol Obstet 1982;155(2):221–4.

91. Rogers DM, Blouin GS, O'Leary JP. Povidone-iodine wound irrigation and wound sepsis. Surg Gynecol Obstet 1983;157(5):426–30.

92. Tatnall FM, Leigh IM, Gibson JR. Assay of antiseptic agents in cell culture: conditions affecting cytotoxicity. J Hosp Infect 1991;17(4):287–96.

93. Brown CD, Zitelli JA. A review of topical agents for wounds and methods of wounding. Guidelines for wound management. J Dermatol Surg Oncol 1993; 19(8):732–7.

94. Leyden JJ, Kligman AM. Rationale for topical antibiotics. Cutis 1978;22(4): 515–20, 22–8.

95. Watcher MA, Wheeland RG. The role of topical agents in the healing of full-thickness wounds. J Dermatol Surg Oncol 1989;15(11):1188–95.

96. Forbes GB. Staphylococcal infection of operation wounds with special reference to topical antibiotic prophylaxis. Lancet 1961;2:505.

97. Fielding G, Rao A, Davis NC, et al. Prophylactic topical use of antibiotics in surgical wounds: a controlled clinical trial using "Polybactrin". Med J Aust 1965;2(4):159–61.

98. Gisby J, Bryant J. Efficacy of a new cream formulation of mupirocin: comparison with oral and topical agents in experimental skin infections. Antimicrob Agents Chemother 2000;44(2):255–60.

99. Wahdan HA. Causes of the antimicrobial activity of honey. Infection 1998;26(1): 26–31.

100. Moore OA, Smith LA, Campbell F, et al. Systematic review of the use of honey as a wound dressing. BMC Complement Altern Med 2001;1(2).
101. Fraser JF, Bodman J, Sturgess R, et al. An in vitro study of the anti-microbial efficacy of a 1% silver sulphadiazine and 0.2% chlorhexidine digluconate cream, 1% silver sulphadiazine cream and a silver coated dressing. Burns 2004;30(1):35–41.
102. Singer AJ, Dagum AB. Current management of acute cutaneous wounds. N Engl J Med 2008;359(10):1037–46.
103. Chung JY, Herbert ME. Myth: silver sulfadiazine is the best treatment for minor burns. West J Med 2001;175(3):205–6.
104. Rode H, Hanslo D, de Wet PM, et al. Efficacy of mupirocin in methicillin-resistant *Staphylococcus aureus* burn wound infection. Antimicrob Agents Chemother 1989;33(8):1358–61.
105. Sinha R, Agarwal RK, Agarwal M. Povidone iodine plus neosporin in superficial burns—a continuing study. Burns 1997;23(7–8):626–8.
106. Subrahmanyam M. A prospective randomised clinical and histological study of superficial burn wound healing with honey and silver sulfadiazine. Burns 1998; 24(2):157–61.
107. Kwakman PH, Van den Akker JP, Guclu A, et al. Medical-grade honey kills anti-biotic-resistant bacteria in vitro and eradicates skin colonization. Clin Infect Dis 2008;46(11):1677–82.
108. Feng QL, Wu J, Chen GQ, et al. A mechanistic study of the antibacterial effect of silver ions on *Escherichia coli* and *Staphylococcus aureus*. J Biomed Mater Res 2000;52(4):662–8.
109. MacKeen PC, Person S, Warner SC, et al. Silver-coated nylon fiber as an anti-bacterial agent. Antimicrob Agents Chemother 1987;31(1):93–9.
110. George A, Rubin G. A systematic review and meta-analysis of treatments for impetigo. Br J Gen Pract 2003;53(491):480–7.
111. Mertz PM, Marshall DA, Eaglstein WH, et al. Topical mupirocin treatment of impetigo is equal to oral erythromycin therapy. Arch Dermatol 1989;125(8): 1069–73.
112. Rist T, Parish LC, Capin LR, et al. A comparison of the efficacy and safety of mu-pirocin cream and cephalexin in the treatment of secondarily infected eczema. Clin Exp Dermatol 2002;27(1):14–20.
113. O'Meara SM, Cullum NA, Majid M, et al. Systematic review of antimicrobial agents used for chronic wounds. Br J Surg 2001;88(1):4–21.
114. Saji M, Taguchi S, Uchiyama K, et al. Efficacy of gentian violet in the eradication of methicillin-resistant *Staphylococcus aureus* from skin lesions. J Hosp Infect 1995;31(3):225–8.
115. Walker JR, Shafiq NA, Allen RG. Bacterial cell division regulation: physiological effects of crystal violet on *Escherichia coli* lon + and lon − strains. J Bacteriol 1971;108(3):1296–303.
116. Natarajan S, Williamson D, Grey J, et al. Healing of an MRSA-colonized, hydroxyurea-induced leg ulcer with honey. J Dermatolog Treat 2001;12(1):33–6.
117. Kanj LF, Phillips TJ. Management of leg ulcers. Fitzpatrick's J Clin Dermatol 1994;52–60.
118. Chaiyakunapruk N, Veenstra DL, Lipsky BA, et al. Vascular catheter site care: the clinical and economic benefits of chlorhexidine gluconate compared with povidone iodine. Clin Infect Dis 2003;37(6):764–71.
119. Chaiyakunapruk N, Veenstra DL, Lipsky BA, et al. Chlorhexidine compared with povidone-iodine solution for vascular catheter-site care: a meta-analysis. Ann Intern Med 2002;136(11):792–801.

120. Zinner SH, Denny-Brown BC, Braun P, et al. Risk of infection with intravenous indwelling catheters: effect of application of antibiotic ointment. J Infect Dis 1969;120(5):616–9.
121. Maki DG, Band JD. A comparative study of polyantibiotic and iodophor ointments in prevention of vascular catheter-related infection. Am J Med 1981; 70(3):739–44.

Antibiotics for Gram-Positive Bacterial Infections: Vancomycin, Teicoplanin, Quinupristin/ Dalfopristin, Oxazolidinones, Daptomycin, Dalbavancin, and Telavancin

Michael D. Nailor, PharmD[a,b], Jack D. Sobel, MD[c,*]

KEYWORDS

- Gram positive bacteria • Vancomycin • Daptomycin
- Linezolid • Quinupristin • Dalfopristin • MRSA • VRE

VANCOMYCIN

Vancomycin is a glycopeptide antibiotic that was isolated in 1956 from the actinomycete *Streptomyces orientalis*. It consists of a seven-membered peptide chain and two sugar moieties, vancosamine and glucose.[1] The clinical use of vancomycin became widespread in 1958 with the emergence of penicillinase-producing staphylococci, but the drug fell into disuse 2 years later with the advent of methicillin. Early

[a] Department of Internal Medicine, Wayne State University, Detroit, MI 48201, USA
[b] University of Connecticut School of Pharmacy, 69 North Eagleville Road Unit 3092, Storrs, CT 06269, USA
[c] Division of Infectious Diseases, Department of Internal Medicine, Wayne State University, 320 E. Canfield, Detroit, MI 48201, USA
* Corresponding author. Harper University Hospital, 3990 John R Street, Detroit, MI 40201, USA
E-mail address: jsobel@intmed.wayne.edu (J.D. Sobel).

Infect Dis Clin N Am 23 (2009) 965–982
doi:10.1016/j.idc.2009.06.010
0891-5520/09/$ – see front matter © 2009 Elsevier Inc. All rights reserved.

preparations of vancomycin contained fermentation byproducts, resulting in marked toxicity. It is one of most widely used antibiotics in the United States for the treatment of serious gram-positive infections, particularly those involving methicillin-resistant Staphylococcus aureus (MRSA).[2]

Mechanism of Action

Vancomycin exhibits concentration-independent bactericidal activity by the inhibition of bacterial cell wall synthesis. Specifically, it complexes with the D-alanyl-D-alanine portion of peptide precursor units, inhibiting peptidoglycan polymerase and transpeptidation reactions. This prevents the cross-linking of the cell wall peptidoglycan, which occurs during the second stage of cell wall synthesis. Because β-lactams inhibit cell wall biosynthesis in the third phase, there is no cross-resistance between the drugs and no competition for binding sites. Like penicillin, vancomycin requires actively growing bacteria to exert its effect. Also, vancomycin is capable of injuring protoplasts by altering the permeability of their cytoplasmic membrane and selectively inhibiting RNA synthesis.[3,4] Vancomycin exhibits minimal concentration-dependent killing action, but a moderately long in vitro postantibiotic effect.[5]

Antimicrobial Activity

Virtually all Staphylococcus aureus strains are susceptible to vancomycin. In addition, the vast majority of coagulase-negative staphylococci are susceptible. Vancomycin-resistant enterococci (VRE) bloodstream isolates have increased over the years, and in 2002, 17.7% of all enterococci isolates were resistant to vancomycin. Vancomycin resistance was more frequent among Enterococcus faecium isolates, at 60.9%, whereas in the more frequently isolated E. faecalis, resistance was detected in only 2.5% of cases.[6]

Vancomycin is bactericidal for most gram-positive organisms, with minimum inhibitory concentrations (MICs) in the range of 1 to 4 μg/mL.[2] However, against enterococci, vancomycin is only bacteriostatic.

Vancomycin-aminoglycoside combinations are synergistic for the majority of Staphylococcus aureus strains, whether they are methicillin susceptible or methicillin resistant.[7] In addition, substantial improvements in cure rates for Staphylococcus epidermidis prosthetic valve endocarditis are achieved by adding rifampin, gentamicin, or both to vancomycin.[8] Barring the presence of high-level gentamicin-resistant isolates (MIC > 500 μg/mL), the combination of vancomycin-gentamicin is also synergistic for enterococci.

Vancomycin is bactericidal against a variety of other gram-positive aerobic and anaerobic organisms, including Corynebacterium spp, Bacillus spp, pneumococci, viridans streptococci, and clostridia, including Clostridium difficile. Most Listeria monocytogenes, lactobacilli, actinomycetes, and anaerobic streptococci are also susceptible.

Leuconostoc and Pediococcus species, which cause serious infections in immunocompromised patients, are resistant to vancomycin. Vancomycin has no activity against gram-negative organisms.

Pharmacokinetics, Dosing, and Administration

The 24-hour area under the curve (AUC)-MIC ratio is probably the most important pharmacokinetic (PK)-pharmacodynamic (PD) parameter correlating with the efficacy of vancomycin.[9] Vancomycin has a large volume of distribution, with therapeutic levels achievable in ascitic, pericardial, pleural, and synovial fluids. Vancomycin penetrates poorly into the aqueous humor and bile. Penetration into cerebrospinal fluid is poor, except for cases in which the meninges are inflamed, in cases in which cerebrospinal fluid concentrations range from 7% to 21% of concomitant serum levels.[10–12] The bone-to-serum ratio of vancomycin concentration is 10%, which increases to 20% to 30% in infected bone.[13] Relatively poor penetration of vancomycin into respiratory secretions (eg, epithelial lining fluid) is reported (25% of plasma concentrations in pneumonia), in part as a function of high protein binding (50%–60%).[14]

Vancomycin retains activity at a pH between 6.5 and 8, and concentrations achieved in abscess fluid approach those obtained in serum.[15,16] Vancomycin is eliminated by glomerular filtration, with 80% to 90% of an administered dose appearing in the urine within 24 hours. The serum half-life in adults who have normal renal function is 4 to 8 hours after intravenous injection.[11] Several nomograms exist for initiating vancomycin dosing and adjusting dosage in renal insufficiency.[17,18] However, because nomograms assume a fixed volume of distribution and wide variations can occur, serum levels should be monitored. Desired peak and trough levels have traditionally ranged from 30 to 40 μg/mL and 5 to 10 μg/mL, respectively; however, numerous recent guidelines advocate higher desired trough levels of from 15 to 20 μg/mL.[19–21] Unfortunately, there are limited human data that document superior efficacy for vancomycin or the possibility that increases in trough levels can result in increased toxicity. Vancomycin has an alpha-phase (mostly distribution) half-life of 30 minutes; therefore, if peaks are drawn, the samples should be collected approximately 1 hour postinfusion, using a 1-hour infusion.

Unlike previous recommendations of 1 g every 12 hours as a standard initiation dose, typical adult dosing is now highly variable as a result of variation in desired target trough concentrations. Vancomycin dosages should be calculated using actual body weight[21]; however, caution should be used for individuals weighing more than 120 kg. Elderly patients might only require 1 g every 24 hours, whereas younger patients might require 1.5 g every 8 hours or more to achieve serum trough concentrations of 15 to 20 μg/mL, depending on renal function and weight. Additionally, using loading doses (eg, 25 mg/kg) may also be helpful in quickly achieving desired trough levels that may prevent elevations in MRSA MICs, or tolerance, from occurring during therapy.[22] Although the AUC/MIC ratio is now considered the most predictive pharmacodynamic parameter for vancomycin, (specifically a target AUC/MIC ratio of ≥400), the ratio's clinical utility does not appear practical.[21] Continuous infusion regimens do not appear to offer any therapeutic advantage.[20] Regardless of the dosing interval selected, critically ill patients should have their trough concentrations measured within the first day of therapy, even if the levels are not believed to be at steady state, to ensure that adequate levels are achieved quickly. Determining trough serum vancomycin concentrations is the most practical and accurate method for monitoring vancomycin effectiveness.[21] The recommended intravenous dosing schedules for pediatric patients vary according to age and site of infection.[23] In newborns, vancomycin is given at a dosage of 15 mg/kg every 12 hours for the first week of life, or every 8 hours in newborns 8 to 30 days of age; 10–15 mg/kg every 6 hours is recommended for older infants and children. For central nervous system infections, 15 mg/kg every 6 hours is recommended. The volume of distribution is increased and the elimination phase is prolonged in adults compared with children.

Vancomycin cannot be administered intramuscularly because it causes severe pain at the injection site. Orally administered vancomycin is poorly absorbed from the gastrointestinal tract. However, patients who have renal impairment and inflamed bowel can have significant absorption.[24] The oral drug in a dosage of 125 to 500 mg every 6 hours is used to treat C difficile enterocolitis, with stool concentrations of vancomycin ranging from 100 to 800 μg/g for the 125-mg dose.[25] Vancomycin is rapidly absorbed into the general circulation after intraperitoneal administration and can be used to treat gram-positive bacterial infections related to continuous ambulatory peritoneal dialysis (CAPD). Therapeutic serum levels of vancomycin are attainable using this method.[26]

Hemodialytic removal of vancomycin depends on a variety of factors, including the filter being used, the flow rates, and the time on the dialysis circuit.[27] With the advent of high-flux filters, previous recommendations regarding vancomycin dosages of just 500 mg every week[5] may be outdated. Some patients now require 1 g of vancomycin after each dialysis session. Dosing recommendations at institutions should be individualized, and therapeutic drug monitoring should be used. Care should be taken so that levels are not obtained too soon after dialysis to avoid misinterpreting falsely low vancomycin levels. In such settings, falsely low vancomycin levels result from drug redistribution from tissues back into the serum after rapid removal of the drug in the serum during dialysis.[27]

Clinical Indications

Vancomycin is the drug of choice for methicillin-resistant strains of coagulase-negative and coagulase-positive staphylococcal infections, including bacteremia, endocarditis, pneumonia, cellulitis, and osteomyelitis.[15,28] For patients who are allergic to semisynthetic penicillins or cephalosporins, vancomycin is an alternative for methicillin-susceptible staphylococcal infections. However, in cases of serious infections caused by methicillin-susceptible organisms such as endocarditis, vancomycin may be less effective than semisynthetic antistaphylococcal penicillins[29] and should not be used for convenience alone. Some methicillin-susceptible strains that are deficient in autolysins may be tolerant to vancomycin, in which case the addition of gentamicin, rifampin, or both should be considered.

Vancomycin should be combined with gentamicin, rifampin, or both agents when treating prosthetic-device-related *Staphylococcus epidermidis* infections because cure rates are improved by using such combinations.[8] Foreign bodies may need to be removed if the patient has not responded to antibiotics or if infection relapses. *Staphylococcus epidermidis* infections of long-term intravenous catheters can usually be cured without removal of the device. Administration of the antibiotic should be rotated to alternating lumens in the case of multilumen catheters. Central nervous system shunt infections can often be treated using a combination of intravenous and intraventricular vancomycin, but in some cases, removal of the foreign body is necessary.[30] Vancomycin can be given intrathecally or intraventricularly at dosages of 3 to 5 mg per day in children if necessary.[31] In adults higher daily doses of 10 to 20 mg are needed.

Vancomycin is also the drug of choice for infections caused by penicillin-resistant streptococci, *Corynebacterium* group jeikeium, *Bacillus* spp, and penicillin-resistant enterococci. Accordingly, given the recent increased frequency of penicillin-resistant pneumococcal disease, vancomycin is now recommended as initial therapy for cases of proved, suspected, or possible pneumococcal meningitis, in combination with a third-generation cephalosporin, until susceptibility data are available. In cases of serious enterococcal infections, vancomycin should be combined with an aminoglycoside (gentamicin or streptomycin) unless high-level aminoglycoside resistance (MIC > 500 or 2000 μg/mL, respectively) is present.

In the treatment of *C difficile* enterocolitis, the use of oral vancomycin should be reserved for patients who do not respond to therapy using metronidazole, for patients who have severe, life-threatening infections, for patients who cannot tolerate metronidazole, and for those who have relapsing disease and who require long courses or multiple repeated courses of therapy. Although vancomycin has the advantages of poor systemic absorption and fewer side effects, concern about the emergence of VRE isolates should limit its use to treat this condition. If oral vancomycin is used, it should not be combined with cholestyramine because that agent binds vancomycin.

Resistance

VRE are becoming an alarming problem. In all National Nosocomial Infections Surveillance System–participating hospitals, resistance frequency has increased, regardless of the hospital's size or teaching affiliation.[32,33] The VanA phenotype (vancomycin MIC > 256, teicoplanin resistant) is encoded by a gene located on a plasmid that is easily transferable to other enterococci using conjugation. The VanB phenotype is also transferable, and it codes for vancomycin resistance; however, these isolates retain susceptibility to teicoplanin. The transfer to and expression of enterococcal vancomycin-resistant genes in Staphylococcus aureus has been accomplished in the laboratory,[34] heightening concern that widespread vancomycin resistance in staphylococci will eventually emerge. The use of vancomycin and cephalosporin is a well-recognized risk factor for infection by VRE.[35] Thus, any program to control resistance must consider reducing unnecessary use of these antibiotics.

Reports to the US Centers for Disease Control and Prevention of glycopeptide-resistant enterococci (GRE) indicate an increase of more than 25 fold in the prevalence of GRE between 1989 and 1993.[28] The proportion of health care–associated GRE infections in intensive care units rose to 14%; although E faecalis is isolated at about four times the frequency of E faecium, the latter is responsible for most episodes of GRE.[28] Huycke and colleagues[28] reported that although vancomycin resistance varied between 1.3% and 2.3% between the years 1995 and 1997 in cases of E faecalis infection, resistance increased from 28% to 52% in E faecium during the same period. Although carriage of these organisms by health care professionals has been described, most infections arise from the patient's own flora. As could be expected, vancomycin use is believed to contribute to the increase in GRE[36]; however, the use of other antibiotics, such as third-generation cephalosporins, also has contributed to GRE selection.[37] Additional factors associated with the emergence of GRE are shown in Box 1.

Selection pressure by overuse of vancomycin can be enormous. Ena and colleagues[39] described a 20-fold increase in the use of vancomycin between 1981 and 1991 in a 900-bed university teaching hospital. In only one-third of cases was

---

Box 1
Factors associated with emergence of glycopeptide-resistant enterococci[38]

1. Current or recent vancomycin use
2. Gastrointestinal tract colonization by GRE
3. Duration of hospital stay
4. Proximity to patients who are infected by GRE
5. Intrahospital transfer of patients between wards or floors
6. Prior use of certain broad spectrum antimicrobials (antianaerobes).
7. Location in an intensive care unit
8. Hemodialysis, ventilator, catheter, and other invasive device use.
9. Large hospital size
10. Intra-abdominal surgery.

vancomycin used for specific culture-directed therapy. The remainder of the cases were divided between prophylactic use and empiric therapy. In addition, the authors found a failure to make adjustments in therapy in the majority of cases in which vancomycin use for prophylactic or empiric reasons was initiated. Strong efforts should be made to control vancomycin use in all medical centers, as recommended by the US Centers for Disease Control and Prevention report from the Hospital Infection Control Practices Advisory Committee.[38]

Methicillin-resistant *Staphylococcus epidermidis* infections that are clinically unresponsive to vancomycin therapy have been described. One such infection occurred in a patient who was treated using vancomycin for more than two months for CAPD-associated peritonitis.[40] Heterogeneous resistance was found, with an MIC range to vancomycin of 2 to 16 μg/mL. Population analysis showed some colonies that had vancomycin MICs of 25 to 50 μg/mL.

An analysis of a large surveillance database of 35,458 *Staphylococcus aureus* strains by Jones[41] found that the MIC required to inhibit the growth of 90% of organisms (MIC_{90}) for vancomycin is 1 μg/mL. Some researchers are reporting that a greater percentage of their MRSA isolates have elevated MICs to vancomycin but are still within the susceptible range, a phenomenon known as MIC creep.[41,42] The most alarming aspect of these findings is that infections caused by MRSA that have vancomycin MICs of 2 μg/mL have worse surrogate outcomes.[43,44] Recently, a study showed that after adjusting for a number of variables, mortality was also worse in the elevated MIC group.[45] These reports have formed the basis for consensus recommendations that trough serum concentrations should always be maintained at greater than 10 μg/mL to avoid the development of resistance and possibly improve clinical outcome.[21] Accordingly, total trough serum vancomycin concentrations of 15 to 20 μg/mL are recommended.[21] Unfortunately, there is also a lack of data on antibiotic therapy that is superior to vancomycin for these infections. One center reported the emergence of daptomycin-nonsusceptible isolates when patients were switched to daptomycin as a result of elevated vancomycin MICs.[46] Patients in that report had a mean duration of vancomycin therapy of 4 days prior to switching to daptomycin, which may have contributed to the development of daptomycin-nonsusceptible isolates.

Glycopeptide-intermediate-resistant *Staphylococcus aureus* (GISA) was first described in Japan in May 1996, in a child who had an MRSA wound infection that was clinically unresponsive to vancomycin.[47–49] According to the National Committee for Clinical Laboratory Standards, vancomycin-susceptible strains of *Staphylococcus aureus* have MICs of 2 μg/mL or less, GISA strains of 4 to 8 μg/mL, and resistant strains of 16 μg/mL or greater.[50]

Strains of apparently vancomycin-susceptible MRSA have also been detected that display subpopulations that have reduced sensitivity to vancomycin; they have been termed heterogeneous heteroresistant, vancomycin-intermediate *Staphylococcus aureus* (hVISA). Similar to cases of infection by MRSA that have MICs of 2 μg/mL to vancomycin, poor outcomes have been reported.[51] In some centers, rates of hVISA have been steadily rising since 1986, to as high as 8.3% between 2003 and 2007. However, there seems to be a lack of correlation between the trends for hVISA and vancomycin-intermediate *Staphylococcus aureus* (VISA) because the same researchers noted that the lowest rates of VISA, at 0.3%, were detected during the period from 2003 to 2007, which was down from 2.3% in the period preceding it.[52] Because this analysis was done retrospectively and vancomycin had been used as a mainstay of therapy in the hospitals reporting these results, it is unclear whether continued vancomycin use to treat infections caused by hVISA will promote the formation of VISA.

In 2002, the first naturally occurring vancomycin-resistant *Staphylococcus aureus* (VRSA) infection was described in a patient who had a nonhealing foot wound and who was receiving long-term hemodialysis in Michigan at an outpatient dialysis center.[53] Approximately 1 month later, an independent second case of VRSA was reported in an outpatient in Pennsylvania who also had nonhealing foot wounds.[54] Upon further analysis, it was determined that the VRSA from the Michigan patient carried the VanA gene coding for high-level vancomycin resistance and was most likely acquired from coexisting *E faecalis* present in the foot wound.[53] The first patient was cured of VRSA using a combination of antibiotic therapy (trimethoprim and sulfame-thoxazole) and aggressive foot care.[53] The second patient was transiently colonized and did not require antimicrobial treatment. Common to both patients were repeated infections by *Staphylococcus aureus* and enterococci. An extensive contact tracing failed to show any spread beyond the index cases. However, if spread had occurred, the public health consequences of these difficult-to-treat, gram-positive infections would have been enormous.

Toxicity and Adverse Reactions

The "red man" syndrome is a nonimmunologically mediated histamine release associated with rapid infusion of vancomycin. Clinical signs and symptoms include pruritis, erythema and flushing of the upper torso, angioedema, and occasionally, hypotension. Slow administration (for at least 1 hour) and the administration of prophylactic antihistamines given two hours prior to infusion can protect against the development of this side effect.[55] A rapid bolus of vancomycin can also result in muscle spasms of the chest and back, which is known as the "pain and spasm" syndrome. Ototoxicity, which may continue to progress after discontinuation of therapy, may occur when serum levels of vancomycin are excessively high but rarely occurs when peak serum levels are 40 to 50 μg/mL or less. Deafness may be proceeded by tinnitus and high-tone hearing loss. Nephrotoxicity is similarly rare when vancomycin is used alone and at conventional dosages (eg, 1 g every 12 hours). Ototoxicity and nephrotoxicity may be potentiated when vancomycin and aminoglycosides are used in combination.[56] A recent retrospective report called into question the use of higher doses of vancomycin in light of the higher rates of nephrotoxicity seen in patients who received 4 g or more of vancomycin.[57] Care should be used when extrapolating these data because there may have been an unseen selection bias of giving patients higher doses of vancomycin when they were perceived by a clinician as having a more severe disease state, and the patients' underlying condition may have also contributed to the perceived toxicity.

Vancomycin-induced neutropenia is dose- and time-dependent, rare, and reversible after the drug is discontinued. It typically occurs when the duration of therapy exceeds 14 days.[58] Skin rash and drug fever occur in 4% to 5% of patients.[59]

TEICOPLANIN

Teicoplanin is a glycopeptide antibiotic with activity similar to that of vancomycin.[60] It is not commercially available in the United States.

QUINUPRISTIN/DALFOPRISTIN (SYNERCID)

Quinupristin-dalfopristin is a combination of two naturally occurring compounds isolated from *Streptomyces pristinaspiralis*.[61] This streptogramin class is water soluble[62] and contains quinupristin and dalfopristin in a 30:70 weight/weight ratio.[63]

Mechanism of Action

Quinupristin-dalfopristin exerts its activity through the inhibition of protein synthesis. Quinupristin and dalfopristin sequentially bind to different sites on the 50S ribosome, resulting in a stable, ternary drug-ribosome complex and interfering with different targets of 23S RNA. Newly synthesized peptide chains cannot be extruded from this complex.[61,64]

Pharmacokinetics, Dosing, and Administration

Quinupristin and dalfopristin are metabolized quickly after intravenous administration. Neither component is extensively protein bound. The recommended dosage is 7.5 mg/kg every 8 hours by the intravenous route for infections by VRE. The interval may be lengthened to every 12 hours for complicated skin and skin structure infections. There are no adjustments necessary for renal or hepatic impairment.[61] The combination has a postantibiotic effect for 6 to 8 hours. High intracellular concentrations are seen.[65] Excretion is primarily by way of the biliary tract. The drug combination is a potent inhibitor of the cytochrome P450 enzymes, with the potential for drug interactions.

Clinical Activity

The spectrum of activity of quinupristin-dalfopristin is similar to that of vancomycin. In a study of nearly 30,000 clinical isolates in the United States, susceptibility was seen for 97.7% of *Streptococcus pneumoniae* (including penicillin-resistant isolates), 97% of other streptococcal spp, 99% to 99.9% of *Staphylococcus aureus*, and 98% to 100% of coagulase-negative staphylococci. *E faecium* susceptibility varied by participating study region.[63] Overall, 0.2% of *E faecium* isolates were resistant to quinupristin/dalfopristin, with MICs greater than 4 µg/mL. The drug has no activity against *E faecalis*. It is bacteriostatic for *E faecium* and *Legionella* spp.[65] Gram-negative anaerobes such as *Fusobacterium* spp and *Bacteroides* spp are also susceptible.[61] VRSA isolates retained susceptibility to quinupristin-dalfopristin. In a study of 274 South African enterococcal isolates, 19.7% of *E faecium* strains were resistant. *Staphylococcus aureus* MICs were similar to those for vancomycin.[66] The main use for quinupristin-dalfopristin is in the treatment of vancomycin-resistant *E faecium*, and potentially for the treatment of GISA and VRSA. One case of successful therapy for VRE *faecium* prosthetic valve endocarditis has been described.[67]Superinfection by *E faecalis* during therapy has also been described.[68]

Resistance

Resistance may develop as the result of decreased ribosomal binding of either component, through enzymatic modification, or through efflux mechanisms and altered target.[61,69] A patient who developed quinupristin-dalfopristin–resistant *E faecium* bacteremia while receiving therapy using quinupristin-dalfopristin has been described.[70] In addition to clinical failures, resistant isolates have been recovered from human stool samples.[69] No cross-resistance to other currently available antimicrobials occurs. When used in combination with doxycycline, resistance to the streptogramin may be prevented.[71]

Toxicity and Adverse Events

Side effects of quinupristin-dalfopristin include venous irritation and elevation of conjugated bilirubin. The most troublesome side effect seen is the development of arthralgias and myalgias, which can be severe.

OXAZOLIDINONES

The oxazolidinones are a synthetic class of antimicrobial agents that were discovered in 1987. Although there are a number compounds in development, linezolid is the only commercially available product.

Mechanism of Action

Linezolid exerts its effect early in protein synthesis by inhibiting the initiation complex at the 30S ribosome.[72,73] The agent interacts with a translational component that is either directly or indirectly involved in binding mRNA during the start of translation.[73] Because of this unique action, no cross-resistance with other currently available antimicrobials occurs.

Antimicrobial Activity

The antimicrobial spectrum of the oxazolidinones is similar to that of vancomycin, with activity against most gram-positive organisms, including MRSA and penicillin-resistant pneumococci.[74,75] The compounds also have activity against gram-negative anaerobes and mycobacteria.[75] They are bacteriostatic for enterococci and staphylococci, but bactericidal for *Streptococcus pyogenes* and *Bacteroides fragilis*.[76]

Pharmacokinetics, Dosing, and Administration

Maximum peak plasma levels are achieved within 1 to 2 hours after administration. Linezolid has 100% oral bioavailability.[77,78] Linezolid differs from vancomycin by its enhanced penetration into respiratory secretions. Rapid penetration into bone, fat, and muscle is also reported, achieving levels of 4 μg/mL or greater in excess of the MIC of most susceptible organisms.[79] Urinary concentrations of linezolid are high, achieving bactericidal activity against urinary pathogens such as enterococci.[80] There is a short postantibiotic effect of about 1 hour; however, inhibition of virulence-factor expression by gram-positive cocci continues after exposure to subinhibitory concentrations of linezolid.[81] No synergy with aminoglycosides for gram-positive bacteria exists. Isolates of enterococci and streptococci are considered sensitive if their MICs are 2 μg/mL or less, and 4 μg/mL or less for staphylococci. The recommended dosage is 600 mg every 12 hours. The 24-hour AUC-MIC ratio is the pharmacodynamic parameter that bests predicts clinical efficacy.[9]

Clinical Indications

Although initially used to mainly treat patients who were infected by VRE, linezolid's role in treating MRSA infections has grown significantly. Linezolid is currently used for the treatment of pneumonia and skin and skin-structure infections caused by MRSA.[74,82] The high penetration of the drug into respiratory secretions is believed to contribute to linezolid being a very effective agent for the treatment of pneumonia caused by *Staphylococcus aureus* and *Streptococcus pneumoniae*.[83] A recent retrospective analysis of 339 patients who had documented *Staphylococcus aureus* pneumonia, including 160 patients who had MRSA pneumonia, suggested the superior efficacy of linezolid rather than vancomycin.[84] Additional prospective studies are required to confirm these findings. Similarly, several reports of superior activity for ceftriaxone in bacteremic pneumococcal pneumonia have appeared.[85,86]

Given the excellent bioavailability of linezolid and its activity against MRSA and methicillin-resistant, coagulase-negative staphylococci, reports have appeared of efficacy and cost-savings accompanying the early switch and early discharge of patients who were treated using oral linezolid.[87–90] These studies, combined with the prevalence of community-acquired MRSA skin and skin-structure infections, have greatly increased the use of linezolid. It is apparent that parenteral linezolid is now being considered as a first-line therapy for multisite infections caused by MRSA organisms without vancomycin resistance. Although evidence of clinical equivalence has been published, many experts continue to reserve linezolid for vancomycin-resistant organisms, refractory infections, and vancomycin-intolerant patients.

Resistance

In gradient plate experiments, there was no increase in the MICs to linezolid upon serial passage of either MRSA or methicillin-resistant *Staphylococcus epidermidis* strains.[91–94] The previously described VRSA isolates retained susceptibility to linezolid. However, linezolid resistance has been described in enteroccci, even in patients who had no prior exposure to this novel antibiotic.[93,94] Additionally, reports of MRSA resistant to linezolid have emerged.[95]

Toxicity and Adverse Events

Increases in the levels of hepatic enzymes and creatinine can occasionally occur. Skin rash has been reported. Linezolid has the potential for monoamine oxidase inhibition. In preclinical animal studies, reversible time- and dose-dependent myelosuppression occurred, particularly thrombocytopenia. Gerson and colleagues[96] concluded that hematological abnormalities associated with linezolid use were mild and reversible and not significantly different from those of comparator drugs. Thrombocytopenia occurred in 2.2% of patients, usually after 2 weeks of therapy. Long-term use is, however, associated with an incidence of up to 10%. In a study of 686 seriously ill patients who had nosocomial pneumonia, observed in multiple intensive care units, patients treated using linezolid rarely developed thrombocytopenia, which was no more frequent than with the use of vancomycin.[97]

DAPTOMYCIN

Daptomycin is a naturally occurring cyclic lipopeptide antibiotic that is a fermentation byproduct of *Streptomyces roseosporus*.[98] It consists of a 10-membered amino acid ring with a 10-carbon decanoic acid attached to a terminal L-tryptophan.[98]

Mechanism of Action

Daptomycin is rapidly bactericidal in a novel, concentration-dependent manner. It exhibits its action by binding to the cell membrane in a calcium-dependent manner, causing depolarization of the bacterial membrane potential, resulting in the termination of bacterial DNA, RNA, and protein synthesis and the termination of intracellular potassium release, thus causing cell death.[99]

Antimicrobial Activity

The spectrum of activity includes *Staphylococcus aureus*, streptococci, and enterococcal species, including those with multidrug resistance.[100,101] This includes vancomycin-, quinupristin-dalfopristin–, and linezolid-resistant gram-positive organisms. Daptomycin also demonstrates clinical activity against vancomycin-resistant *Leuconostoc* spp.[102] Neither *Listeria* nor *Clostridium* spp are susceptible. Daptomycin in combination with gentamicin is synergistic in killing staphylococci and enterococci.[99] Data regarding the addition of rifampin have been positive or indifferent.[103]

Pharmacokinetics, Dosing, and Administration

Daptomycin is available in intravenous form. It is administered once daily and exhibits linear pharmacokinetics at doses of up to 12 mg/kg.[99] Daptomycin is highly protein bound (92%) and is excreted in the kidney as intact drug.[99] Dosage adjustment for patients who have a creatinine clearance of less than 30 mL/min is recommended. It has a postantibiotic effect that lasts for about 2.5 to 5 hours.[104] Bactericidal activity is dose-dependent. Streptococci and staphylococci are considered sensitive if the MIC is 1 μg/mL or less, and enterococci are considered sensitive when the MIC is 4 μg/mL or less.

Clinical Indications

Daptomycin is approved by the US Food and Drug Administration for the treatment of complicated skin and soft-tissue infections caused by staphylococci (methicillin-susceptible *Staphylococcus aureus* and MRSA), *Streptococcus* spp, and *E faecalis*, at a dose of 4 mg/kg/day administered intravenously. A trial was completed that led to its approval for use in *Staphylococcus aureus* bloodstream infections, including right-sided endocarditis, using daptomycin at 6 mg/kg/day.[105] In the MRSA arm (99 patients) of this trial, success rates were numerically higher but not statistically significant in favor of daptomycin rather than the comparator vancomycin with 4 days of gentamicin. The toxicity of daptomycin was less than that of the vancomycin-genta-micin combination. Among patients who had treatment failure, six daptomycin-treated patients and one vancomycin-gentamicin–treated patient developed reduced susceptibility to their primary therapy. The length of bacteremia infection was similar between the two groups. Patients should not be treated using daptomycin for pneumonia because the drug binds to surfactant, inhibiting its activity.

Resistance

VRSA and VRE isolates are susceptible to daptomycin. However, some hVISA and VISA isolates have shown reduced susceptibility to daptomycin without previous exposure to daptomycin but with exposure to vancomycin.[106–108] Resistance in MRSA has rarely been reported. However, only recently have the various automated systems used by many hospitals incorporated daptomycin into standard panels. One health system recently reported reduced susceptibility to daptomycin for MRSA isolates.[109] All of the isolates that showed reduced susceptibility had vancomycin MICs of 2 μg/mL. The correlation of MRSA with reduced susceptibility to vancomycin and reduced cross-susceptibility to daptomycin requires further study.

Toxicity and Adverse Events

Two major causes of toxicity for daptomycin are elevated levels of creatine phospho-kinase and myopathy, both of which resolve after discontinuation of the drug. Weekly monitoring of creatine phosphokinase values during daptomycin therapy and discontinuation if creatine phosphokinase elevation is 5 times the upper limit of normal or greater is recommended. These effects are more common when divided doses are used compared with once-daily dosing.[110] Constipation and other gastrointestinal side effects have also been noted to occur.

DALBAVANCIN AND TELAVANCIN

Dalbavancin and telavancin are two new antimicrobial agents that are structurally and mechanistically related to vancomycin. Neither agent is currently licensed by the US Food and Drug Administration. Their respective spectrums of activity are similar to those of vancomycin, with the most notable exception being that these two agents have lower MICs against MRSA isolates, with MICs of 2 μg/mL to vancomycin and to VISA isolates. Both agents also have lower MICs to VRE isolates, but the MICs are considerably higher for non–vancomycin-resistant isolates. Both agents have longer half-lives than vancomycin, which allows for simpler dosing regimens. In clinical trials, dalbavancin has been tested using once-weekly infusions, whereas telavancin has been studied using daily infusions. Studies have been completed that used both agents for the treatment of skin and soft-tissue infections. If approved by the Food and Drug Administration, the clinical role for both agents will likely be in the treatment of infections caused by *Staphylococcus aureus* that have reduced susceptibility to vancomycin or to simplify the intravenous regimens for patients who are being discharged and will receive long-term outpatient antimicrobial therapy.[111–114]

SUMMARY

Gram-positive bacteria have shown a propensity to develop resistance to all of the available antibiotics in use. Additionally, the superiority data for any one agent rather than another is lacking, with the possible exception of linezolid, rather than vancomycin, for the treatment of MRSA pneumonia. Selecting the appropriate therapy is also complicated by differences in local susceptibility patterns, particularly as they relate to diminished susceptibility to vancomycin and daptomycin, site of infection, propensity to induce resistance, toxicity, dosage form availability, and only if the proceeding factors are similar, costs. Despite the increasing prevalence of gram-positive infections, judicious use of these agents and strict infection-control practices to preserve the activity of these agents is warranted.

REFERENCES

1. Pfeiffer RR. Structural features of vancomycin. Rev Infect Dis 1981;Nov–Dec (Suppl 3):S205–9.
2. Moellering RC Jr. Vancomycin: a 50-year reassessment. Clin Infect Dis 2006; 42(Suppl 1):S3–4.
3. Jordan DC, Inniss WE. Selective inhibition of ribonucleic acid synthesis in *Staphylococcus aureus* by vancomycin. Nature 1959;184(Suppl 24):1894–5.
4. Jordan DC, Mallory HDC. Site of action of vancomycin on *Staphylococcus aureus*. Antimicrob Agents Chemother 1964;4:489–94.
5. Cunha BA, Quintiliani R, Deglin JM, et al. Pharmacokinetics of vancomycin in anuria. Rev Infect Dis 1981;Nov–Dec(Suppl 3):S269–72.
6. Biedenbach DJ, Moet GJ, Jones RN. Occurrence and antimicrobial resistance pattern comparisons among bloodstream infection isolates from the SENTRY Antimicrobial Surveillance Program (1997–2002). Diagn Microbiol Infect Dis 2004;50:59–69.
7. Watanakunakorn C, Guerriero JC. Synergism between vancomycin and gentamicin or tobramycin for methicillin-susceptible and methicillin-resistant *Staphylococcus aureus* strains. Antimicrob Agents Chemother 1982;22:903–5.
8. Karchmer AW, Archer GC, Dismukes WE. *Staphylococcus epidermidis* causing prosthetic valve endocarditis: microbiologic and clinical observation as a guide to therapy. Ann Intern Med 1983;98:447–55.
9. Craig WA. Basic pharmacodynamics of antibacterials with clinical application to the use of ß-lactam, glycopeptides and linezolid. Infect Dis Clin North Am 2003; 17:479–501.

10. Hawley HB, Gump DW. Vancomycin therapy of bacterial meningitis. Am J Dis Child 1973;126:261–4.
11. Matzke GR, Zhanel GG, Guay DRP. Clinical pharmacokinetics of vancomycin. Clin Pharm 1986;11:257–82.
12. Redfield DC, Underman A, Norman D, et al. Cerebrospinal fluid penetration of vancomycin in bacterial meningitis. In: Nelson JD, Grassi C, editors, Current chemotherapy and infectious disease, vol. 1. Washington, DC: American Society for Microbiology; 1980. p. 638–41.
13. Graziani AL, Lawson LA, Gibson GA, et al. Vancomycin concentrations in infected and non-infected human bone. Antimicrob Agents Chemother 1988;32: 1320–2.
14. Lamer C, de Beco V, Soler P, et al. Analysis of vancomycin entry into pulmonary lung fluid by bronchoalveolar lavage in critically ill patients. Antimicrob Agents Chemother 1993;37:281–6.
15. Geraci JE, Heilman FR, Nichols DR, et al. Antibiotic therapy of bacterial endocarditis: VII. Vancomycin for acute micrococcal endocarditis: preliminary report. Proc Staff Meet Mayo Clin 1958;33:172–81.
16. Torres JR, Sanders CV, Lewis AC. Vancomycin concentration in human tissues: preliminary report. J Antimicrob Chemother 1979;5:475–7.
17. Lake KD, Peterson CD. Evaluation of a method for initiating vancomycin therapy. Experience in 205 patients. Pharmacotherapy 1988;8:284–6.
18. Moellering RC Jr, Krogstad DJ, Greenblatt DJ. Vancomycin therapy in patients with impaired renal function: a nomogram for dosage. Ann Intern Med 1981; 94:343–6.
19. American Thoracic Society and Infectious Diseases Society of America. Guidelines for the management of adults with hospital-acquired, ventilator-associated, and healthcare-associated pneumonia. Am J Respir Crit Care Med 2005;171: 388–416.
20. Tunkel AR, Hartman BJ, Kaplan SL, et al. Practice guidelines for the management of bacterial meningitis. Clin Infect Dis 2004;39:1267–84.
21. Rybak M, Lomaestro B, Rotschafer JC, et al. Therapeutic monitoring of vancomycin in adult patients: a consensus review of the American Society of Health-System Pharmacists, the Infectious Diseases Society of America, and the Society of Infectious Diseases Pharmacists. Am J Health Syst Pharm 2009;66:82–98.
22. Rybak MJ. The pharmacokinetic and pharmacodynamic properties of vancomycin. Clin Infect Dis 2006;42:S35–9.
23. Schaad VB, McCracken GH, Nelson JD. Clinical pharmacology and efficacy of vancomycin in pediatric patients. J Pediatr 1980;96:119–26.
24. Spitzer PG, Eliopoulos GM. Systemic absorption on enteral vancomycin in a patient with pseudomembranous colitis. Ann Intern Med 1984;100(4):533–4.
25. Tedesco F, Markham R, Gurwith M, et al. Oral vancomycin for pseudomembranous colitis. Lancet 1978;2:226–8.
26. Morse GD, Nairn DK, Walshe JJ. Once weekly intraperitoneal therapy for gram-positive peritonitis. Am J Kidney Dis 1987;4:300–5.
27. Pallotta KE, Manley HJ. Vancomycin use in patients requiring hemodialysis: a literature review. Semin Dial 2008;21:63–70.
28. Huycke MM, Sahm DF, Gilmore MS. Multiple-drug resistant enterococci: the nature of the problem and an agenda for the future. Emerg Infect Dis 1998;4:239–49.
29. Small PM, Chambers HF. Vancomycin for Staphylococcus aureus endocarditis in intravenous drug abusers. Antimicrob Agents Chemother 1990;34:1227–31.

30. Swayne R, Rampling A, Newsome SWB. Intraventricular vancomycin for treatment of shunt-associated ventriculitis. J Antimicrob Chemother 1987;19:249–53.
31. Gump DW. Vancomycin for treatment of bacterial meningitis. Rev Infect Dis 1981;Nov–Dec(Suppl 3):S289–92.
32. National Nosocomial Infections Surveillance System (NNIS). Nosocomial enterococci resistant to vancomycin—United States, 1989–1993. Morb Mortal Wkly Rep 1993;42:597–9.
33. Moellering RC Jr. The enterococcus: a classic example of antimicrobial resistance on therapeutic options. J Antimicrob Chemother 1991;28:1–12.
34. Noble WC, Virani Z, Cree RGA. Co-transfer of vancomycin and other resistance genes from *Enterococcus faecalis* NCTC 12201 to *Staphylococcus aureus.* FEMS Microbiol Lett 1992;72:195–8.
35. Frieden TR, Munsiff SS, Low DE, et al. Emergence of vancomycin-resistant enterococci in New York City. Lancet 1993;342:76–9.
36. Boyce JM. Vancomycin-resistant enterococcus. Detection, epidemiology, and control measures. Infect Dis Clin North Am 1997;11:367–84.
37. Fridkin SK, Edwards JR, Courvall JM, et al. The effect of vancomycin and third-generation cephalosporins on prevalence of vancomycin-resistant enterococci in 126 U.S. adult intensive care units. Ann Intern Med 2001;135:175–83.
38. Centers for Disease Control and Prevention. Preventing the spread of vancomycin resistance—report from the Hospital Infection Control Practices Advisory Committee. Federal Register 1994.
39. Ena J, Dick RW, Jones RN. The epidemiology of intravenous vancomycin usage in a university hospital. JAMA 1993;269:598–602.
40. Sieradzki K, Roberts RB, Serur D, et al. Heterogeneously vancomycin-resistant *Staphylococcus epidermidis* strain causing recurrent peritonitis in a dialysis patient during vancomycin therapy. J Clin Microbiol 1999;37:39–44.
41. Jones RN. Microbiological features of vancomycin in the 21st century: minimum inhibitory concentration creep, bactericidal/static activity, and applied breakpoints to predict clinical outcomes or detect resistant strains. Clin Infect Dis 2006;42(Suppl 1):S13–24.
42. Steinkraus G, White R, Friedrich L. Vancomycin MIC creep in non-vancomycin–intermediate *Staphylococcus aureus* (VISA), vancomycin-susceptible clinical methicillin-resistant *S. aureus* (MRSA) blood isolates from 2001–05. J Antimicrob Chemother 2007;60:788–94.
43. Howden BP, Ward PB, Charles PG, et al. Treatment outcomes for serious infections caused by methicillin-resistant *Staphylococcus aureus* with reduced vancomycin susceptibility. Clin Infect Dis 2004;38:521–8.
44. Lodise TP, Graves J, Evans A, et al. Relationship between vancomycin MIC and failure among patients with methicillin-resistant *Staphylococcus aureus* bacteremia treated with vancomycin. Antimicrob Agents Chemother 2008; 52:3315–20.
45. Soriano A, Marco F, Martinez JA, et al. Influence of vancomycin minimum inhibitory concentration on the treatment of methicillin-resistant *Staphylococcus aureus* bacteremia. Clin Infect Dis 2008;46(2):193–200.
46. Nailor MD, Zhao JJ, Salimnia H. Daptomycin for methicillin-resistant Staphylococcus aureus bacteremia with elevated vancomycin minimum inhibitory concentrations [abstract]. IDSA/ICAAC: K3488, 2008.
47. Centers for Disease Control and Prevention. Reduced susceptibility of *Staphylococcus aureus* to vancomycin—Japan, 1996. Morb Mortal Wkly Rep 1997;46: 624–6.

48. Hiramatsu K, Aritaka N, Hanaki H, et al. Dissemination in Japanese hospitals of strains of *Staphylococcus aureus* heterogeneously resistant to vancomycin. Lancet 1997;350:1670–3.

49. Smith TL, Pearson ML, Wilcox KR, et al. Emergence of vancomycin resistance in *Staphylococcus aureus*. N Engl J Med 1999;340:493–501.

50. Tenover FC, Moellering RC. The rationale for revising the clinical and laboratory standards institute vancomycin minimal inhibitory concentration interpretive criteria for *Staphylococcus aureus*. Clin Infect Dis 2007;44(9):1208–15.

51. Charles PG, Ward PB, Johnson PD, et al. Clinical features associated with bacteremia due to heterogeneous vancomycin-intermediate *Staphylococcus aureus*. Clin Infect Dis 2004;38:448–51.

52. Rybak MJ, Leonard SN, Rossi KL, et al. Characterization of vancomycin-hetero-resistant *Staphylococcus aureus* from the metropolitan area of Detroit, Michigan, over a 22-year period (1986–2007). J Clin Microbiol 2008;46:2950–4.

53. Chang S, Sievert D, Hageman J, et al. Infection with vancomycin-resistant *Staphylococcus aureus* containing the vanA resistance gene. N Engl J Med 2003;348(14):1342–7.

54. Centers for Disease Control and Prevention Public Health Dispatch: vancomycin-resistant *Staphylococcus aureus*—Pennsylvania, 2002. 51(40), 2002.

55. Polk RE, Healy DP, Schwartz LP, et al. Vancomycin and the red man syndrome: pharmacodynamics of histamine release. J Infect Dis 1988;157:502–7.

56. Sorrell TC, Collignon PJ, et al. A prospective study of adverse reactions associated with vancomycin therapy. J Antimicrob Chemother 1985;16(2):235–41.

57. Lodise TP, Lomaestro B, Graves J, et al. Larger vancomycin doses are associated with an increased incidence of nephrotoxicitiy. Antimicrob Agents Chemother 2008;52:1330–6.

58. Adrouny A, Meguerditchian S, Koo CH, et al. Agranulocytosis related to vancomycin therapy. Am J Med 1986;81:1059–61.

59. Cook FV, Farrar WE. Vancomycin revisited. Ann Intern Med 1978;88:813–8.

60. Lundstrom TS, Sobel JD. Antibiotics for gram-positive bacterial infections: vancomycin, teicoplanin, quinupristin/dalfopristin and linezolid. In: D. Kaye, editor. WB Saunders Co, Philadelphia. Infect Dis Clin North Am 2000;14(2):463–74.

61. Chant C, Rybak MJ. Quinupristin/dalfopristin (RP 59500): a new streptogramin antibiotic. Ann Pharmacother 1995;29:1022–7.

62. Nichterlein T, Kretschmar M, Hof H. RP 59500, a streptogramin derivative, is effective in murine listeriosis. J Chemother 1996;8:107–12.

63. Jones RN, Ballow CH, Biedenbach DJ, et al. Antimicrobial activity of quinupristin-dalfopristin (RP 59500, Synercid) tested against over 28,000 recent clinical isolates from 200 medical centers in the United States and Canada. Diagn Microbiol Infect Dis 1998;30:437–51.

64. Hussain Qadri SM, Ueno Y, Abu Mostafa FM, et al. In vitro activity of quinupristin/dalfopristin, RP 59500, against gram-positive clinical isolates. Chemotherapy 1997;43:94–9.

65. Schulin T, Wennersten CB, Ferraro MJ, et al. Susceptibilities of *Legionella spp.* to newer antimicrobials in vitro. Antimicrob Agents Chemother 1998;42:1520–3.

66. Struwig MC, Botha PL, Chalkley LJ. In vitro activities of 15 antimicrobial agents against clinical isolates of South African enterococci. Antimicrob Agents Chemother 1998;42:2752–5.

67. Furlong WB, Rakowski TA. Therapy with RP 59500 (quinupristin/dalfopristin) for prosthetic valve endocarditis due to enterococci with VanA/VanB resistance patterns. Clin Infect Dis 1997;25:163–4.

68. Chow JW, Davidson A, Sanford E III, et al. Superinfection with *Enterococcus faecalis* during quinupristin/dalfopristin therapy. Clin Infect Dis 1997;24:91–2.
69. Hershberger E, Donabedian S, Konstantinou K, et al. Quinupristin-dalfopristin resistance in gram-positive bacteria: mechanism of resistance and epidemiology. Clin Infect Dis 2004;38:92–8.
70. Chow JW, Donabedian SM, Zervos MJ. Emergence of increased resistance to quinupristin/dalfopristin during therapy for *Enterococcus faecium* bacteremia. Clin Infect Dis 1997;24:90–1.
71. Aeschlimann JR, Zervos MJ, Rybak MJ. Treatment of vancomycin-resistant *Enterococcus faecium* with RP59500 (quinupristin-dalfopristin) administered by intermittent or continuous infusion, alone, or in combination with doxycycline, in an in vitro pharmacodynamic infection model with simulated endocardial vegetation. Antimicrob Agents Chemother 1998;42:2710–7.
72. Muller M, Sehimz KL. Oxazolidinones: a novel class of antibiotics. Cell Mol Life Sci 1999;56:280–5.
73. Tucker JA, Allwine DA, Grega KC, et al. Piperazinyl oxazolidinone antibacterial agents containing a pyridine, diazine, or triazene heteroaromatic ring. J Med Chem 1998;41:3727–35.
74. Clemett D, Markham A. Linezolid. Drugs 2000;59:815–27.
75. Dresser LD, Rybak MJ. The pharmacologic and bacteriologic properties of oxazolidinones, a new class of synthetic antimicrobials. Pharmacotherapy 1998;18:456–62.
76. Zurenko GE, Yagi BH, Schaadt RD, et al. In vitro activities of U-100592 and U-100766, novel oxazolidinone antibacterial agents. Antimicrob Agents Chemother 1996;40:839–45.
77. Patel R, Rouse MS, Piper KE, et al. In vitro activity of linezolid against vancomycin-resistant enterococci, methicillin-resistant *Staphylococcus aureus*, and penicillin-resistant *Streptococcus pneumoniae*. Diagn Microbiol Infect Dis 1999;34:119–22.
78. Pawsey SD, Dalry-Yates PT, Wajszczuk CP, et al. U-100766 safety, toleration and pharmacokinetics after oral and intravenous administration. In: Program and abstracts of the first European Congress of Infections [abstract]. Berlin. sy13.4, 1997.
79. Lovering AM, Zhang J, Bannister GC, et al. Penetration of linezolid into bone, fat, muscle and haematoma of patients undergoing routine hip replacement. J Antimicrob Chemother 2002;50:73–7.
80. Wagenlehner FME, Wydra S, Onda H, et al. Concentrations in plasma, urinary excretion, and bactericidal activity of linezolid (600 milligrams) versus those of ciprofloxacin (500 milligrams) in healthy volunteers receiving a single oral dose. Antimicrob Agents Chemother 2003;47:3789–94.
81. Gemmell CG, Ford CW. Virulence factor expression by gram-positive cocci exposed to subinhibitory concentrations of linezolid. J Antimicrob Chemother 2002;50:665–72.
82. Noskin G, Siddique F, Stosor V, et al. Successful treatment of persistent vancomycin-resistant *Enterococcus faecium* bacteremia with linezolid and gentamicin. Clin Infect Dis 1999;28:689–90.
83. Conte JE, Golden JA, Kipps J, et al. Intrapulmonary pharmacokinetics of linezolid. Antimicrob Agents Chemother 2002;46:1475–80.
84. Wunderink RG, Rello J, Cammarata SK, et al. Linezolid vs vancomycin: Analysis of two double-blind studies of patients with methicillin-resistant *Staphylococcus aureus* nosocomial pneumonia. Chest 2003;124:1789–97.

85. Birmingham MC, Rayner CR, Meagher AK, et al. Linezolid for the treatment of multidrug-resistant, gram-positive infections: experience from a compassionate use program. Clin Infect Dis 2003;36:159–68.
86. Moise PA, Forrest A, Birmingham MC, et al. The efficacy and safety of linezolid as treatment for *Staphylococcus aureus* infections in compassionate use patients who are intolerant of, or who have failed to respond to, vancomycin. J Antimicrob Chemother 2002;50:1017–26.
87. Lipsky BA, Itani K, Norden C, et al. Treating foot infections in diabetic patients: a randomized, multicenter; open-label trial of linezolid versus ampicillin-sulbactam/amoxicillin-clavulanate. Clin Infect Dis 2004;38(1):17–24.
88. Parodi S, Rhew DC, Goetz MB. Early switch and early discharge opportunities in intravenous vancomycin treatment of suspected methicillin-resistant staphylococcal species infections. J Manag Care Pharm 2003;9:317–26.
89. Shorr AF, Susla GM, Kollef MH. Linezolid for treatment of ventilator-associated pneumonia: a cost-effective alternative to vancomycin. Crit Care Med 2004;32: 137–43.
90. Li JZ, Willke RJ, Rittenhouse BE, et al. Effect of linezolid versus vancomycin on length of hospital stay in patients with complicated skin and soft tissue infections caused by known or suspected methicillin-resistant staphylococci: results from a randomized clinical trial. Surg Infect 2003;4(1):57–70.
91. Brickner SJ, Hutchinson DK, Burbachyn MR, et al. Synthesis and antibacterial activity of U-100592 and U-100766, two oxazolidinone antibacterial agents for the potential treatment of multidrug-resistant gram-positive bacterial infections. J Med Chem 1996;39:673–9.
92. Kaatz GW, Seo SM. In vitro activities of oxazolidinone compounds U-100592 and U-100766 against staphylococcus species. Antimicrob Agents Chemother 1996;40:799–801.
93. Rahim S, Pillai SK, Gold HS, et al. Linezolid-resistant, vancomycin-resistant *Enterococcus faecium* infection in patients without prior exposure to linezolid. Clin Infect Dis 2003;36:E146–8.
94. Schwartz MD, Shive DK, Sheikh ZHA. Delayed discovery of linezolid-resistant, vancomycin-resistant *Enterococcus faecium*: lessons learned. Clin Infect Dis 2004;38:155–6.
95. Wilson P, Andrews JA, Charlesworth R. Linezolid resistance in clinical isolates of *Staphylococcus aureus*. J Antimicrob Chemother 2003;51:186–8.
96. Gerson SL, Kaplan SL, Bruss JB, et al. Hematologic effects of linezolid: summary of clinical experience. Antimicrob Agents Chemother 2002;46: 2723–6.
97. Nasraway SA, Shorr AF, Kuter DJ. Linezolid does not increase the risk of thrombocytopenia in patients with nosocomial pneumonia: comparative analysis of linezolid and vancomycin use. Clin Infect Dis 2003;37:1609–16.
98. Thorne GM, Adler J. Daptomycin: a novel lipopeptide antibiotic. Clin Microbiol Newslett 2002;24:33–40.
99. Tally FP, DeBruin MF. Development of daptomycin for gram-positive infections. J Antimicrob Chemother 2000;46:523–6.
100. Critchley IA, Draghi DC, Sahm DF, et al. Activity of daptomycin against susceptible and multidrug-resistant gram-positive pathogens collected in the SECURE study (Europe) during 2000–2001. J Antimicrob Chemother 2003;51:639–49.
101. Pankuch GA, Jacobs MR, Appelbaum PC. Bactericidal activity of daptomycin against *Streptococcus pneumoniae* compared with eight other antimicrobials. J Antimicrob Chemother 2003;51:443–6.

102. Golan Y, Poutsiaka D, Tozzi S, et al. Daptomycin for line-related *Leuconostoc* bacteremia. J Antimicrob Chemother 2001;47:364–5.
103. Credito K, Lin G, Appelbaum PC. Activity of daptomycin alone and in combination with rifampin and gentamicin against *Staphylococcus aureus* assessed with time-kill methodology. Antimicrob Agents Chemother 2007;51:1504–7.
104. Bush LM. In vitro post-antibiotic effect of daptomycin (LY-146032) against *Enterococcus faecalis* and methicillin-susceptible and methicillin-resistant *Staphylococcus aureus* strains. Antimicrob Agents Chemother 1989;33: 1198–2000.
105. Fowler VG, Boucher HW, Corey GR, et al. Daptomycin versus standard therapy for bacteremia and endocarditis caused by *Staphylococcus aureus*. N Engl J Med 2006;355:653–65.
106. Sakoulas G, Adler J, Thauvin-Eliopoulos C, et al. Induction of daptomycin heterogeneous susceptibility in *Staphylococcus aureus* by exposure to vancomycin. Antimicrob Agents Chemother 2006;50:1581–5.
107. Jevitt LA, Smith AJ, Williams PP, et al. In vitro activities of daptomycin, linezolid, and quinupristin-dalfopristin against a challenge panel of staphylococci and enterococci, including vancomycin-intermediate *Staphylococcus aureus* and vancomycin-resistant *Enterococcus faecium*. Microb Drug Resist 2003;9: 389–93.
108. Patel JB, Jevitt LA, Hagerman J, et al. An association between reduced susceptibility to daptomycin and reduced susceptibility to vancomycin in *Staphylococcus aureus*. Clin Infect Dis 2006;42(11):1652–3.
109. Fairfax MR, Nailor MD, Painter T. et al. Vancomycin and daptomycin susceptibility testing of Staphylococcus aureus in a clinical laboratory. IDSA/ICAAC C1–140, 2008.
110. Dvorchil BH, Brazier D, DeBruin MF, et al. Daptomycin pharmacokinetics and safety following administration of escalating doses once daily to healthy subjects. Antimicrob Agents Chemother 2003;47:1318–23.
111. Bailey J, Summers KM. Dalbavancin: a new lipoglycopeptide antibiotic. Am J Health Syst Pharm 2008;65:599–610.
112. Lin S, Carver PL, DePestel DD. Dalbavancin: a new option for the treatment of gram-positive infections. Ann Pharmacother 2006;40:449–60.
113. Attwood RJ, LaPlante KL. Telavancin: a novel lipoglycopeptide antimicrobial agent. Am J Health Syst Pharm 2007;64:2335–48.
114. Drew RH. Emerging options for treatment of invasive, multidrug-resistant *Staphylococcus aureus* infections. Pharmacotherapy 2007;27:227–49.

Newer Beta-lactam Antibiotics: Doripenem, Ceftobiprole, Ceftaroline, and Cefepime

Jose A. Bazan, DO[a], Stanley I. Martin, MD[b], Kenneth M. Kaye, MD[c],*

KEYWORDS

• Beta-lactam • Doripenem • Ceftobiprole
• Ceftaroline • Cefepime

Beta-lactam (β-lactam) antibiotics have been, and remain, the cornerstone of therapy for many life-threatening infections. Over the years, newer formulations have allowed clinicians to better provide broad empiric coverage and to use targeted therapy against commonly encountered gram-positive and gram-negative bacteria. For the most part, β-lactam antibiotics have evolved concomitantly with global antimicrobial resistance patterns. However, the emergence of pathogens like methicillin-resistant *Staphylococcus aureus* (MRSA), penicillin-intermediate and penicillin-resistant *Streptococcus pneumoniae*, multidrug-resistant (MDR) *Pseudomonas aeruginosa*, and extended-spectrum β-lactamase (ESBL)–producing gram-negative enteric organisms have provided new challenges, and the evolution of new β-lactams has slowed. This article focuses on the agents doripenem, ceftobiprole, and ceftaroline. At this writing, ceftobiprole and ceftaroline have yet to be approved for use in the United States. In addition, this article summarizes recent developments regarding the potential increased mortality observed with the use of cefepime compared with that of other agents in the treatment of some infections.

---

[a] Clinical and Research Fellow, Division of Infectious Diseases, The Ohio State University Medical Center, N1129 Doan Hall, 410 West 10th Avenue, Columbus, OH 43210, USA
[b] Division of Infectious Diseases, The Ohio State University Medical Center, N1148 Doan Hall, 410 West 10th Avenue, Columbus, OH 43210, USA
[c] Division of Infectious Diseases, Harvard Medical School, Channing Laboratory, Brigham and Women's Hospital, 181 Longwood Avenue, Boston, MA 02115, USA
* Corresponding author.
E-mail address: kkaye@rics.bwh.harvard.edu (K.M. Kaye).

Infect Dis Clin N Am 23 (2009) 983–996
doi:10.1016/j.idc.2009.06.007
0891-5520/09/$ – see front matter © 2009 Elsevier Inc. All rights reserved.

id.theclinics.com

DORIPENEM

Since the introduction of imipenem-cilastatin more than 20 years ago, the use of carbapenems such as meropenem, ertapenem, and most recently doripenem has become more common in the face of infections caused by increasingly MDR bacteria. Doripenem (formerly S-4661), a parenteral 1-β-methyl carbapenem, is the newest agent in the family, and it received approval by the US Food and Drug Administration (FDA) in 2007 for the treatment of complicated intra-abdominal infections (IAIs) and complicated urinary tract infections (UTIs).[1] Doripenem binds to penicillin-binding proteins (PBPs) and leads to the inhibition of bacterial cell wall synthesis.[1,2] Similar to other β-lactams, its bactericidal activity is directly related to the time the concentration of free drug exceeds the minimum inhibitory concentration (MIC) of the bacteria (% fT > MIC).[1,3] Unlike imipenem, its 1-β-methyl side chain confers stability in the face of renal dihydropeptidases.[4]

Similar to other carbapenems, doripenem exhibits a low degree of plasma protein binding. Imipenem-cilastatin, meropenem, and doripenem have ~20%, ~2%, and ~8% protein binding, respectively.[5–7] The metabolization of doripenem occurs through the actions of renal dihydropeptidase-I and undergoes renal excretion by a combination of glomerular filtration and active tubular secretion (78.7% unchanged drug and 18.5% inactive metabolites).[1,7,8] The normal plasma elimination half-life is approximately 1 hour, and the usual dose for patients who have normal renal function is 500 mg infused intravenously (i.v.) for 1 hour every 8 hours.[1,3,7,8] This dosing regimen has been shown to achieve the fT > MIC target of 35% for susceptible organisms that have an MIC that is 1 μg/mL or less. For organisms that have an MIC that is 2 μg/mL or greater, the same target fT > MIC can be achieved by increasing the infusion time (>1 hour) without increasing the total daily dose, given the stability of the drug at room temperature.[3,7,9] Dosing requires adjustment in the setting of moderate renal dysfunction. For patients who have a creatinine clearance (CrCl) of 30 to 50 mL/min, 250 mg i.v. every 8 hours is recommended, and for a CrCl of 10 to 30 mL/min, 250 mg i.v. every 12 hours is recommended.[1,7] There are no established parameters at this time for dosing in patients who have a CrCl of less than 10 mL/min and those undergoing hemodialysis.[1,7]

A number of studies have analyzed the in vitro activity of doripenem against bacterial isolates, using broth microdilution methods. The spectrum of antimicrobial activity of doripenem is similar to that of imipenem-cilastatin and meropenem for gram-positive and gram-negative bacteria.[10–13]

With regard to gram-positive bacteria, doripenem was the most active carbapenem against various isolates of methicillin-sensitive Staphylococcus aureus (MSSA) and methicillin-sensitive coagulase-negative staphylococci (MS-CoNS). It was twofold more active than meropenem or ertapenem against strains of Enterococcus faecalis and non-faecium enterococci, but twofold less active than imipenem-cilastatin.[10] On the other hand, vancomycin-resistant Enterococcus faecium isolates were uniformly resistant to doripenem.[10–14] Excellent in vitro activity has also been demonstrated against penicillin-susceptible, -intermediate, and -resistant Streptococcus pneumoniae, penicillin-susceptible and -resistant Streptococcus viridans, and the various β-hemolytic Streptococcus spp.[10–13]

Doripenem is active against Enterobacteriaceae. Its activity is similar to that of meropenem against wild-type (non-ESBL producing) and derepressed AmpC and ESBL-producing Enterobacteriaceae isolates.[10–14] Doripenem also displays excellent activity against common respiratory pathogens such as Haemophilus influenzae and Moraxella catarrhalis (including β-lactamase-producing strains).[10,12–14] With regard to the nonfermenting, aerobic, gram-negative bacteria, doripenem had the greatest activity against wild-type strains of *P aeruginosa* that had an MIC_{50} and MIC_{90} of 0.5 μg/mL and 8 μg/mL, respectively.[10] In addition, doripenem may still retain activity against strains of *P aeruginosa* that are resistant to other carbapenems. For instance, of 34 *P aeruginosa* strains resistant to carbapenems, 29.4% were susceptible to doripenem, whereas none were susceptible to imipenem-cilastatin, and 2.9% were susceptible to meropenem.[14] Notably, 44.1% of these same strains were sensitive to piperacillin-tazobactam, 29.4% were sensitive to cefepime, and 44.1% were sensitive to amikacin.[14] However, only 6.7% of Class B metallo-β-lactamase–producing strains of *P aeruginosa* strains were sensitive to doripenem.[14] Doripenem was active against 75.8% of wild-type *Acinetobacter baumanii* and 20.8% of carbapenem-resistant *Acinetobacter* spp (MIC_{90} of 16 μg/mL and >32 μg/mL, respectively).[13,14] *Aeromonas* spp isolates were sensitive to doripenem (MIC_{90} of 1 μg/mL), whereas doripenem's activity against strains of *Burkholderia cepacia* was variable and less than that of meropenem but similar to that of imipenem-cilastatin (MIC_{90} of 8 μg/mL). *Stenotrophomonas maltophilia* showed marked resistance to all carbapenems, including doripenem (MIC_{90} >16 μg/mL).[10] Finally, doripenem had good activity against anaerobic isolates of clinical importance such as *Bacteroides* spp, *Prevotella* spp, *Clostridium* spp, *Fusobacterium* spp, and anaerobic gram-positive cocci.[15]

Carbapenems as a class are generally resistant to hydrolysis by β-lactamases. Doripenem demonstrates enhanced stability and resistance to hydrolysis by derepressed AmpC β-lactamases and ESBLs.[16] Currently known mechanisms of decreased microbial susceptibility to doripenem include the production of metallo-β-lactamases such as IMP and VIM, decreased production or absence of the OprD outer membrane porin protein leading to decreased entry of the drug into the cell, and expression of multidrug efflux pumps that promote excretion of the drug out of the cell.[7,16–20] Compared with the other carbapenems, doripenem has a higher threshold for selection of nonsusceptible mutants in vitro, and it seems that high-level resistance may require the coexistence of more than one resistance mechanism.[7,16,17] At this time, some authors have suggested that it is unlikely that such complex alterations and multilevel mechanisms of resistance are selected in vivo during doripenem therapy.[7,16–18,21]

In a phase 3, prospective, multicenter, randomized, double-blind, noninferiority study, doripenem was found to have clinical cure rates comparable to those of meropenem for the treatment of complicated IAIs in the clinically evaluable (86.7% versus 86.6%) and microbiologically evaluable (85.9% versus 85.3%) cases at test-of-cure follow-up. In cases in which *P aeruginosa* was isolated (n = 19), microbial eradication was similar for doripenem and meropenem. Patients who had infected necrotizing pancreatitis and pancreatic abscesses were excluded from the study.[22] Another phase 3, randomized, double-blind, multicenter trial showed that doripenem was noninferior to levofloxacin for the treatment of complicated UTIs. Clinical cure rates in evaluable patients were 95.1% and 90.2% for the doripenem and levofloxacin groups, respectively.[23] Doripenem has also been studied for the treatment of hospital-acquired pneumonia (HAP) and ventilator-associated pneumonia (VAP) in two prospective, randomized, multicenter, and open-label studies.[24,25] Rea-Neto and colleagues[24] showed that doripenem was comparable and noninferior to piperacillin-tazobactam for the treatment of HAP and VAP. Cure rates for clinically evaluable patients were 81.3% and 79.8% for doripenem and piperacillin-tazobactam, respectively. Decreased susceptibility of *P aeruginosa* isolates was seen in 26.9% of patients treated using piperacillin-tazobactam and 7.7% of patients treated using doripenem. The authors acknowledged, however, a low rate of study-drug monotherapy when infection with *P aeruginosa* was suspected and severely ill and immunocompromised patients were excluded.[24] Chastre and colleagues[25] showed that doripenem was noninferior to imipenem-cilastatin in the treatment of VAP, with comparable cure rates of 68.3% versus 64.8% in clinically evaluable patients. All-cause mortality was similar for both treatment arms at 28 days (10.8% for doripenem versus 9.5% for imipenem-cilastatin). In cases in which *P aeruginosa* was isolated at baseline, both treatment arms had similar clinical cure and microbiological eradication rates. There was a trend toward better outcomes for patients who had higher baseline Acute Physiology and Chronic Health Evaluation II (APACHE II) scores, which were more than 20 points higher in the doripenem group than in the imipenem-cilistatin group (70.4% versus 57.7%).[25]

In previous studies, doripenem showed a good safety and tolerability profile compared with drugs studied in other arms. The incidence of study-drug-related adverse events (AEs) ranged from 16% to 32% for doripenem and from 18% to 27% for various comparators. The most commonly reported AEs were nausea, emesis, diarrhea, headaches, phlebitis, rash, and transaminitis. No seizure events that could be directly attributed to doripenem were reported.[22–25] Nevertheless, the epileptogenic potential of some carbapenems in patients who are at risk is a known potential side effect, particularly for imipenem-cilastatin.[26] Doripenem may not be exempt from this risk, according to some postmarketing reports from outside the United States.[1] However, a study evaluating the epileptogenic potential of doripenem administered i.v. or intracisternally in animal models failed to produce seizures.[27]

As the newest member of the carbapenem family, the role of doripenem may mirror that of meropenem more than any other carbapenem. They both have similar spectrums of antimicrobial activity and safety profiles. Based on the aforementioned noninferiority comparative trials, doripenem has a place in the treatment of not only complicated IAIs and complicated UTIs but also other health-care-associated infections such as HAP and VAP that are caused by susceptible pathogens. The true clinical efficacy of doripenem against strains of *Pseudomonas* that are resistant to other carbapenems remains unclear. Another area that may merit future research is the role of doripenem for the treatment of postneurosurgical meningitis caused by MDR gram-negative bacteria.

CEFTOBIPROLE

Since the emergence of the first MRSA isolate in the 1960s, the medical community has witnessed the widespread dissemination of MRSA and the burden that it can create in hospital wards and, most recently, surrounding communities.[28] It has been the rule that β-lactams as a class are ineffective against MRSA because of alterations in the target binding site PBP-2a that is coded by the *mecA* gene of the *mec* type IV staphylococcal cassette chromosome.[29,30] Ceftobiprole-medocaril (formerly BAL 5788, RO-5788) is a new, i.v.–administered, broad-spectrum pyrrolidinone cephalosporin that retains a high degree of affinity for PBP-2a.[31–33] In addition, ceftobiprole also has affinity for PBP-2x in penicillin-resistant *Streptococcus pneumoniae* and for PBP-3 in *Escherichia coli* and *P aeruginosa*.[31,33–35] At the time of writing, ceftobiprole has been approved for use in Canada and Switzerland and is under review by the FDA in the United States.[36]

Ceftobiprole-medocaril, the inactive prodrug, is cleaved to the active compound of ceftobiprole, diacetyl, and carbon dioxide by plasma esterases shortly after infusion. The degree of plasma protein binding has been reported to be ~16% to 38%, whereas the volume of distribution is similar to that of the extracellular fluid compartment in adults at steady state. Ceftobiprole primarily undergoes renal excretion, and the majority of the drug is recovered in the urine (~83% unchanged drug, ~0.3%

prodrug, and ~0.8% inactive metabolites). The activity of ceftobiprole depends on the length of time that the concentration of free drug is more than the MIC of the organism (% f T > MIC), and the mean serum half-life is approximately 3 to 4 hours.[31,37,38] Based on Monte Carlo simulation analysis, the likelihood of achieving the target f T > MIC of 30% and 50% for organisms with an MIC that is 2 µg/mL or less and 1 µg/mL or less, respectively, was greater than 90% with a dosage of 500 mg i.v. over 1 hour every 12-hours. Similarly, the likelihood of achieving the target f T > MIC of 40% and 60% for organisms with an MIC that is 4 µg/mL or less and 2 µg/mL or less, respectively, was greater than 90% with a dosage of 500 mg i.v. over 2 hours every 8 hours.[38,39] The current recommended dosage in the setting of normal renal function is 500 mg i.v. infused for 30 minutes to 2 hours every 8 to 12 hours, depending on the target percentage of f T > MIC desired and type of infection being treated. Thus, treatment of polymicrobial diabetic foot infections and gram-positive or gram-negative HAP or VAP may require 500 mg i.v. for 2 hours every 8 hours, versus treatment of a complicated skin and soft-tissue infection (SSTI) caused by a gram-positive bacteria, which may only require 500 mg i.v. for 1 hour every 12 hours.[31,38–42] Pharmacodynamic studies suggest that dose adjustments are required in the setting of mild to moderate renal dysfunction (CrCl ≤ 50 mL/min; 500 mg i.v. for 2 hours every 12 hours). Further data are needed regarding optimal dosing in the setting of severe renal dysfunction and hemodialysis.[38,39] Ceftobiprole does not undergo significant hepatic metabolism, and no dose adjustments appear to be required in the setting of hepatic dysfunction.[38]

The spectrum of antimicrobial activity of ceftobiprole is among the broadest of all currently available cephalosporins. As part of a longitudinal, global, resistance-surveillance program (SENTRY), Fritsche and colleagues[43] analyzed the in vitro activity of ceftobiprole using broth microdilution methods in 40,675 common bacterial isolates. With regard to gram-positive bacteria, ceftobiprole readily inhibited MSSA and MRSA at concentrations that are 4 µg/mL or less (MIC$_{90}$ 0.5 µg/mL and 2 µg/mL, respectively). The activity of ceftobiprole against MSSA isolates was equal to that of oxacillin and daptomycin, and eightfold greater than that of cefepime and ceftriaxone. Its activity was at least eightfold greater than that of any other β-lactam against MRSA and equal to that of linezolid, but twofold to fourfold less than that of vancomycin, TMP-SMX, or daptomycin. Ceftobiprole inhibited more than 99% of MS-CoNS and methicillin-resistant coagulase-negative staphylococci (MR-CoNS) isolates at concentrations of 0.5 µg/mL and 4 µg/mL, respectively. Its activity against MR-CoNS was comparable to that of vancomycin. Ceftobiprole showed good activity against ampicillin-sensitive, ampicillin-resistant, and vancomycin-resistant strains of Enterococcus faecalis, β-hemolytic Streptococcus spp, Streptococcus viridans Bacillus spp, Listeria spp, and Streptococcus pneumoniae. Ceftobiprole inhibited 100% of penicillin-susceptible and penicillin-resistant Streptococcus pneumoniae at concentrations of 0.25 µg/mL and 2 µg/mL respectively. Ceftobiprole, however, did not show significant activity against Corynebacterium spp. It also has no documented in vitro activity against Enterococcus faecium isolates regardless of their vancomycin or ampicillin susceptibility profiles.[43,44]

With regard to the Enterobacteriaceae, ceftobiprole showed good activity against non-ESBL–producing Escherichia coli, Proteus mirabilis, Citrobacter spp, Serratia spp, and Salmonella spp isolates. Ceftobiprole was less active than cefepime against non-ESBL–producing Klebsiella pneumoniae, Enterobacter spp, and indole-positive Proteus spp, with 76.9%, 85.4%, and 72.2% of respective isolates being inhibited by drug concentrations that were 8 µg/mL or less. Similar to other extended-spectrum cephalosporins, ceftobiprole showed limited activity against ESBL-producing strains of Escherichia coli and Klebsiella pneumoniae.[43]

The in vitro activity of ceftobiprole against nonfermenting, aerobic, gram-negative bacteria such as *P aeruginosa* was generally similar to other agents. Ceftobiprole inhibited 77.9% at concentrations that were 8 μg/mL or less, whereas the percentage susceptible to ceftazidime was 75.5%, imipenem 75.8%, cefepime 79.4%, meropenem 80.9%, piperacillin-tazobactam 84.8%, amikacin 87.4%, and polymixin B 99.8%. Ceftobiprole was active against *Aeromonas* spp, but not against *Stenotrophomonas maltophilia*, *B cepacia*, or *Acinetobacter* spp. It was readily active against wild-type and β-lactamase–producing strains of *H influenzae* and *M catarrhalis*.[43] Finally, it does have some activity against most anaerobic gram-positive cocci such as *Propionibacterium acnes*, non-*difficile Clostridium* spp, and *Porphyromonas* spp. However, *Peptostreptococcus anaerobius, Clostridium difficile, Prevotella* spp, and *Bacteroides* spp were generally tolerant or resistant.[45]

Ceftobiprole is generally resistant to hydrolysis by staphylococcal penicillinases, but not to ESBLs, carbapenemases, or OXA-10 β-lactamases produced by some MDR gram-negative bacteria. However, it is a poor substrate for Class A and SHV-1, and class C AmpC β-lactamases, demonstrating low rates of hydrolysis on exposure.[46]

Ceftobiprole has been evaluated for the treatment of complicated SSTIs in phase 3 clinical trials. A randomized, double-blind, multicenter, noninferiority study compared ceftobiprole with vancomycin for the treatment of complicated SSTIs caused by gram-positive bacteria. The results showed comparable cure rates in clinically evaluable patients (93.3% for ceftobiprole versus 93.5% for vancomycin). In cases of documented MRSA infection, cure rates were similar for both treatment arms (91.8% for ceftobiprole versus 90.0% for vancomycin), including those caused by Panton-Valentin leukocidin (+) strains.[41] A second randomized, double-blind, multi-center, noninferiority trial compared ceftobiprole with vancomycin plus ceftazidime for the treatment of complicated SSTIs. In contrast with the first trial, patients who had diabetic foot infections were included in this study. Among the clinically evaluable patients, cure rates were 90.5% and 90.2% for the ceftobiprole and vancomycin/ceftazidime arms, respectively. Comparable clinical cure rates were found in patients who had documented infections caused by MRSA (89.7% for ceftobiprole versus 86.1% for vancomycin/ceftazidime) and *P aeruginosa* (86.7% for ceftobiprole versus 100% for vancomycin/ceftazidime). Similarly, cure rates for patients who had diabetic foot infections were 86.2% and 81.8% for ceftobiprole and vancomycin/ceftazidime, respectively.[42]

The incidence of at least one AE was 52% for ceftobiprole and 51% for vancomycin in the first study and 56% for ceftobiprole and 57% for vancomycin/ceftazidime group in the second. Nausea (14%), vomiting (7%), taste disturbance (8%), and infusion-site reactions (9%) were the most commonly reported AEs for the ceftobiprole arms.[41,42]

Laboratory studies using a rabbit model of MRSA aortic valve endocarditis and tibial osteomyelitis showed promising results with the use of ceftobiprole.[47,48] In addition, neutropenic-mouse-model studies have shown that ceftobiprole has excellent lung tissue penetration and achieves high concentrations in alveolar epithelial lining fluids that are much more than the MICs for various isolates of *Staphylococcus aureus*, including MRSA.[49]

Phase 3 clinical trials looking at the use of ceftobiprole for the treatment of community-acquired pneumonia, HAP, VAP, and neutropenic fever are currently under way.[31] Additional prospective, randomized, multicenter studies are needed to address the role of ceftobiprole in the treatment of MRSA bacteremia, endocarditis, and bone and joint infections.

Ceftobiprole is the first available β-lactam to show bactericidal activity against MRSA in addition to a wide array of gram-negative pathogens. Given its documented clinical efficacy, microbial eradication rates, and safety profile in phase 3 trials of complicated SSTIs, ceftobiprole will likely be used in the increasingly complex fight against infections caused by MRSA and susceptible gram-negative pathogens.

CEFTAROLINE

Ceftaroline is another β-lactam of the cephalosporin class that retains activity against MRSA. At the time of this writing, ceftaroline remains investigational and is not yet approved for use. Ceftaroline fosamil (formerly PPI-0903M, formerly TAK-599) is a new, water-soluble, i.v.-administered, N-phosphono–type cephalosporin that undergoes hydrolysis of the phosphate group and is rapidly converted to its active compound in vivo after parenteral administration in animal models. In addition, it has a high degree of affinity for PBP-2a, with documented anti-MRSA activity.[50,51] The pharmacokinetic and pharmacodynamic profiles of ceftaroline have been analyzed in murine models of thigh, lung, and aortic valve infection, and in healthy human volunteers and patients who had complicated SSTIs. The results of these studies show that the mean serum half-life is ~2.6 hours, plasma protein binding is less than 20%, and drug clearance occurs mainly by way of renal excretion, with ~75% of the drug recovered in the urine.[52–56] The current dosing regimen used in patients who have normal renal function in phase 2 and 3 clinical trials is 600 mg i.v. infused for 1 hour every 12 hours.[57,58] Dosage adjustments are not required in the setting of mild renal dysfunction (CrCl >50–80 mL/min), but should be undertaken for patients who have moderate renal dysfunction (CrCl >30–50 mL/min; 400 mg i.v. for 1 hour every 12 hours). No specific recommendations regarding dosing in the setting of severe renal dysfunction (CrCl < 30 mL/min) or hemodialysis are available at this time.[56]

Analysis of the in vitro activity of ceftaroline against various clinical and laboratory bacterial isolates from various parts of the world using broth microdilution methods showed that it has excellent activity against MSSA, MRSA, MS-CoNS, and MR-CoNS. Activity was fourfold greater than that of vancomycin and 16 fold greater than that of ceftriaxone or cefepime against MSSA isolates. When tested against 102 MRSA isolates, ceftaroline had an MIC_{90} of 2 μg/mL, which is similar to that of linezolid and slightly higher than that of vancomycin (MIC_{90} of 1 μg/mL). Activity was also documented against vancomycin-intermediate strains of *Staphylococcus aureus*. For 100 isolates of vancomycin-intermediate strains of *Staphylococcus aureus* tested, the ceftaroline MIC_{90} was 2 μg/mL, which is only slightly higher than that of linezolid, which had an MIC_{90} of 1 μg/mL.[59] Similar results were noted in clinical isolates from the United States, in which ceftaroline was the most active cephalosporin against all staphylococci tested.[60] Other gram-positive bacteria that showed susceptibility to ceftaroline included *Streptococcus pneumoniae* (ceftaroline MIC_{90}: penicillin-susceptible, ≤ 0.016 μg/mL; penicillin-intermediate, 0.06 μg/mL; penicillin-resistant, 0.25 μg/mL), β-hemolytic streptococci spp, and *Streptococcus viridans*. Ceftaroline was less active than vancomycin, imipenem-cilastatin, and levofloxacin against *Bacillus* spp. Ceftaroline showed only marginal activity against *Enterococcus faecalis* and was not effective against *Enterococcus faecium* (ceftaroline MIC_{90} for vancomycin-susceptible and vancomycin-resistant strains, >32 μg/mL).[59]

Ceftaroline displayed significant activity against the Enterobacteriaceae. Non-ESBL–producing strains were uniformly susceptible, whereas ESBL-producing strains of *Escherichia coli, K pneumoniae*, and *P mirabilis* were resistant. Among the nonfermenting, gram-negative bacteria, ceftaroline showed only minimal activity against certain isolates of *P aeruginosa* and *A baumanii* (ceftaroline MIC_{50} of 16 and MIC_{90} >32 μg/mL for both organisms) and was not active against *Alcaligenes* spp or

Stenotrophomonas maltophilia. On the other hand, ceftaroline showed excellent activity against *Neisseria meningitidis*, *M catarrhalis*, and both β-lactamase–producing and non–β-lactamase–producing strains of *H influenzae*. In terms of anaerobic activity, it has significant effect against *Peptostreptococcus* spp, *Propionibacterium* spp, and non-*difficile Clostridium* spp. It has minimal to no activity against *Bacteroides fragilis* and *Prevotella* spp.[59]

Phase 2 and 3 clinical trials have been done to compare the safety and efficacy of ceftaroline with that of vancomycin with or without aztreonam for the treatment of SSTIs in randomized and observer-blinded studies. In the phase 2 study, the clinical cure rate was 96.7% for ceftaroline and 88.9% for standard therapy.[57] In the phase 3 study, overall cure rates were 91.1% for ceftaroline and 93.3% for standard therapy in the clinically evaluable patient population. With respect to MRSA, similar clinical and microbiological cure rates were observed for both treatment arms (94.9% and 94.9% for ceftaroline versus 95.1% and 91.8% for vancomycin/aztreonam).[58]

In phase 2 and 3 comparative clinical trials, ceftaroline proved to be a well-tolerated drug and showed a good safety profile.[57,58] In the phase 2 study, the incidence of reported AEs was similar for both treatment groups (61.2% for ceftaroline versus 56.3% for standard therapy), with the great majority of AEs being mild in nature (87.9% for ceftaroline versus 70.8% for standard therapy). The most commonly reported ceftaroline-related AEs in this study were crystalluria (9% for ceftaroline versus 15.6% for standard therapy) and elevated serum creatinine phosphokinase levels (7.5% for ceftaroline and 6.3% for standard therapy).[57] In the phase 3 study, both treatment arms had comparable rates of possibly and probably study-drug-related AEs (43.2% for ceftaroline versus 47% for standard therapy). Similar to the first study, the majority of AEs were mild in nature. The most commonly reported AEs were nausea (5.7% for ceftaroline and 4.6% for standard therapy), headache (5.1% for ceftaroline and 3.7% for standard therapy), and generalized pruritus (3.7% for ceftaroline and 4.6% for standard therapy).[58]

As with ceftobiprole, future clinical trials should help clarify ceftaroline's role among the new anti-MRSA β-lactams and determine its place in the treatment of community- and hospital-acquired infections such as pneumonia, bacteremia, endocarditis, and bone and joint infections.

CEFEPIME

This section on cefepime summarizes recent data from two comprehensive meta-analyses that put into question the safety and efficacy of cefepime and led to an FDA review regarding possible increased mortality risk from the use of cefepime.[61,62] This section also highlights reports of side effects such as neurotoxicity in the setting of renal failure.[63–65]

Since its introduction into clinical use more than a decade ago, cefepime, which is a broad-spectrum, antipseudomonal, fourth generation oxyimino-cephalosporin, has been one of the first-line agents for the empiric treatment of patients who have neutropenic fever. It is currently FDA approved for the treatment of moderate to severe pneumonia, uncomplicated and complicated UTIs, complicated IAIs, and uncomplicated SSTIs caused by susceptible bacteria.[65] Given its broad spectrum of antimicrobial activity, its stability in the face of inducible β-lactamases, and its higher threshold for selection of hyperproducing strains of chromosomally mediated β-lactamases, cefepime has been considered an appropriate agent for the treatment of severe gram-negative infections.[66–68] In addition, it also has superior activity against *Streptococcus pneumoniae* and staphylococci (methicillin-sensitive strains) compared with other extended-spectrum late-generation cephalosporins.[69-71] Cefepime has been for the most part a fairly well-tolerated drug, with most reported AEs being categorized as mild and statistically similar to those for the comparator arms in phase 3 clinical trials.[72] In addition, it has a low incidence of allergic cross-reactivity with penicillin and ceftazidime because of its unique side chain structure.[73] A comprehensive review of cefepime's dosing regimens, pharmacodynamic and pharmacokinetic properties, metabolism and elimination, and spectrum of antimicrobial coverage has been published in *Infectious Disease Clinics of North America*.[74]

In 2002, the FDA reviewed data submitted by the manufacturer of cefepime and approved an addition to cefepime's label warning about the increased risk for neurotoxicity, especially in the setting of renal failure.[64] The data were based on postmarketing reports that included episodes of encephalopathy, myoclonus, and seizures. Most of these cases were in patients who had renal dysfunction for whom administered doses exceeded recommendations. Some events, however, were also reported in patients who received renal-adjusted doses of cefepime. Discontinuation of the offending drug, or hemodialysis in some cases, led to resolution of symptoms in most patients.[63-65]

Recent data from two comprehensive systematic reviews and meta-analyses of randomized controlled trials, both from the same group, have put into question cefepime's efficacy and safety compared with that of other broad-spectrum β-lactams.[61,62] The first meta-analysis reviewed the results of 33 studies to determine if the outcomes of patients who had neutropenic fever were influenced by the choice of initial empiric β-lactam therapy.[61] The primary outcome was all-cause mortality assessed at 30 days posttreatment. The results showed that patients who received cefepime (17 trials, n = 3,123 patients) had a higher and more statistically significant 30 day all-cause mortality compared with patients who received other antipseudomonal β-lactams ($P=.02$). However, no significant differences were noted with regard to secondary outcomes analyzed, such as treatment failure, microbiological failure, infection-related mortality, antibiotic modification, addition of vancomycin, addition of antifungal agents, bacterial superinfections, any other superinfections, or AEs. The authors of that study compared piperacillin-tazobactam with cefepime (4 trials) and found no differences in all-cause mortality. However, they stated that the latter results were hampered by a lack of substantial methodologic data that would allow definitive conclusions for this particular analysis.[61]

The second meta-analysis, by Yahav and colleagues,[62] reviewed the results of 57 studies in which cefepime was compared with other β-lactams to assess all-cause mortality at 30 days posttreatment as the primary outcome. Randomized trials were subdivided based on the comparator drug used and the type of infection for which the patient was being treated. Similar to the first meta-analysis, the authors found that in the 41 studies (38 of which were clinical trials) for which all-cause mortality was available, patients treated using cefepime had an overall higher and more statistically significant all-cause mortality compared with patients treated using other β-lactams, despite similar baseline risk factors for mortality ($P=.005$). This difference was most significant when cefepime was compared with piperacillin-tazobactam (relative risk [RR] 2.14; $P=.01$), but it was seen for all comparator drugs. The authors also concluded that except for cases of UTIs, all-cause mortality was higher for cefepime than for the comparator drugs with regard to the type of infection being treated.[62]

Yahav and colleagues offered some possible explanations for their findings. First, they stated that cefepime-induced neurotoxicity may have been underrecognized in the pool of patients that was analyzed, which in turn may have contributed to the overall higher all-cause mortality observed. Second, they argued that other factors such as inoculum, inadequate targeted-tissue concentrations, and pharmacodynamics (intermittent versus continuous cefepime dosing) may have played a role in the results.[61,62]

These reports have some limitations, however. In particular, complete all-cause mortality results were lacking in some of the trials analyzed, and potential patient selection bias might not have been fully accounted for in the meta-analysis. The FDA is reviewing the safety data on cefepime further and requested support from Bristol-Meyers Squibb, the manufacturer of cefepime (Maxipime), with the goal of reaching a conclusion and releasing further recommendations to the public in the near future.[75,76]

SUMMARY

The advent of novel cephalosporins with anti-MRSA activity such as ceftobiprole and ceftaroline is an exciting new development. MRSA is a major and growing problem in infectious diseases, and the addition of cephalosporins with activity against this organism will be greeted with high anticipation if and when they are FDA approved. Doripenem is also a welcome addition to the carbapenems, and its use will most likely mirror that of meropenem. However, based on the currently available data, it is difficult to recommend the use of doripenem rather than meropenem. Despite the fact the in vitro results seem to suggest that doripenem may retain activity against some carbapenem-resistant strains of *P aeruginosa*, it is not clear whether this has any in vivo clinical relevance. The authors of this article hope that future phase 3 clinical trials will help expand potential FDA-approved indications for these and any other upcoming β-lactams that might be in the early stages of development. The FDA recently updated its recommendations regarding cefepime. The FDA independently conducted both trial-level (n = 88 trials; including 24 neutropenic fever trials) and patient-level (n = 35 trials) meta-analyses and concluded there was no statistically significant difference in 30 day all cause mortality between the cefepime and comparator treatment arms (adjusted risk difference 5-38 per 1000 population, 95% C.I. −1.53–12.28 and 4.83 per 1000 population, 95% C.I. −4.72–14.38 respectively). Based on these findings, the FDA issued a statement that cefepime should retain its status as a first-line treatment option for already approved indications, including the treatment of neutropenic fever. Nevertheless, both the FDA and the manufacturer of cefepime (Bristo-Myers Squibb) will continue to perform independent safety reviews on the drug based on hospital utilization data. According to the FDA, it may take a year before such findings are made public.[75,76,77]

REFERENCES

1. Ortho-McNeil Pharmaceutical. Doribax (doripenem) package insert. Raritan (NJ): Ortho-McNeil Pharmaceutical; 2007.
2. Davies T, Shang W, Bush K, et al. Affinity of doripenem and comparators to penicillin-binding proteins in *Escherichia coli* and *Pseudomonas aeruginosa*. Antimicrob Agents Chemother 2008;52:1510–2.
3. Bhavnani SM, Hammel JP, Cirincione BB, et al. Use of pharmacokinetic–pharmacodynamic target attainment analyses to support phase 2 and 3 dosing strategies for doripenem. Antimicrob Agents Chemother 2005;49:3944–7.
4. Iso Y, Irie T, Nishino Y, et al. A novel 1 β-methylcarbapenem antibiotic, S-4661. Synthesis and structure-activity relationships of 2-(5-substituted pyrrolidin-3-ylthio)-1 β-methylcarbapenems. J Antibiot 1996;49:199–209.
5. Rogers JD, Meisinger MA, Ferber F, et al. Pharmacokinetics of imipenem and cilastatin in volunteers. Rev Infect Dis 1985;7(Suppl 3):S435–46.

6. Moon YSK, Chung KC, Gill MA. Pharmacokinetics of meropenem in animals, healthy volunteers, and patients. Clin Infect Dis 1997;24(Suppl 2):S249–55.

7. Greer ND. Doripenem (Doribax): the newest addition to the carbapenems. Proc (Bayl Univ Med Cent) 2008;21:337–41.

8. Cirillo I, Mannens G, Janssen C, et al. The disposition, metabolism, and excretion of 14C-doripenem after a single 500-mg intravenous infusion in healthy men. Antimicrob Agents Chemother 2008;52:3478–83.

9. Lister PD. Carbapenems in the USA: focus on doripenem. Expert Rev Anti Infect Ther 2007;5:793–809.

10. Fritsche TR, Stilwell MG, Jones RN. Antimicrobial activity of doripenem (S-4661): a global surveillance report (2003). Clin Microbiol Infect 2005;11:974–84.

11. Ge Y, Wikler MA, Sahm DF, et al. In vitro antimicrobial activity of doripenem, a new carbapenem. Antimicrob Agents Chemother 2004;48:1384–96.

12. Tsuji M, Ishii Y, Ohno A, et al. In vitro and in vivo antibacterial activities of S-4661, a new carbapenem. Antimicrob Agents Chemother 1998;42:94–9.

13. Jones RN, Huynh HK, Biedenbach DJ, et al. Doripenem (S-4661), a novel carbapenem: comparative activity against contemporary pathogens including bactericidal action and preliminary in vitro methods evaluations. J Antimicrob Chemother 2004;54:144–54.

14. Jones RN, Huynh HK, Biedenbach DJ. Activities of doripenem (S-4661) against drug-resistant clinical pathogens. Antimicrob Agents Chemother 2004;48:3136–40.

15. Wexler HM, Engel AE, Glass D, et al. In vitro activities of doripenem and comparator agents against 364 anaerobic clinical isolates. Antimicrob Agents Chemother 2005;49:4413–7.

16. Mushtaq S, Ge Y, Livermore DM. Doripenem versus *Pseudomonas aeruginosa* in vitro: activity against characterized isolates, mutants, and transconjugants and resistance selection potential. Antimicrob Agents Chemother 2004;48:3086–92.

17. Sakyo S, Tomita H, Tanimoto K, et al. Potency of carbapenems for the prevention of carbapenem-resistant mutants of *Pseudomonas aeruginosa*. J Antibiot (Tokyo) 2006;59:220–8.

18. Kohler T, Michea-Hamzehpour M, Epp SF, et al. Carbapenem activities against *Pseudomonas aeruginosa*: respective contributions of OprD and efflux systems. Antimicrob Agents Chemother 1999;43:424–7.

19. Livermore DM. Of *Pseudomonas aeruginosa*, porins, pumps, and carbapenems. J Antimicrob Chemother 2001;47:247–50.

20. Masuda N, Sakagawa E, Ohya S, et al. Substrate specificities of MexAB-OprM, MexCD-OprJ, and MexXY-OprM efflux pumps in *Pseudomonas aeruginosa*. Antimicrob Agents Chemother 2000;44:3322–7.

21. Carmeli Y, Troillet N, Eliopoulos GM, et al. Emergence of antibiotic-resistant *Pseudomonas aeruginosa*: comparison of risks associated with different antipseudomonal agents. Antimicrob Agents Chemother 1999;43:1379–82.

22. Lucasti C, Jasovich A, Umeh O, et al. Efficacy and tolerability of IV doripenem versus meropenem in adults with complicated intra-abdominal infection: a phase III, prospective, multicenter, randomized, double-blind, noninferiority study. Clin Ther 2008;30:868–83.

23. Naber K, Redman R, Kotey P, et al. Intravenous therapy with doripenem versus levofloxacin with an option for oral step-down therapy in the treatment of complicated urinary tract infections and pyelonephritis. Int J Antimicrob Agents 2007; 29(Suppl 2):S212 [abstract form only].

24. Rea-Neto A, Niederman M, Lobo SM, et al. Efficacy and safety of intravenous doripenem vs. piperacillin/tazobactam in nosocomial pneumonia: a randomized, open-label, multicenter study. Curr Med Res Opin 2008;24:2113–26.

25. Chastre J, Wunderink R, Prokocimer P, et al. Efficacy and safety of intravenous infusion of doripenem versus imipenem in ventilator-associated pneumonia: a multicenter, randomized study. Crit Care Med 2008;36:1089–96.

26. Norrby SR. Neurotoxicity of carbapenem antibacterials. Drug Saf 1996;15:87–90.

27. Horiuchi M, Kimura M, Tokumura M, et al. Absence of convulsive liability of doripenem, a new carbapenem antibiotic, in comparison with β-lactam antibiotics. Toxicology 2006;222:114–24.

28. Chambers HF. The changing epidemiology of Staphylococcus aureus? Emerg Infect Dis 2001;7:178–82.

29. Livermore DM. Can beta-lactams be re-engineered to beat MRSA? Clin Microbiol Infect 2006;12(Suppl 2):11–6.

30. De Lecastre H, De Jonge BL, Matthews PR, et al. Molecular aspects of methicillin resistance in Staphylococcus aureus. J Antimicrob Chemother 1994;33:7–24.

31. Anderson SD, Gums JG. Ceftobiprole: an extended-spectrum anti-methicillin resistant Staphylococcus aureus cephalosporin. Ann Pharmacother 2008;42:806–16.

32. Adis R&D profile. Ceftobiprole medocaril. Drugs R D 2006;7:305–11.

33. Chambers HF. Solving staphylococcal resistance to beta-lactams. Trends Microbiol 2003;11:145–8.

34. Davies TA, Page MG, Shang W, et al. Binding of ceftobiprole and comparators to the penicillin-binding proteins of Escherichia coli, Pseudomonas aeruginosa, Staphylococcus aureus, and Streptococcus pneumoniae. Antimicrob Agents Chemother 2007;51:2621–4.

35. Georgopapadakou NH. Penicillin-binding proteins and bacterial resistance to β-lactams. Antimicrob Agents Chemother 1993;37:2045–53.

36. Wikipedia-free encyclopedia Ceftobiprole. Available at: http://en.wikipedia.org/wiki/ceftobiprole. Accessed December 9, 2008.

37. Murthy B, Schmitt-Hoffman A. Pharmacokinetics and pharmacodynamics of ceftobiprole, an anti-MRSA cephalosporin with broad-spectrum activity. Clin Pharmacokinet 2008;47:21–33.

38. Lodise TP, Patel N, Renaud-Mutart A, et al. Pharmacokinetic and pharmacodynamic profile of ceftobiprole. Diagn Microbiol Infect Dis 2008;61:96–102.

39. Lodise TP, Pypstra R, Kahn JB, et al. Probability of target attainment for ceftobiprole as derived from a population pharmacokinetic analysis of 150 subjects. Antimicrob Agents Chemother 2007;51:2378–87.

40. Mouton JW, Schmitt-Hoffman A, Shapiro S, et al. Use of Monte Carlo simulations to select therapeutic doses and provisional breakpoints of BAL9141. Antimicrob Agents Chemother 2004;48:1713–8.

41. Noel GJ, Strauss RS, Amsler K, et al. Results of a double-blind, randomized trial of ceftobiprole treatment of complicated skin and skin structure infections caused by gram-positive bacteria. Antimicrob Agents Chemother 2008;52:37–44.

42. Noel GJ, Bush K, Bagchi P, et al. A randomized double-blind trial comparing ceftobiprole medocaril to vancomycin plus ceftazidime in the treatment of patients with complicated skin and skin structure infections. Clin Infect Dis 2008;46:647–55.

43. Fritsche TR, Sader HS, Jones RN. Antimicrobial activity of ceftobiprole, a novel anti-methicillin–resistant Staphylococcus aureus cephalosporin, tested against contemporary pathogens: results from the SENTRY antimicrobial surveillance program (2005–2006). Diagn Microbiol Infect Dis 2008;61:86–95.

44. Arias CA, Singh KV, Panesso D, et al. Time-kill and synergism studies of ceftobiprole against *Enterococcus faecalis*, including β-lactamase–producing and vancomycin-resistant isolates. Antimicrob Agents Chemother 2007;51:2043–7.
45. Goldstein EJ, Citron DM, Merriam CV, et al. In vitro activity of ceftobiprole against aerobic and anaerobic strains isolated from diabetic foot infections. Antimicrob Agents Chemother 2006;50:3959–62.
46. Queenan AM, Shang W, Kania M, et al. Interactions of ceftobiprole with β-lactamases from molecular classes A to D. Antimicrob Agents Chemother 2007;51:3089–95.
47. Chambers HF. Evaluation of ceftobiprole in a rabbit model of aortic valve endocarditis due to methicillin-resistant and vancomycin-intermediate *Staphylococcus aureus*. Antimicrob Agents Chemother 2005;49:884–8.
48. Yin LY, Calhoun JH, Thomas JK, et al. Efficacies of ceftobiprole medocaril and comparators in a rabbit model of osteomyelitis due to methicillin-resistant *Staphylococcus aureus*. Antimicrob Agents Chemother 2008;52:1618–22.
49. Laohavaleeson S, Tessier PR, Nicolau DP. Pharmacodynamic characterization of ceftobiprole in experimental pneumonia caused by phenotypically diverse *Staphylococcus aureus* strains. Antimicrob Agents Chemother 2008;52:2389–94.
50. Ishikawa T, Matsunaga N, Tawada H, et al. TAK-599, a novel n-phosphono type prodrug of anti-MRSA cephalosporin T-91825: synthesis, physicochemical and pharmacological properties. Bioorg Med Chem 2003;11:2427–37.
51. Iizawa Y, Nagai J, Ishikawa T, et al. In vitro antimicrobial activity of T-91825, a novel anti-MRSA cephalosporin, and in vivo anti-MRSA activity of its prodrug, TAK-599. J Infect Chemother 2004;10:146–56.
52. Andes D, Craig WA. Pharmacodynamics of a new cephalosporin, PPI-0903 (TAK-599), active against methicillin-resistant *Staphylococcus aureus* in murine thigh and lung infection models: identification of an in vivo pharmacokinetic–pharmacodynamic target. Antimicrob Agents Chemother 2006;50:1376–83.
53. Jacqueline C, Caillon J, Le Mabecque V, et al. In vivo efficacy of ceftaroline (PPI-0903), a new broad-spectrum cephalosporin, compared with linezolid and vancomycin against methicillin-resistant and vancomycin-intermediate *Staphylococcus aureus* in a rabbit endocarditis model. Antimicrob Agents Chemother 2007;51:3397–400.
54. Ge Y, Hubbel A. Poster.A-1935, 46th Intersci Conf Antimicrob Agents Chemother 2006.
55. Ge Y, Liao S, Talbot GH. Poster A-34, 47th Intersci Conf Antimicrob Agents Chemother 2007.
56. Ge Y, Liao S, Thye DA, et al. Poster A-35, 47th Intersci Conf Antimicrob Agents Chemother 2007.
57. Talbot GH, Thye D, Das A, et al. Phase 2 study of ceftaroline versus standard therapy in treatment of complicated skin and skin structure infections. Antimicrob Agents Chemother 2007;51:3612–6.
58. Corey R, Wilcox M, Talbot GH, et al. Poster L-1515a, 48th Intersci Conf Antimicrob Agents Chemother/Infec Dis Soc Am 2008.
59. Sader HS, Fritsche TR, Kaniga K, et al. Antimicrobial activity and spectrum of PPI-0903M (T-91825), a novel cephalosporin, tested against a worldwide collection of clinical strains. Antimicrob Agents Chemother 2005;49:3501–12.
60. Ge Y, Biek D, Talbot GH, et al. In vitro profiling of ceftaroline against a collection of recent bacterial clinical isolates from across the United States. Antimicrob Agents Chemother 2008;52:3398–407.

61. Paul M, Yahav D, Fraser A, et al. Empirical antibiotic monotherapy for febrile neutropenia: systematic review and meta-analysis of randomized controlled trials. J Antimicrob Chemother 2006;57:176–89.
62. Yahav D, Paul M, Fraser A, et al. Efficacy and safety of cefepime: a systematic review and meta-analysis. Lancet Infect Dis 2007;7:338–48.
63. B. Braun Medical Inc. Y36-002-592: cefepime for injection; proposed package insert. issued:xxx. Available at: http://www.fda.gov/OHRMS/DOCKETS/dockets/06p0461/06p-0461-cp00001-04-attachment-03-vol1.pdf. Accessed December 7, 2008.
64. U.S. Food and Drug Administration. FDA drug warning. NDA 50–679/S-009, S-0014, and S-018.Available at: http://www.fda.gov/cder/foi/appletter/2002/50679 slr009,014,018ltr.pdf. Accessed October 13, 2008.
65. Bristol-Myers Squibb. Maxipime (cefepime) package insert. Princeton (NJ): Bristol-Myers Squibb; 2007.
66. Sanders CC. Cefepime: the next generation? Clin Infect Dis 1993;17:369–79.
67. Sanders WE Jr, Tenney JH, Kessler RE. Efficacy of cefepime in the treatment of infections due to multiply resistant Enterobacter species. Clin Infect Dis 1996; 23:454–61.
68. Acar J. Rapid emergence of resistance to cefepime during treatment. Clin Infect Dis 1998;26:1484–6.
69. Wynd MA, Paladino JA. Cefepime: a fourth generation parenteral cephalosporin. Ann Pharmacother 1996;30:1414–24.
70. Kessler RE, Bies M, Buck RE, et al. Comparison of a new cephalosporin, BMY-28142, with other broad spectrum beta-lactam antibiotics. Antimicrob Agents Chemother 1985;27:207–16.
71. Conrad DA, Scribner RK, Weber AH, et al. In vitro activity of BMY-28142 against pediatric pathogens, including isolates from cystic fibrosis sputum. Antimicrob Agents Chemother 1985;28:58–63.
72. Neu HC. Safety of cefepime: a new extended-spectrum parenteral cephalosporin. Am J Med 1996;100(6A):68S–75S.
73. Pichichero ME. Use of selected cephalosporins in penicillin-allergic patients: a paradigm shift. Diagn Microbiol Infect Dis 2007;57(Suppl 3):S13–8.
74. Martin SI, Kaye KM. Beta-lactam antibiotics: newer formulations and newer agents. Infect Dis Clin North Am 2004;18:603–19.
75. U.S. Food and Drug Administration. Early communication about ongoing safety review: cefepime (marketed as Maxipime). Available at: http://www.fda.gov/cder/drug/early_comm/cefepime.htm. Accessed October 19, 2008.
76. U.S. Food and Drug Administration. Update of safety review: follow-up to the November 14, 2007, communication about the ongoing safety review of cefepime (marketed as Maxipime). Available at: http://www.fda.gov/cder/drug/early_comm/cefepime_update_200805.htm. Accessed October 19, 2008.
77. U.S. Food and Drug Administration. FDA Alert June 17, 2009; Information for Healthcare Professionals: Cefepime (marketed as Maxipime). Available at: http://www.fda.gov/drugs/DrugSafety/PostmarketDrugSafetyInformationforPatientsand Providers/DrugsSafetyInformationforHealthcareProfessionals/ucm167254.htm. Accessed July 27, 2009.

Macrolides, Ketolides, and Glycylcyclines: Azithromycin, Clarithromycin, Telithromycin, Tigecycline

Jerry M. Zuckerman, MD[a,b,*], Fozia Qamar, MD[b],
Bartholomew R. Bono, MD[a,b]

KEYWORDS

- Macrolides • Ketolides • Glycylcyclines
- Antimicrobials • Review

Erythromycin, the first macrolide antibiotic discovered, has been used since the early 1950s for the treatment of upper respiratory tract and skin and soft tissue infections caused by susceptible organisms, especially in patients who are allergic to penicillin. Several drawbacks, however, have limited the use of erythromycin, including frequent gastrointestinal intolerance and a short serum half-life. Advanced macrolide antimicrobials synthesized by altering the erythromycin base have resulted in compounds with broader activity, more favorable pharmacokinetics and pharmacodynamics, and better tolerability. In 1991 and 1992, the US Food and Drug Administration (FDA) approved two of these agents, clarithromycin (Biaxin) and azithromycin (Zithromax), for clinical use. Since their introduction, these advanced macrolides have been used extensively for the treatment of respiratory tract infections, sexually transmitted diseases, and infections caused by *Helicobacter pylori* and *Mycobacterium avium* complex (MAC).

Ketolides, a new class of macrolides, share many of the characteristics of the advanced macrolides. Their in vitro spectrum of activity also includes gram-positive organisms (*Streptococcus pneumoniae, Streptococcus pyogenes*) that are macrolide

[a] Jefferson Medical College, 1025 Walnut Street, Philadelphia, PA 19107, USA
[b] Division of Infectious Diseases, Department of Medicine, Albert Einstein Medical Center, Klein Building, Suite 331, 5501 Old York Road, Philadelphia, PA 19141, USA
* Corresponding author. Division of Infectious Diseases, Department of Medicine, Albert Einstein Medical Center, Klein Building, Suite 331, 5501 Old York Road, Philadelphia, PA 19141.
E-mail address: zuckermj@einstein.edu (J.M. Zuckerman).

Infect Dis Clin N Am 23 (2009) 997–1026
doi:10.1016/j.idc.2009.06.013
0891-5520/09/$ – see front matter © 2009 Elsevier Inc. All rights reserved.

id.theclinics.com

resistant. Telithromycin (Ketek), specifically developed for the treatment of respiratory tract infections, received FDA approval in 2004. In 2007, because of increasing reports of hepatotoxicity, the FDA withdrew two of telithromycin's treatment indications, limiting its approval to the treatment of mild to moderate community-acquired pneumonia.

Glycylcyclines are a new class of antimicrobial agents developed to overcome tetracycline-specific resistance mechanisms (efflux pumps and ribosomal protection). Tigecycline (Tygacil), a derivative of minocycline, is the first antimicrobial in this class to receive FDA approval. Tigecycline is active in vitro against a broad spectrum of bacteria, including multidrug-resistant (MDR) organisms, and is indicated for the treatment of complicated skin and skin structure infections, complicated intra-abdominal infections and community-acquired pneumonia. This article reviews the pharmacokinetics, antimicrobial activity, clinical use, and adverse effects of these antimicrobial agents.

CHEMISTRY

Erythromycin is a macrolide antibiotic whose structure consists of a macrocyclic 14-membered lactone ring attached to two sugar moieties (a neutral sugar, cladinose, and an amino sugar, desosamine). In the acidic environment of the stomach, it is rapidly degraded to the 8,9-anhydro-6,9-hemiketal and then to the 6,9,9,12-spiroketal form. The hemiketal intermediate may be responsible for the gastrointestinal adverse effects associated with erythromycin.[1]

Clarithromycin (6-O-methylerythromycin) is synthesized by substituting a methoxy group for the C-6 hydroxyl group of erythromycin. This substitution creates a more acid-stable antimicrobial and prevents the degradation of the erythromycin base to the hemiketal intermediate, which results in improved oral bioavailability and reduced gastrointestinal intolerance.[2] Clarithromycin is available as immediate-release tablets (250 or 500 mg), extended-release tablets (500 mg), and granules for oral suspension (125 or 250 mg/5 mL).

Azithromycin (9-deoxo-9a-aza-9a-methyl-9a-homoerythromycin) is formed by inserting a methyl-substituted nitrogen in place of the carbonyl group at the 9a position of the aglycone ring. The resulting dibasic 15-membered ring macrolide derivative is more appropriately referred to as an azalide. This change produces a compound that is more acid stable and has a longer serum half-life ($t_{1/2}$), increased tissue penetration, and greater activity against gram-negative organisms compared with erythromycin.[2] Azithromycin is available as 250- or 500-mg immediate-release tablets, 2-g microsphere extended-release powder, oral suspension (100–200 mg/5 mL), and intravenous preparation (lypholized 500 mg/10 mL vial).

Ketolides are synthesized by two changes in the 14-membered erythronolide A ring: substituting a keto function for the alpha-L-cladinose moiety at position 3 and replacing the hydroxyl group at position 6 with a methoxy group.[3] These changes promote greater acid stability and prevent induction of macrolide-lincosamide-streptogramin B (MLS$_B$) resistance.[4] Telithromycin is synthesized by cycling of the C11-12 positions to form a carbamate ring with an imidazo-pyridyl group attachment that enhances binding to the bacterial ribosome and in vitro activity.[5] Telithromycin is available in 300- or 400-mg tablets.

Tigecycline is synthesized by the addition of a *tert*-butyl-glycylamido group to the C-9 position of minocycline. This addition overcomes the efflux pump and ribosomal protection mechanisms that confer resistance to tetracycline and extends its antimicrobial activity against a variety of bacteria.[6] Tigecycline is only available as an intravenous preparation (lyophilized 50 mg/vial).

MECHANISM OF ACTION AND RESISTANCE

The macrolides and ketolides are bacteriostatic antimicrobials. They reversibly bind to domain V of 23S ribosomal RNA (rRNA) of the 50s subunit of the bacterial ribosome inhibiting RNA-dependent protein synthesis.[7,8] The ketolides bind with a 10- to 100-fold higher affinity to the ribosome than erythromycin. The ketolides also have a greater affinity for binding to domain II of the 23S rRNA, which enables it to maintain antimicrobial activity against bacterial strains that are macrolide resistant because of alterations in the domain V binding site.[4]

Macrolide resistance in streptococci arises from either an alteration of the drug-binding site on the ribosome by methylation (MLS_B resistance) or by active drug efflux. The efflux mechanism is mediated by the macrolide efflux (*mef*) genes and is specific for 14- and 15-membered macrolides.[3] Macrolide resistance is usually low level (minimum inhibitory concentrations [MICs] 1–32 mg/L), and in vitro susceptibility to ketolides, lincosamides, and streptogramins is maintained.[9] Methylation of an adenine residue in domain V of the 23S rRNA, mediated by the erythromycin ribosome methylase (*erm*) genes, prevents binding of the macrolides and ketolides to domain V and results in high level macrolide resistance (MIC $\geq$ 64 mg/L). Ketolides presumably maintain their antimicrobial activity by virtue of their ability to bind to an alternative site—domain II of the 23S rRNA.[10] Methylase may be either induced or constitutively expressed, and resistance to erythromycin implies cross-resistance to clarithromycin and azithromycin. Clarithromycin and azithromycin can induce methylase production but telithromycin does not.[11] Decreased susceptibility to telithromycin in streptococci has been associated with a variety of mutations in the *erm*(B) gene and its promoter region, ribosomal proteins L4 and L22, and in the 23S rRNA.[12–14]

Tigecycline is also a bacteriostatic antibiotic. It reversibly binds to the 30S ribosomal subunit inhibiting protein synthesis. Glycylcyclines bind with a fivefold higher affinity to the ribosome compared with tetracyclines.[15] This enhanced ribosomal binding enables tigecycline to overcome resistance caused by ribosomal protection. Tigecycline also maintains activity against bacteria-containing tetracycline-specific efflux pumps by failing to be recognized as a substrate.[16] Susceptibility to tigecycline is reduced, however, by the overexpression of multidrug efflux pumps (eg, MexXY, AcrAB) that may be found in gram-negative organisms. These multidrug efflux pumps are naturally expressed in *Pseudomonas aeruginosa*.[16,17] Reduced susceptibility of *Acinetobacter spp* to tigecycline has been reported in isolates with a resistance-nodulation-division-type multicomponent efflux transporter.[18]

PHARMACOKINETICS

The structural alterations to the erythromycin base used to synthesize the advanced macrolides and ketolides result in improved pharmacokinetic properties. Compared with erythromycin, clarithromycin and azithromycin are more acid stable and have greater oral bioavailability (55% and 37%, respectively).[2] The peak plasma concentration of clarithromycin immediate-release tablets is increased by 24% when administered with food, but the overall bioavailability is unchanged.[19] The bioavailability of the extended-release formulation, however, is decreased by 30% when administered in the fasting state and should be administered with food.[20] The bioavailabilities of the tablet, sachet, or suspension formulations of azithromycin are not affected by meals.[21] The absorption of azithromycin 2-g extended-release microsphere formulation is increased with food and should be administered on an empty stomach to ensure appropriate (slower) absorption from the gastrointestinal tract.[22] Oral absorption of an 800-mg dose of telithromycin is excellent (90%); however, 33% of the dose undergoes first-pass metabolism, which results in an absolute oral bioavailability of 57%.[23] The bioavailability, rate, and extent of absorption of telithromycin are unaffected by food.[24]

The single-dose pharmacokinetics of erythromycin, clarithromycin, azithromycin, and telithromycin are summarized in **Table 1**. Several differences between the pharmacokinetics of these antimicrobials are apparent. First, the peak serum concentration (C_{max}) of azithromycin after a 500-mg dose is fivefold lower than that achieved with a comparable dose of clarithromycin or telithromycin. Although azithromycin concentrations are low in the serum, tissue concentrations are significantly higher, as discussed later. Second, the terminal half-life of azithromycin and telithromycin are long enough to allow once-daily dosing. Twice-daily dosing of the immediate-release formulation of clarithromycin is necessary based on the terminal half-life of 4 to 5 hours.[2] Protein binding is higher for clarithromycin and telithromycin (60%–70%) compared with azithromycin (7%–50%).

Clarithromycin is metabolized to an active metabolite, 14-hydroxyclarithromycin. Larger doses of clarithromycin result in nonlinear increases in the $t_{1/2}$ and in the area under the plasma concentration-time curve (AUC) of clarithromycin because of saturation of the metabolic pathway.[25] Steady-state peak plasma concentrations of 3 to 4 mg/L are achieved within 3 days with clarithromycin, 500 mg, every 8 to 12 hours and the elimination half-life increases to 5 to 7 hours.[19] Although steady-state peak plasma concentrations are lower and achieved later with the extended-release formulation of clarithromycin than a comparable daily dose of the immediate-release formulations, the 24-hour AUC is equivalent between the two formulations, supporting the once-daily dosing of the extended-release formulation.[20]

The azithromycin 2-g extended-release microsphere formulation has a slower rate of absorption compared with an equivalent dose of the immediate-release tablet, which results in a mean peak serum concentration that is 57% lower and a t_{max} that is 2.5 hours later.[22] The mean relative bioavailability of the extended-release form was 82.8%. When compared with a 3-day regimen of 500-mg azithromycin immediate-release tablets in healthy subjects, a 2-g single dose of extended-release azithromycin on day 1 had a C_{max} and 24-hour AUC that were two- and threefold higher, respectively. Overall AUC for the 5-day study period was equivalent for the two dosing regimens.[26] Daily doses of telithromycin, 800 mg, result in a steady-state peak plasma concentration of 2.27 mg/L and a terminal half-life of 9.81 hours.[27]

Tigecycline is only available in an injectable formulation. The recommended dosage is an initial load of 100 mg, followed by a maintenance dose of 50 mg every 12 hours

Table 1
Comparative pharmacokinetics of macrolide antibiotics[a]

Parameter	Erythromycin Base	Azithromycin	Clarithromycin	14-Hydroxy-Clarithromycin	Telithromycin
Bioavailability %	25	37	55	35	57
C_{max} (mg/L)	0.3–0.9	0.4	2.1–2.4	0.6	1.9–2.0
t_{max} (h)	3–4	2	2	2–3	1.0
$t_{1/2}$ (h)	2–3	40–68	3–5	4–7	7.16–13
AUC (mg/L × h)	8	3.4	19	5.7	7.9–8.25

Abbreviations: AUC, area under plasma concentration time curve; C_{max}, peak serum concentration; t_{max}, time to peak serum concentration; $t_{1/2}$, serum half-life.
[a] Mean values after a single 500-mg oral dose (800-mg dose for telithromycin).
Data from Zhanel GG, Dueck M, Hoban DJ, et al. Review of macrolides and ketolides: focus on respiratory tract infections. Drugs 2001;61(4):443–98.

infused over 30 to 60 minutes. Pooled data from healthy volunteers showed that the C_{max} after a single 100-mg dose was 1.45 mg/L and 0.90 mg/L after 30- and 60-minute infusions, respectively. The C_{max} at steady state was 0.87 mg/L and 0.63 mg/L after 30- and 60-minute infusions, respectively, and the 24-hour AUC was 4.70 mg/L × h. The serum half-life was 27.1 hours after a single 100-mg dose and increased to 42.2 hours with multiple doses of 50 mg twice daily. The pharmacokinetics of tigecycline are not affected by the presence of food or differences in sex or age.[28-30]

The macrolides and ketolides are lipophilic and are extensively distributed in body fluids and tissues. Mean tissue concentrations are 2- to 20-fold greater than serum concentrations for clarithromycin and are 10- to 100-fold greater than serum concentrations for azithromycin.[31,32] Tissue concentrations do not peak until 48 hours after administration of azithromycin and persist for several days afterwards.[2] Twenty-four hours after the last dose of drug administration, concentrations of clarithromycin and azithromycin in lung epithelial cell lining fluid exceeded serum concentrations by 20-fold.[33] Measurements at this interval also revealed that alveolar macrophage concentrations were 400 times (clarithromycin) and 800 times (azithromycin) greater than their respective serum concentrations. Telithromycin also has excellent penetration into bronchopulmonary tissues. Levels in alveolar macrophages (median concentration 81 mg/L) significantly exceeded plasma levels 8 hours after dosing and maintained elevated levels 24 and 48 hours after dosing (23 mg/L and 2.15 mg/L, respectively).[34] Concentrations of telithromycin in bronchial mucosa and epithelial lining fluid exceeded for 24 hours the mean MIC_{90} of *S pneumoniae, Moraxella catarrhalis,* and *Mycoplasma pneumoniae.*[35] In these studies, 24 hours after the last dose of drug administration, concentrations of telithromycin in lung epithelial cell lining fluid were 12-fold, and in alveolar macrophages the levels were 400-fold greater than their respective serum concentrations.

Tigecycline is also distributed widely in tissues, with a steady-state volume of distribution of 7 to 10 L/kg.[30] At steady-state levels, the tigecycline AUC_{0-12h} in alveolar cells and epithelial lining fluid was 78-fold higher and 32% higher compared with serum.[36] Tissue levels of tigecycline were higher in the gallbladder (38-fold), lung (8.6-fold), and colon (2.1-fold) compared with serum levels 4 hours after a single 100-mg dose. Synovial fluid and bone concentrations, however, were 0.58 and 0.35 lower, respectively, relative to serum.[37] Tissue penetration of tigecycline into skin blister fluid was 74% of serum concentration.[38]

Clarithromycin is metabolized in the liver by the cytochrome P450 3A4 (CYP3A4) enzymes to the active 14-hydroxy form and six additional products. Thirty percent to 40% of an oral dose of clarithromycin is excreted in the urine either unchanged or as the active 14-hydroxy metabolite.[39] The remainder is excreted into the bile. In patients with moderate to severe renal impairment (ie, creatinine clearance < 30 mL/min), the dose should be reduced.[39] In patients with moderate to severe hepatic impairment and normal renal function, there is less metabolism of clarithromycin to the 14-hydroxy form, which results in decreased peak plasma concentrations of the metabolite and increased renal excretion of unchanged clarithromycin. Dosing modifications do not seem to be necessary for these patients.[40]

Azithromycin elimination occurs primarily in the feces as the unchanged drug, and urinary excretion is minimal.[41] Unlike clarithromycin, azithromycin does not interact with the cytochrome P450 system.[42] In patients with mild or moderate hepatic impairment, dosing modifications do not seem to be necessary.[42,43]

Telithromycin is eliminated via multiple pathways, including unchanged drug in feces (7%) and urine (13%) and the remainder via hepatic metabolism by the CYP 3A4 and 1A isoenzymes.[44] Four metabolites of telithromycin do not have appreciable antibacterial activity.[10] Plasma concentrations and AUC were 1.4- and 1.9-fold higher in patients with creatinine clearance less than 30 mL/min. In patients with mild to moderate renal impairment, there was no significant change in the pharmacokinetics of telithromycin.[10] Dosing modifications are not necessary when administering telithromycin to patients with hepatic impairment because pharmacokinetics do not change significantly as the result of a compensatory increase in renal excretion.[45]

Tigecycline is not extensively metabolized and is primarily eliminated unchanged via biliary excretion. In healthy male volunteers who received ^{14}C-tigecycline, 59% of the radioactive dose was recovered in the feces and 33% recovered in the urine.[46] Secondary elimination pathways include renal excretion of unchanged drug and, to a lesser degree, metabolism to glucuronide conjugates and N-acetyl-9-aminominocycline. Dose adjustment is not necessary based on age, sex, renal impairment, or mild to moderate hepatic impairment (Child Pugh class A-B).[28,30] In patients with severe hepatic impairment (Child Pugh class C), the maintenance dose should be reduced by 50%.[47]

SPECTRUM OF ACTIVITY

The Clinical and Laboratory Standards Institute provides guidelines for the interpretation of in vitro MICs for clarithromycin, azithromycin, and telithromycin. The FDA established breakpoints for tigecycline (**Table 2**).[47,48] The breakpoints for azithromycin are based on expected tissue concentrations, whereas the breakpoints for clarithromycin are based on achievable serum concentrations. In vitro susceptibility testing does not account for the antimicrobial activity of the active 14-hydroxy metabolite and may underestimate the activity of clarithromycin.[49] In vitro MIC measurements also do not account for the pharmacodynamic properties of an antimicrobial (eg, tissue penetration, intracellular half-life, postantibiotic effect) and may not predict its relative efficacy at the site of infection.

Comparative in vitro susceptibility data for erythromycin, clarithromycin, azithromycin, and telithromycin are shown in **Table 3**. Compared with erythromycin, clarithromycin demonstrates equal or better in vitro activity against gram-positive organisms, whereas azithromycin is two- to fourfold less active.[53] Azithromycin and clarithromycin are generally inactive against methicillin-resistant staphylococci. Telithromycin is more active in vitro against S pneumoniae compared with clarithromycin

Table 2
Susceptibility test result interpretative criteria

	Clarithromycin		Azithromycin		Telithromycin		Tigecycline	
	S	R	S	R	S	R	S	R
S aureus	≤2	≥8	≤2	≥8	≤1	≥4	≤0.5	N/A
Streptococcus spp, including pneumoniae	≤0.25	≥1	≤0.50	≥2	≤1	≥4	≤0.25	N/A
Enterococcus faecalis	N/A	N/A	N/A	N/A	N/A	N/A	≤0.25	N/A
Haemophilus spp	≤8	≥32	≤4	NA	≤4	≥16	N/A	N/A
Enterobacteriaceae	N/A	N/A	N/A	N/A	N/A	N/A	≤2	≥8
Anaerobes	N/A	N/A	N/A	N/A	N/A	N/A	≤4	≥16

Values expressed as MIC (mg/L).
Data from Tygacil (tigecycline) prescribing information. 2008;2008(11/28); Clinical and Laboratory Standards Institute. Performance standards for antimicrobial susceptibility Testing; Eighteenth Informational Supplement; 2008.

Table 3
Comparative in vitro activities of macrolide/ketolide antibiotics*

Organism	Erythromycin	Azithromycin	Clarithromycin	Telithromycin
Gram-positive aerobes				
Streptococcus pyogenes				
erythromycin susceptible	0.06–0.12	0.12–0.25	0.06–0.12	0.03
*erm*A resistance	1–32	16–32	2–16	0.015–0.25
*erm*B resistance	> 64	> 64	> 64	> 8
*mef*A resistance	8–16	8	8–16	0.25–1
Streptococcus pneumoniae				
erythromycin sensitive	0.03–0.12	0.06–0.25	0.03–0.12	0.008–0.03
erythromycin resistant *erm*B	≥32	≥64	≥64	0.125–0.5
erythromycin resistant *mef*A	8–16	8–16	8	0.25–1
Gram-negative aerobes				
Haemophilus influenzae	8	2–4	4–16	2–4
Moraxella catarrhalis	0.125–0.25	0.06–0.12	0.12–0.25	0.12
Legionella pneumophila	0.12–2	0.25–2	0.06–0.25	0.015–0.06
Neisseria gonorrhoeae	0.5	0.25		0.12
Other pathogens				
Chlamydophila pneumoniae	0.06–0.25	0.125–0.25	0.03–0.06	0.06–0.25
Mycoplasma pneumoniae	≤0.015–0.06	≤0.015	≤0.015–0.03	≤0.015

* Values expressed as MIC 90 (mg/L). Ranges indicate the different values reported in references. *Data from* references.[3,44,50–52]

and azithromycin and maintains activity against strains that are macrolide resistant.[54] In one study, the MIC_{90} for telithromycin against *S pneumoniae* strains with the *mef*A gene was 0.25 mg/L or less, compared with 1 to 4 mg/L for macrolides. Against strains expressing the *erm*B gene, telithromycin had an MIC_{90} of 0.5 mg/L, whereas the macrolides had an MIC_{90} of more than 64 mg/L.[55] Telithromycin MIC_{90} increased from 0.015 mg/L to 0.25 mg/L and 0.5 mg/L for penicillin-intermediate and penicillin-resistant pneumococcal strains, respectively.[56] Telithromycin is also two- to eightfold more active against erythromycin-susceptible strains of *S aureus* compared with clarithromycin and azithromycin. Telithromycin maintains activity against macrolide-resistant strains of *S aureus* that have an inducible MLS_B gene but not against strains in which resistance is constitutively expressed.[57]

The newer macrolides demonstrate enhanced activity against respiratory pathogens. The MIC against *H influenzae* for clarithromycin, combined with its active metabolite, 14-hydroxyclarithromycin, is two- to fourfold lower compared with erythromcyin.[58] Azithromycin and telithromycin are more active against *H influenzae* with an MIC four- to eightfold lower compared with erythromycin.[59] Clarithromycin seems more active in vitro than azithromycin and erythromycin against *Legionella pneumophila* and *Chlamydophila pneumoniae*, whereas azithromycin demonstrates better activity against *M catarrhalis* and *M pneumoniae*.[53,60] Telithromycin has excellent in vitro activity against *Mycoplasma*, *Chlamydia*, and *Legionella* and is more active compared with the macrolides.[44]

Azithromycin has activity against enteric pathogens, including *Escherichia coli*, *Salmonella spp*, *Yersinia enterocolitica*, and *Shigella spp*.[53] Clarithromycin and telithromycin have no in vitro activity against these gram-negative organisms.

Azithromycin is more active against *Campylobacter jejuni* than erythromycin or clarithromycin, whereas clarithromycin has greater activity against *H pylori*.[61,62]

Azithromycin and clarithromycin have similar or increased in vitro activity against genital pathogens compared with erythromycin. *Neisseria gonorrhoeae, Haemophilus ducreyi*, and *Ureaplasma urealyticum* are susceptible to both antibiotics, with azithromycin demonstrating lower MICs.[61,62] Clarithromycin is approximately tenfold more active than erythromycin against *Chlamydia trachomatis*, whereas azithromycin's activity is similar to that of erythromycin.[61,62] Only azithromycin demonstrated in vitro activity against *Mycoplasma hominis*.[49]

Tigecycline has a broad spectrum of activity against aerobic and anaerobic grampositive and -negative pathogens, including micro-organisms that demonstrate resistance to multiple classes of antimicrobials. In addition to the Clinical and Laboratory Standards Institute breakpoints listed in **Table 2**, the MICs indicating susceptibility to tigecycline are 0.25 mg/L or less for vancomycin-susceptible *Enterococcus faecalis*, 2 mg/L or less for *Enterobacteriaceae* and 4 mg/L or less for anaerobes. *P aeruginosa* isolates are intrinsically resistant to tigecycline. Tigecycline also has limited activity against *Proteus spp* and *Providencia spp*.[63]

The Tigecycline Evaluation and Surveillance Trial evaluated the in vitro activity of tigecycline against a large population of organisms.[64,65] Overall, the global in vitro susceptibility data showed that tigecycline was highly active against most gram-positive isolates, including 100% of the methicillin-susceptible *S aureus*, 99% of the methicillin-resistant *S aureus*, and 98% of the vancomycin-resistant enterococcus isolates tested. Ninety-five percent of *Enterobacteriaceae* were susceptible to tigecycline at the FDA susceptibility breakpoint of 2 mg/L or less. Tigecycline maintained in vitro activity against MDR gram-negative organisms, including *E coli* and *Klebsiella spp* isolates expressing extended-spectrum β-lactamases and carbapenemase-producing strains of *Enterobacteriaceae*.[66] Tigecycline demonstrated excellent activity against *Acinetobacter baumanii* with MIC 50/90 results of 0.5/2 mg/L.[67,68] Tigecycline also was active against community-acquired infectious agents such as *S pneumoniae* and *H influenzae* regardless of penicillin susceptibility or β-lactamase production, with MIC 90 values of less than 0.5 mg/L.[69,70]

CLINICAL USE: MACROLIDES AND KETOLIDES
Respiratory Tract Infections

Upper respiratory tract infections
Clarithromycin, azithromycin, and telithromycin are effective against the most frequently isolated bacterial causes of pharyngitis, otitis media, and sinusitis. A 5-day course of the extended-release formulation of clarithromycin, azithromycin, or telithromycin is equally as effective as a 10-day course of penicillin for the treatment of streptococcal pharyngitis.[2,71,72] In comparative trials, clarithromycin has proved to be equivalent to amoxicillin, amoxicillin-clavulanate, and cefaclor for the treatment of acute otitis media in children.[73,74] Otitis media in children was also treated equally well with azithromycin (3 or 5 days) versus 10 days of amoxicillin/clavulanate or cefaclor or 5 days of cefdinir.[75,76] One study showed greater efficacy with a 10-day course of high-dose amoxicillin/clavulanate compared with a 5-day course of azithromycin.[77] A single oral dose of azithromycin at 30 mg/kg was as effective as a 10-day course of high-dose amoxicillin.[78]

For the treatment of acute sinusitis, clarithromycin had equivalent efficacy compared with cefuroxime axetil, levofloxacin, or ciprofloxacin.[79–81] Once-daily dosing of the extended-release formulation of clarithromycin was comparable to amoxicillin/clavulanate in the treatment of acute maxillary sinusitis.[82] Studies for acute sinusitis treatment with azithromycin concluded that a 3-day regimen (500 mg daily) was equally efficacious as a 10-day course of amoxicillin-clavulanate, and a single dose of the 2-g azithromycin extended-release microsphere formulation had a similar cure rate as a 10-day course of levofloxacin.[83,84] A 5-day course of telithromycin was equally effective as a 10-day course of high-dose amoxicillin-clavulanate, cefuroxime axetil, or moxifloxacin.[85–87]

Currently, clarithromycin is approved for the treatment of pharyngitis caused by *S pyogenes*; the recommended dose is 250 mg every 12 hours for 10 days. Dosage for treatment of acute maxillary sinusitis is either 500 mg every 12 hours with the immediate-release tablets for 14 days or 2 × 500 mg every 24 hours with the extended-release tablets for 7 days. For children, the recommended dose is 7.5 mg/kg every 12 hours. Azithromycin is approved as a second-line agent for the treatment of pharyngitis. The recommended adult dose is 500 mg on the first day followed by 250 mg once daily on days 2 through 5. For children, the following azithromycin dosing regimens can be used for the treatment of otitis media: 30 mg/kg as a single dose, 10 mg/kg once daily for 3 days, or 10 mg/kg on the first day followed by 5 mg/kg on days 2 through 5. Azithromycin is also approved for the treatment of acute bacterial sinusitis; the adult dose is either 500 mg daily for 3 days or a single 2-g dose of the extended-release formulation and for children it is 10 mg/kg once daily for 3 days. Telithromycin is not FDA approved for the treatment of upper respiratory tract infections.

Lower respiratory tract infections

Various trials have demonstrated the efficacy of clarithromycin, azithromycin, and telithromycin for treatment of lower respiratory tract infections, including acute bronchitis, acute exacerbation of chronic bronchitis (AECB), and community-acquired pneumonia. Most studies involved patients who were not hospitalized. Studies have shown equal efficacy of clarithromycin compared with ceftibuten, cefaclor, cefuroxime axetil, and cefixime for the treatment of lower respiratory tract infections.[88] Comparable efficacy was also demonstrated between the once-daily dosing of the extended-release formulation of clarithromycin and the twice-daily dosing of the immediate-release formulation for the treatment of lower respiratory tract infections.[89,90] Clinical cure rates for the treatment of AECB were similar between a 10-day course of clarithromycin compared with levofloxacin or cefuroxime axetil and a 5- or 7-day course of extended-release tablets of clarithromycin compared with telithromycin or amoxicillin/clavulanic acid.[91–94] In a comparative trial between 5 days of gemifloxacin and 7 days of clarithromycin, clinical and bacteriologic cures were similar, but significantly more patients in the gemifloxacin group remained free of AECB recurrences.[95] For the outpatient treatment of community-acquired pneumonia, equivalent efficacy has been shown between (1) clarithromycin 500 mg twice daily for 10 days and moxifloxacin or gatifloxacin and (2) clarithromycin extended-release tablets (2 × 500 mg tablets once daily for 7 days) and levofloxacin or trovafloxacin.[96–99]

Azithromycin (500 mg on day 1 followed by 250 mg daily for 4 days) was equivalent to cefaclor in patients with outpatient community-acquired pneumonia.[100] Outcomes for the treatment of community-acquired pneumonia were also similar between a 3-day course of azithromycin (1 g daily) and a 7-day course of amoxicillin-clavulanate.[101] Two comparative trials showed that the efficacy of a single 2-g dose of azithromycin extended-release microsphere formulation was equivalent to a 7-day course of extended-release clarithromycin or levofloxacin for the treatment of mild to moderate community-acquired pneumonia in adults.[102,103]

In an analysis of randomized controlled trials comparing azithromycin with alternative antimicrobials, azithromycin was found to have comparable clinical cure rates for the treatment of acute bronchitis and AECB and superior efficacy in the treatment of community-acquired pneumonia.[104,105] For the treatment of AECB, azithromycin (500 mg daily for 3 days) was as efficacious as clarithromycin (500 mg twice daily for 10 days).[106] Equivalent efficacy was also demonstrated between a 3- or 5-day course of azithromycin with either a 5-day course of moxifloxacin or a 7-day course of levofloxacin for the treatment of AECB.[107,108] The clinical efficacy of telithromycin has been demonstrated in the outpatient treatment of community-acquired pneumonia in open-label studies and comparator trials. Telithromycin was equally effective when compared with a 10-day course of high-dose amoxicillin, twice-daily clarithromycin, or a 7- to 10-day course of trovafloxacin.[109–111] Clinical cure rates and bacterial eradication were comparable in patients treated with either a 5- or 7-day course of telithromycin or a 10-day course of clarithromycin.[112] Pooled analysis from clinical trials showed that telithromycin was effective in community-acquired pneumonia caused by erythromycin-resistant *S pneumoniae* infections, including bacteremic patients.[113,114] For the treatment of AECB, a 5-day course of telithromycin was equally effective as a 10-day course with cefuroxime axetil, clarithromycin, or amoxicillin-clavulanate.[115,116] In several studies, however, eradication rates for *H influenzae* were lower for telithromycin (66%) than comparators (88%).[117]

Azithromycin and clarithromycin have been shown to be effective in the treatment of community-acquired pneumonia in patients who require hospitalization. Monotherapy with intravenous azithromycin was equally effective as a respiratory fluoroquinolone or a β-lactam plus macrolide regimen for patients hospitalized with community-acquired pneumonia.[118–120] Recent comparative trials showed equivalent efficacy between respiratory fluoroquinolones and ceftriaxone plus azithromycin or clarithromycin in patients with community-acquired pneumonia who required hospitalization.[121–123] Other studies imply an advantage in dual empiric therapy, including a macrolide, in reducing mortality in patients with community-acquired pneumonia or bacteremic pneumococcal pneumonia.[124–126] Azithromycin monotherapy successfully treated 96% of patients (22/23) hospitalized with legionella pneumonia with a mean total duration of antibiotic therapy (intravenous plus oral) of 7.92 days.[127] To date, limited data have been published on the use of telithromycin with a β-lactam antimicrobial for the treatment of community-acquired pneumonia in hospitalized patients.

Pneumococcal resistance to macrolides is prevalent. Surveillance studies in the United States revealed that 28% to 34% of *S pneumoniae* isolates are macrolide resistant.[128–130] Telithromycin resistance was infrequent in these studies. In the United States, 60% of the macrolide-resistant isolates exhibited low-level erythromycin resistance (16 mg/L) via expression of the *mef*(A) gene, and nearly 20% expressed the *mef*(A) gene and the *erm*(B) gene, resulting in high-level resistance.[131] The prevalence of macrolide resistance among *S pneumoniae* isolates varies greatly among geographic regions, with the highest prevalence of resistance reported from Asia.[132] Telithromycin resistance among *S pneumoniae* isolates has been reported in a small number of case series. One surveillance study of *S pneumoniae* isolates from Taiwan revealed that 2% were resistant to telithromycin and 96% were macrolide resistant.[13,14,133,134]

Despite the high prevalence of macrolide resistance, reported clinical failures have been limited to small case series. In a prospective cohort study of patients who were discharged from emergency departments and prescribed clarithromycin for the treatment of community-acquired pneumonia, macrolide resistance among *S pneumoniae* isolates did not affect outcomes.[135] A matched-case control study of patients with bacteremic pneumococcal infections investigated whether development of breakthrough bacteremia during macrolide treatment was related to macrolide susceptibility of the isolate.[136] Breakthrough bacteremia with an erythromycin-resistant isolate occurred in 18 (24%) of 76 patients taking a macrolide, compared with none of the 136 matched patients with bacteremia with an erythromycin-susceptible isolate. Given the possibility of treatment failure, most guidelines recommend combining a macrolide with a β-lactam if risk factors are present for drug-resistant S pneumoniae. Telithromycin maintains in vitro activity against macrolide-resistant isolates. Whether this translates into a therapeutic advantage in the empiric treatment of respiratory tract infections, especially when drug-resistant S pneumoniae is of concern, needs to be determined.

Practice guidelines from the Infectious Diseases Society of America (IDSA) and American Thoracic Society (ATS) provide recommendations for the empiric treatment of community-acquired pneumonia based on the clinical setting, presence of comorbidities, severity of disease, and risk for drug-resistant S pneumoniae.[137] Only treatment options that include a macrolide are discussed, and the reader is referred to the guidelines for alternative options. In the outpatient setting, recommended antimicrobial therapy for patients who were previously healthy and have no risk factors for drug-resistant S pneumoniae includes any macrolide (erythromycin, azithromycin, clarithromycin). Recommended outpatient therapy for individuals who have comorbid conditions, have received antibiotics within the previous 3 months, or have other risk factors for drug-resistant S pneumoniae includes a macrolide in combination with a β-lactam. The IDSA/ATS guidelines suggest that in regions in which high-level (MIC ≥ 16 mg/L) macrolide resistance among S pneumoniae exceeds 25%, alternative antimicrobials should be considered in lieu of the macrolides. For patients who require hospitalization, a macrolide combined with a β-lactam is one of the preferred regimens recommended. Azithromycin monotherapy is not endorsed as a routine treatment option. The use of telithromycin is not addressed in the practice guidelines because at the time of publication, telithromycin's safety profile was being re-evaluated by the FDA.

The approved dose of azithromycin for treatment of lower respiratory tract infections is 500 mg the first day followed by 250 mg for days 2 through 5. An alternative regimen for the treatment of AECB is 500 mg daily for 3 days. The recommended treatment of community-acquired pneumonia with the extended-release microsphere formulation of azithromycin is a single 2-g dose. The recommended dose of intravenous azithromycin for the treatment of community-acquired pneumonia is 500 mg daily for at least 2 days followed by oral azithromycin 500 mg daily to complete a 7- to 10-day course. Clarithromycin immediate- and extended-release tablets are approved for treatment of community-acquired pneumonia and AECB. The dose of the immediate-release tablets is 250 mg twice daily for 7 to 14 days. The dose should be increased to 500 mg if H influenzae is being treated. The dose of the extended-release formulation is 2 × 500 mg tablets daily for 7 days. Telithromycin is FDA approved for the treatment of community-acquired pneumonia (including infections caused by multidrug-resistant S pneumoniae) at a dose of 800 mg daily for 7 to 10 days.

Sexually Transmitted Diseases

The use of the advanced macrolides in the treatment of sexually transmitted diseases has focused primarily on azithromycin. The prolonged tissue half-life of azithromycin allows single-dose treatment courses, directly observed therapy, and improved patient compliance. A meta-analysis of randomized clinical trials concluded that a single 1-gram dose of azithromycin was equally efficacious and had similar tolerability as a standard 7-day regimen of doxycycline for the treatment of uncomplicated urethritis or cervicitis caused by C trachomatis.[138] Another meta-analysis for treatment of *C trachomatis* infection during pregnancy found similar efficacy between a single 1-gram dose of azithromycin compared with erythromycin or amoxicillin.[139] Guidelines published by the US Public Health Service (USPHS) currently recommend either doxycycline, 100 mg twice daily for 7 days, or azithromycin, 1 g as a single dose, for either chlamydial infections or nongonococcal urethritis among adolescents and adults.[140] In a comparative study for the treatment of chronic prostatitis caused by *C trachomatis*, azithromycin (500 mg daily for 3 days on a weekly basis for 3 weeks) resulted in a significantly higher eradication rate and clinical cure compared with ciprofloxacin (500 mg twice daily for 20 days).[141] Another trial showed equivalent outcomes between azithromycin (1 g weekly for 4 weeks) and doxycycline (100 mg twice daily for 28 days).[142] A single 1-g dose of azithromycin is also one of the recommended treatments for genital ulcer disease caused by *H ducreyi* (chancroid).[140]

Azithromycin has in vitro activity against *N gonorrhoeae,* and a single 2-g oral dose was found to be equally efficacious as ceftriaxone, 250 mg intramuscularly, in the treatment of uncomplicated gonorrhea.[143] Gastrointestinal side effects occurred in 35% of patients who received azithromycin. The increased rate of side effects and greater expense of a 2-g azithromycin dose precluded the USPHS from recommending its use for the treatment of uncomplicated gonorrhea.[140] If chlamydia infection is not ruled out in a patient with uncomplicated gonococcal urethritis or cervicitis, then either a single 1-g dose of azithromycin or 7-day course of doxycycline should be used in addition to the gonorrhea treatment regimen. Azithromycin with or without metronidazole has been shown to have similar clinical response rates to comparative agents (metronidazole + doxycycline + cefoxitin + probenicid or doxycycline + amoxicillin/clavulanate) in the treatment of pelvic inflammatory disease.[144] The USPHS does not currently recommend this regimen for the treatment of pelvic inflammatory disease. Azithromycin resistance among gonococcal isolates is low in the United States, but 5.2% of isolates in Scotland had reduced susceptibility to azithromycin.[145,146]

The use of azithromycin for the treatment of early syphilis also has been evaluated. A meta-analysis of four randomized controlled trials for the treatment of early syphilis concluded that azithromycin achieved a higher cure rate compared with penicillin G benzathine.[147] A large comparative trial compared the efficacy of a single 2-g dose of azithromycin with an intramuscular injection of 2.4 million U of penicillin G benzathine. Cure rates at 3-, 6-, and 9-months were similar between the two treatment groups.[148] Recently, a 23S rRNA gene mutation in *Treponema pallidum* conferring resistance to azithromycin was identified in 32 of 114 isolates (28%) obtained from four sexually transmitted disease clinics located in either the United States or Ireland. The USPHS does not currently recommend the use of azithromycin for the treatment of syphilis in the United States.[140]

Helicobacter Pylori *Infections*

Antibiotic therapy for *H pylori*–associated peptic ulcer disease decreases ulcer recurrence and promotes healing. Triple-therapy regimens that consist of clarithromycin, amoxicillin, or metronidazole and an antisecretory agent for 7 to 14 days are preferable for the treatment of *H pylori* infections.[149,150] These combinations maximize *H pylori* eradication, minimize the risk of antimicrobial resistance, and allow shorter and simplified treatment courses, which results in improved compliance. Clinical efficacy of different triple-therapy clarithromycin-based regimens for 7 to 14 days had cure rates of 70% to 80% based on intention-to-treat analyses.[151–153] One meta-analysis and a recent randomized trial found that a 14-day course of clarithromycin triple therapy was more effective than a 7-day treatment course.[154,155] Sequential therapy involving a proton pump inhibitor plus amoxicillin for 5 days followed by a proton pump inhibitor, clarithromycin, and tinidazole for 5 days for the treatment of *H pylori* was evaluated, mainly in Italy. Eradication rates of *H pylori* with the sequential regimen were 90% or more and were more effective than standard clarithromycin-based triple-therapy regimens.[156,157] A recent meta-analysis concluded that sequential therapy seems to be superior to standard triple therapy, with crude eradication rates of *H pylori* of 93.4% and 76.9%, respectively.[158]

Clarithromycin resistance rates vary in different regions of the world and, within a region, among different population subgroups.[159] In the United States, the clarithromycin resistance rate among *H pylori* isolates was reported to be 13%.[160] In a 15-year interval, the frequency of primary clarithromycin resistance in Italy increased from 10.2% (1989–1990) to 21.3% (2004–2005).[161] *H pylori* resistance to clarithromycin has been shown to be associated with any previous use of macrolides.[162] Pretreatment clarithromycin resistance has a negative impact on treatment efficacy (55% reduction in cure rates) and is associated with failure to eradicate *H pylori*.[163,164]

In the United States, the American College of Gastroenterology practice guidelines recommend a clarithromycin-based regimen as one of two primary treatment options for *H pylori* infection. The recommended regimen includes a proton pump inhibitor, clarithromycin (500 mg twice daily), and either amoxicillin (1000 mg twice daily) or metronidazole (500 mg twice daily) given for 14 days. The alternative primary therapy recommended is a non–clarithromycin-based regimen that includes a proton pump inhibitor or ranitidine, bismuth subsalicylate, metronidazole, and tetracycline for 10 to 14 days. Until validation studies are conducted in other countries, the American College of Gastroenterology recommends that the sequential regimen outlined previously be considered as an alternative to the other standard first-line therapy options.[149]

MAC

Clarithromycin and azithromycin have both been shown to be effective in preventing and treating disseminated MAC disease in HIV-infected patients. Azithromycin is effective as prophylaxis against disseminated MAC disease in patients with CD4 counts of less than 100 cells/mm^3. In a comparative trial with rifabutin, the 1-year incidence rate of disseminated MAC disease was 15.3% in the rifabutin group (300 mg/d) compared with 7.6% in the azithromycin group (1200 mg weekly).[165] Combination of azithromycin and rifabutin decreased the 1-year incidence rate of MAC to 2.8%, but 22.7% of patients discontinued therapy because of drug-related toxicity compared with 13.5% of patients who received azithromycin alone. Azithromycin resistance was seen in 11% of isolates obtained from patients who developed breakthrough disease. Similarly, clarithromycin was shown to be effective for MAC prophylaxis. In a comparative trial, clarithromycin (500 mg twice daily) was more effective in preventing MAC bacteremia than rifabutin (300 mg daily), with rates of 9% and 15%, respectively.[166] Clarithromycin resistance was reported in 29% of the patients with breakthrough MAC bacteremia while on clarithromycin prophylaxis. Current USPHS/IDSA guidelines recommend either azithromycin, 1200 mg weekly, or clarithromycin, 500 mg twice daily, as the preferred regimens for MAC prophylaxis in HIV-infected individuals with a CD4 count of less than 50 cells/mm^3.[167]

The effectiveness of clarithromycin in combination with other antibiotics, especially ethambutol, for treatment of disseminated MAC disease in HIV-infected patients has been demonstrated in several randomized trials. A regimen of clarithromycin, rifabutin, and ethambutol was more effective in clearing MAC bacteremia and improving survival than a four-drug regimen of rifampin, ethambutol, clofazamine, and ciprofloxacin.[168] Another trial compared dosing regimens of clarithromycin in combination with ethambutol plus either rifabutin or clofazamine. Mortality was significantly higher at 4.5 months in patients who received clarithromycin at a dose of 1 g twice daily rather than the lower dose of 500 mg twice daily.[169] In another trial that compared clarithromycin with rifabutin, ethambutol, or both, eradication of MAC bacteremia occurred in 40% to 50% of patients at 12 weeks of treatment.[170] Response rates were not statistically different between the various treatment arms at 12 weeks. The relapse rate (24%) was higher in patients treated with clarithromycin and rifabutin than patients who received clarithromycin plus ethambutol (relapse rate 7%) or clarithromycin plus ethambutol plus rifabutin (relapse rate 6%).

Azithromycin, 600 mg daily, was compared with clarithromycin, 500 mg twice daily, for the treatment of disseminated MAC disease.[171] Both were administered with ethambutol 15 mg/kg/d. Two consecutive sterile blood cultures at 24 weeks were obtained in 46% (31/68) of patients in the azithromycin group compared with 56% (32/57) in the clarithromycin group. There was no difference in mortality between the two treatment groups. Another study that used the same regimens found that clarithromycin was significantly better and more rapid in clearance of MAC bacteremia.[172] Current recommendations for the treatment of disseminated MAC disease are to use at least two or more antimycobacterial drugs. Clarithromycin is the preferred first agent. Azithromycin is an alternative when drug interactions or intolerance preclude the use of clarithromycin.[167]

Clarithromycin and azithromycin are also useful in the treatment of pulmonary MAC infections in HIV-negative patients. In noncomparative studies, sputum conversion rates at 6 months were comparable between azithromycin- and clarithromycin-containing regimens (67 versus 74%).[173,174] The development of clarithromycin-resistant isolates was associated with microbiologic relapse. Intermittent treatment regimens also have been studied. Sixty-five percent of patients achieved treatment success with azithromycin-containing treatment regimens administered three times per week.[175] Clarithromycin-containing regimens administered three times weekly resulted in a 78% sputum conversion to acid fast bacilli culture negative.[176] Three times weekly clarithromycin therapy was less effective in patients with MAC infection and cavitary lung disease.[177] The current ATS/IDSA guidelines recommend a three times weekly regimen, including clarithromycin, 1000 mg, or azithromycin, 500 mg, with ethambutol and rifampin for patients with nodular/bronchiectatic MAC lung disease. For patients with fibrocavitary or severe nodular/bronchiectatic MAC lung disease, the recommended regimen is daily dosing of clarithromycin, 500 to 1000 mg, or azithromycin, 250 mg, with ethambutol and rifampin.[178]

CLINICAL USE: TIGECYCLINE

Tigecycline is FDA approved for the treatment of complicated skin and skin structure infections or complicated intra-abdominal infections. Two double-blind multicenter studies were conducted to evaluate the efficacy and safety of tigecycline monotherapy versus the combination of vancomycin and aztreonam for the treatment of hospitalized adults with complicated skin and skin structure infections.[179–181] Tigecycline monotherapy was demonstrated to be noninferior to the combination of vancomycin and aztreonam; test-of-cure rates in the clinical evaluable population were 86.5% and 88.6%, respectively. Outcomes were similar between the two groups regardless of the type of skin and soft tissue infection present or bacterial species isolated. In another trial that compared tigecycline to vancomycin for the treatment of complicated skin and skin structure infections caused by methicillin-resistant S aureus, the clinical cure rates in the microbiologically evaluable population were 86.4% and 86.9% for tigecycline and vancomycin, respectively.[182]

The efficacy of tigecycline was compared with imipenem/cilastatin in patients with complicated intra-abdominal infections in two double-blind randomized multicenter studies.[183-185] In the microbiologically evaluable population, clinical cure rates were similar between tigecycline and imipenem/cilastin (80.2% and 81.5%, respectively). Tigecycline cure rates were 80.6% versus 82.4% for imipenem/cilastatin, a statistically noninferior result. More than 80% of E coli and Klebsiella spp (the most frequently isolated gram-negative aerobes) were eradicated by tigecycline; 78% of Streptococcus spp and 70% of B fragilis were also eradicated.

Tigecycline has been evaluated against levofloxacin for the treatment of hospitalized patients with community-acquired pneumonia in two phase III, multicenter, double-blind studies. Pooled clinical cure rates were similar between the two treatment groups (89.7% and 86.3%). There were no significant differences in length of hospital stay, median duration of study antibiotic therapy, or hospital readmissions.[186,187] Tigecyline received FDA approval for the treatment of community-acquired pneumonia in March, 2009.

Several studies evaluated the efficacy of tigecycline for the treatment of infections caused by MDR gram-negative organisms. Twenty-three of 33 patients treated with tigecycline had resolution of their infection caused by either a carbapenem-resistant or extended-spectrum beta lactamase-producing or MDR Enterobacteriaceae.[188] An open-label, Phase 3, noncomparative, multicenter study assessed the efficacy in hospitalized patients with serious infections primarily caused by complicated intra-abdominal infections, complicated skin and skin structure infections, or hospital-acquired pneumonia caused by resistant gram-negative organisms. In the microbiologically evaluable population, the clinical cure rate was 72.2% and the microbiologic eradication rate was 66.7%. The most commonly isolated resistant gram-negative pathogens were A baumanii (47%), E coli (25%), K pneumoniae (16.7%) and Enterobacter spp (11%).[189] In a retrospective study of 29 patients who received tigecycline for the treatment of acinetobacter infections, only 8 (28%) demonstrated clinical improvement or cure. None of the isolates was fully susceptible to tigecycline (median MIC 4 mg/L).[190] In a small retrospective review of patients with serious infections caused by MDR gram-negative bacilli, pretherapy MIC values for tigecycline predicted clinical success.[191,192]

ADVERSE EFFECTS

Gastrointestinal intolerance is the primary adverse side effect of the newer macrolides and ketolides, but they occur at a significantly reduced rate when compared with erythromycin. The most common adverse effects reported with azithromycin were diarrhea (3.6%), nausea (2.6%), abdominal pain (2.5%), and headache or dizziness (1.3%). Laboratory abnormalities were infrequent and minor, including transient increases in transaminases in 1.5% of patients. Only 0.7% of patients discontinued azithromycin therapy compared with 2.6% of patients who receive comparative medications.[193] Gastrointestinal adverse effects (primarily diarrhea) occurred in 17% of patients treated with the 2-g extended-release microsphere formulation of azithromycin.[83,102] Adverse events related to the intravenous infusion of azithromycin were pain at the injection site (6.5%) and local inflammation (3.1%).[194] The most common adverse reactions reported with clarithromycin were similar (eg, nausea, 3.8%; diarrhea, 3.0%; abdominal pain, 1.9%; and headache, 1.7%).[195] There was no difference in the spectrum and frequency of adverse reactions between the extended-release or immediate-release formulations of clarithromycin.[20] Gastrointestinal adverse events with the extended-release formulation tended to be less severe and resulted in fewer discontinuations of the medication. Laboratory abnormalities were also rare and included abnormal liver function test results and decreased white blood cell counts. Overall, less than 3% of patients receiving clarithromycin withdrew from studies because of adverse effects. Clarithromycin has been associated with teratogenic effects in animal studies and should not be used in pregnant patients.

In phase 3 clinical trials with telithromycin, the most common adverse effects reported were diarrhea (10.8%), nausea (7.9%), headache (5.5%), dizziness (3.7%), and vomiting (2.9%). These adverse effects were generally mild to moderate in severity and the number of patients discontinuing telithromycin (4.4%) was similar to those receiving comparator agents (4.3%).[196] In a large study to assess clinical safety, more than 12,000 subjects with either community-acquired pneumonia or AECB received a course of telithromycin. Diarrhea occurred in 3.5% of study patients and gastrointestinal side effects occurred in 10.6%. Transient blurred vision occurred in 0.6% of telithromycin-treated patients.[10] Clinical trials have shown a small increase (1.5 ms) in the QTc interval with telithromycin. No significant clinical effect on the QT interval in healthy adults was observed.[197] Because of the potential risk of ventricular arrhythmias, however, telithromycin should be avoided in patients with congenital prolongation of the QT interval and patients with ongoing proarrhythmic conditions.[196]

During clinical trials for treatment of community-acquired pneumonia, patients receiving telithromycin had a greater incidence of transient rises in hepatic transaminases compared with patients receiving alternative antibiotics.[3] In the large clinical safety study mentioned previously, no clinically significant hepatic events were reported. An increase in alanine aminotransferase of more than 3 times upper limit of normal occurred in 1% of patients receiving telithromycin compared with 0.8% in patients receiving amoxicillin-clavulanic acid.[10] Site investigations identified serious irregularities in the conduct of the trial, however, which raised concerns about the integrity of the study results.[198]

Postmarketing surveillance reports described severe cases of hepatotoxicity in patients who received telithromycin. In a case series of 3 patients who developed acute hepatitis within days of receiving telithromycin therapy, one patient died and one required liver transplantation. Liver histology revealed inflammation consistent with a hypersensitivity reaction.[199] By the end of 2006, telithromycin was implicated in 53 cases of hepatotoxicity, which included some fatalities.[198] Telithromycin also was associated with myasthenia gravis exacerbations, including fatal and life-threatening acute respiratory failure.[191,200] On February 12, 2007, the FDA removed telithromycin's indication for the treatment of acute sinusitis and AECB and limited its approved indication to the treatment of community-acquired pneumonia alone. The FDA also issued a black box warning of the risk of respiratory failure in patients with myasthenia gravis and strengthened the warnings concerning the risk of acute hepatic failure and liver injury, which may be fatal.[201]

The most common side effects associated with tigecycline use in clinical trials were nausea and vomiting, both of which were mild to moderate in intensity and transient.[181,185] Overall, 29.5% of tigecycline recipients experienced nausea and 19.7% experienced vomiting. Diarrhea occurred in 13% of patients. Antimicrobial discontinuation as a result of an adverse event in these trials was similar between tigecycline recipients (5%) and the comparator antimicrobials (4.7%). There have been case reports of acute pancreatitis in patients treated with tigecycline.[202] Because tigecycline is structurally similar to tetracyclines, it may have the same safety concerns.[47] Tigecycline is labeled as a pregnancy category class D drug. Animal studies have shown that it crosses the placenta and is found in fetal tissues. Safety and efficacy of tigecycline in children younger than age 18 has not been established. As with tetracyclines, its use during tooth development may be associated with permanent tooth discoloration.

DRUG INTERACTIONS

Several reviews have discussed drug interactions between either clarithromycin or azithromycin and other agents.[42,203] Clarithromycin, like erythromycin, is oxidized by the cytochrome P450 system, primarily the CYP3A4 subclass of hepatic enzymes. This converts clarithromycin to a nitrosalkalane metabolite that forms an inactive metabolite/enzyme complex by binding to the iron of the CYP3A4 enzyme. This interaction inhibits the CYP3A4 enzymes and results in decreased clearance of other agents given concurrently that are metabolized by the same enzyme system. Clarithromycin is a less potent inhibitor of the CYP 3A4 enzymes than erythromycin and azithromycin interferes poorly with this system.[42]

Appropriate dose reductions and clinical and therapeutic drug level monitoring are necessary when drugs metabolized by the CYP3A enzymes are given concurrently with clarithromycin. The concurrent use of cisapride, pimozide, terfenadine, and aztemizole with clarithromycin is contraindicated because of the possible cardiotoxic effects of these agents and the occurrence of torsades de pointes. The concomitant administration of clarithromycin with ergotamine or dihydroergotamine is contraindicated because of the risk of acute ergot toxicity. Other medications such as benzodiazepines (eg, triazolam, midazolam, alprazolam), HMG-CoA reductase inhibitors (eg, lovastatin, simvastatin, atorvastatin), class 1A antiarrhythmic agents (eg, quinidine, disopyramide), theophylline, carbamazepine, warfarin, sildenafil, colchicine, and cyclosporine should be used cautiously when given with clarithromycin.[19] These drug-drug interactions are less likely to occur with azithromycin, because it is not a potent inhibitor of the CYP3A enzymes. There are case reports of toxicity related to coadministration of azithromycin and lovastatin, warfarin, cyclosporine, disopyramide and theophylline, however.[42,204] Clarithromycin and azithromycin have been associated with digoxin toxicity.[205]

The potential for telithromycin to inhibit the cytochrome P450 3A4 pathway is comparable to clarithromycin, although metabolism of telithromycin does not result in the formation of nitrosalkalene metabolite. Telithromycin also competitively inhibits the CYP2D6 system. The concomitant administration of telithromycin with cisapride or pimozide is contraindicated. The use of HMG-CoA reductase inhibitors (simvastatin, lovastatin, or atorvastatin), rifampin, or ergot alkaloid derivatives with telithromycin should be avoided. Caution should be used when administering telithromycin with digoxin, midazolam, metoprolol, oral anticoagulants, or other drugs metabolized by the CYP3A4 enzymes.[196]

Tigecycline does not interact with cytochrome P450 enzymes, making pharmacokinetic drug interactions uncommon. No significant drug interactions were noted during concomitant administration of tigecycline and digoxin or warfarin.[206,207]

SUMMARY

The advanced macrolides (azithromycin and clarithromycin) and ketolides (telithromycin) are structural analogs of erythromycin that have similar mechanisms of action. These antimicrobials have several distinct advantages over erythromycin, including improved oral bioavailability, longer half-life (allowing once- or twice-daily administration), higher tissue concentrations, enhanced antimicrobial activity, and reduced gastrointestinal adverse effects. Clarithromycin and azithromycin have been used extensively for the treatment of upper and lower respiratory tract infections. Despite the increasing prevalence of macrolide resistance among S pneumoniae, clinical failures have been reported infrequently. Treatment guidelines have solidified the roles of azithromycin in the treatment of certain sexually transmitted diseases and clarithromycin for the treatment of *H pylori*–associated peptic ulcer disease. Azithromycin and clarithromycin have been used successfully to prevent and treat MAC infections.

Telithromycin has been shown to be clinically effective in the treatment of outpatient respiratory diseases. Because of safety concerns, however, especially the possibility of hepatotoxicity, the approved indication for telithromycin is limited to the treatment of community-acquired pneumonia. Tigecycline, a derivative of minocycline, has a broad spectrum of antimicrobial activity, including activity against many MDR pathogens. Tigecycline, available only as an intravenous preparation, is indicated for the treatment of complicated skin and skin structure and intra-abdominal infections. It is also approved for the treatment of community-acquired pneumonia. The role for tigecycline in the treatment of other types of infections with MDR organisms needs to be determined.

REFERENCES

1. Omura S, Tsuzuki K, Sunazuka T, et al. Macrolides with gastrointestinal motor stimulating activity. J Med Chem 1987;30(11):1941–3.
2. Piscitelli SC, Danziger LH, Rodvold KA. Clarithromycin and azithromycin: new macrolide antibiotics. Clin Pharm 1992;11(2):137–52.
3. Shain CS, Amsden GW. Telithromycin: the first of the ketolides. Ann Pharmacother 2002;36(3):452–64.
4. Douthwaite S, Champney WS. Structures of ketolides and macrolides determine their mode of interaction with the ribosomal target site. J Antimicrob Chemother 2001;48(Suppl T1):1–8.
5. Champney WS, Tober CL. Superiority of 11,12 carbonate macrolide antibiotics as inhibitors of translation and 50S ribosomal subunit formation in *Staphylococcus aureus* cells. Curr Microbiol 1999;38(6):342–8.
6. Frampton JE, Curran MP. Tigecycline. Drugs 2005;65(18):2623–35.
7. Sturgill MG, Rapp RP. Clarithromycin: review of a new macrolide antibiotic with improved microbiologic spectrum and favorable pharmacokinetic and adverse effect profiles. Ann Pharmacother 1992;26(9):1099–108.
8. Hansen LH, Mauvais P, Douthwaite S. The macrolide-ketolide antibiotic binding site is formed by structures in domains II and V of 23S ribosomal RNA. Mol Microbiol 1999;31(2):623–31.
9. Tait-Kamradt A, Clancy J, Cronan M, et al. mefE is necessary for the erythromycin-resistant M phenotype in *Streptococcus pneumoniae*. Antimicrob Agents Chemother 1997;41(10):2251–5.
10. Ketek (telithromycin): briefing document for the FDA Anti-Infective Drug Products Advisory Committee Meeting, January 8, 2003. Gaithersburg, MD.
11. Bonnefoy A, Girard AM, Agouridas C, et al. Ketolides lack inducibility properties of MLS(B) resistance phenotype. J Antimicrob Chemother 1997;40(1):85–90.
12. Malhotra-Kumar S, Lammens C, Chapelle S, et al. Macrolide- and telithromycin-resistant *Streptococcus pyogenes*, Belgium, 1999–2003. Emerg Infect Dis 2005; 11(6):939–42.
13. Al-Lahham A, Appelbaum PC, van der Linden M, et al. Telithromycin-nonsusceptible clinical isolates of *Streptococcus pneumoniae* from Europe. Antimicrob Agents Chemother 2006;50(11):3897–900.
14. Wolter N, Smith AM, Farrell DJ, et al. Telithromycin resistance in *Streptococcus pneumoniae* is conferred by a deletion in the leader sequence of erm(B) that increases rRNA methylation. Antimicrob Agents Chemother 2008;52(2):435–40.

15. Bergeron J, Ammirati M, Danley D, et al. Glycylcyclines bind to the high-affinity tetracycline ribosomal binding site and evade Tet(M)- and Tet(O)-mediated ribosomal protection. Antimicrob Agents Chemother 1996;40(9):2226–8.

16. Hirata T, Saito A, Nishino K, et al. Effects of efflux transporter genes on susceptibility of *Escherichia coli* to tigecycline (GAR-936). Antimicrob Agents Chemother 2004;48(6):2179–84.

17. Dean CR, Visalli MA, Projan SJ, et al. Efflux-mediated resistance to tigecycline (GAR-936) in *Pseudomonas aeruginosa* PAO1. Antimicrob Agents Chemother 2003;47(3):972–8.

18. Peleg AY, Adams J, Paterson DL. Tigecycline efflux as a mechanism for nonsusceptibility in *Acinetobacter baumannii*. Antimicrob Agents Chemother 2007; 51(6):2065–9.

19. Abbott Laboratories. Biaxin (Clarithromycin): prescribing information. 2008;2008 (12/23).

20. Guay DR, Gustavson LE, Devcich KJ, et al. Pharmacokinetics and tolerability of extended-release clarithromycin. Clin Ther 2001;23(4):566–77.

21. Foulds G, Luke DR, Teng R, et al. The absence of an effect of food on the bioavailability of azithromycin administered as tablets, sachet or suspension. J Antimicrob Chemother 1996;37(Suppl C):37–44.

22. Chandra R, Liu P, Breen JD, et al. Clinical pharmacokinetics and gastrointestinal tolerability of a novel extended-release microsphere formulation of azithromycin. Clin Pharmacokinet 2007;46(3):247–59.

23. Perret C, Lenfant B, Weinling E, et al. Pharmacokinetics and absolute oral bioavailability of an 800-mg oral dose of telithromycin in healthy young and elderly volunteers. Chemotherapy 2002;48(5):217–23.

24. Bhargava V, Lenfant B, Perret C, et al. Lack of effect of food on the bioavailability of a new ketolide antibacterial, telithromycin. Scand J Infect Dis 2002;34(11): 823–6.

25. Ferrero JL, Bopp BA, Marsh KC, et al. Metabolism and disposition of clarithromycin in man. Drug Metab Dispos 1990;18(4):441–6.

26. Liu P, Allaudeen H, Chandra R, et al. Comparative pharmacokinetics of azithromycin in serum and white blood cells of healthy subjects receiving a single-dose extended-release regimen versus a 3-day immediate-release regimen. Antimicrob Agents Chemother 2007;51(1):103–9.

27. Namour F, Wessels DH, Pascual MH, et al. Pharmacokinetics of the new ketolide telithromycin (HMR 3647) administered in ascending single and multiple doses. Antimicrob Agents Chemother 2001;45(1):170–5.

28. Muralidharan G, Fruncillo RJ, Micalizzi M, et al. Effects of age and sex on single-dose pharmacokinetics of tigecycline in healthy subjects. Antimicrob Agents Chemother 2005;49(4):1656–9.

29. Muralidharan G, Micalizzi M, Speth J, et al. Pharmacokinetics of tigecycline after single and multiple doses in healthy subjects. Antimicrob Agents Chemother 2005;49(1):220–9.

30. Meagher AK, Ambrose PG, Grasela TH, et al. The pharmacokinetic and pharmacodynamic profile of tigecycline. Clin Infect Dis 2005;41(Suppl 5):S333–40.

31. Foulds G, Shepard RM, Johnson RB. The pharmacokinetics of azithromycin in human serum and tissues. J Antimicrob Chemother 1990;25(Suppl A): 73–82.

32. Fraschini F, Scaglione F, Pintucci G, et al. The diffusion of clarithromycin and roxithromycin into nasal mucosa, tonsil and lung in humans. J Antimicrob Chemother 1991;27(Suppl A):61–5.

33. Rodvold KA, Gotfried MH, Danziger LH, et al. Intrapulmonary steady-state concentrations of clarithromycin and azithromycin in healthy adult volunteers. Antimicrob Agents Chemother 1997;41(6):1399–402.
34. Muller-Serieys C, Soler P, Cantalloube C, et al. Bronchopulmonary disposition of the ketolide telithromycin (HMR 3647). Antimicrob Agents Chemother 2001; 45(11):3104–8.
35. Khair OA, Andrews JM, Honeybourne D, et al. Lung concentrations of telithromycin after oral dosing. J Antimicrob Chemother 2001;47(6):837–40.
36. Conte JE Jr, Golden JA, Kelly MG, et al. Steady-state serum and intrapulmonary pharmacokinetics and pharmacodynamics of tigecycline. Int J Antimicrob Agents 2005;25(6):523–9.
37. Rodvold KA, Gotfried MH, Cwik M, et al. Serum, tissue and body fluid concentrations of tigecycline after a single 100 mg dose. J Antimicrob Chemother 2006; 58(6):1221–9.
38. Sun HK, Ong CT, Umer A, et al. Pharmacokinetic profile of tigecycline in serum and skin blister fluid of healthy subjects after multiple intravenous administrations. Antimicrob Agents Chemother 2005;49(4):1629–32.
39. Hardy DJ, Guay DR, Jones RN. Clarithromycin, a unique macrolide: a pharmacokinetic, microbiological, and clinical overview. Diagn Microbiol Infect Dis 1992; 15(1):39–53.
40. Chu SY, Granneman GR, Pichotta PJ, et al. Effect of moderate or severe hepatic impairment on clarithromycin pharmacokinetics. J Clin Pharmacol 1993;33(5): 480–5.
41. Ballow CH, Amsden GW. Azithromycin: the first azalide antibiotic. Ann Pharmacother 1992;26(10):1253–61.
42. Westphal JF. Macrolide -induced clinically relevant drug interactions with cytochrome P-450A (CYP) 3A4: an update focused on clarithromycin, azithromycin and dirithromycin. Br J Clin Pharmacol 2000;50(4):285–95.
43. Mazzei T, Surrenti C, Novelli A, et al. Pharmacokinetics of azithromycin in patients with impaired hepatic function. J Antimicrob Chemother 1993;31(Suppl E): 57–63.
44. Zhanel GG, Dueck M, Hoban DJ, et al. Review of macrolides and ketolides: focus on respiratory tract infections. Drugs 2001;61(4):443–98.
45. Cantalloube C, Bhargava V, Sultan E, et al. Pharmacokinetics of the ketolide telithromycin after single and repeated doses in patients with hepatic impairment. Int J Antimicrob Agents 2003;22(2):112–21.
46. Hoffmann M, DeMaio W, Jordan RA, et al. Metabolism, excretion, and pharmacokinetics of [14C]tigecycline, a first-in-class glycylcycline antibiotic, after intravenous infusion to healthy male subjects. Drug Metab Dispos 2007;35(9): 1543–53.
47. Tygacil (tigecycline) prescribing information. 2008;2008(11/28).
48. Clinical and Laboratory Standards Institute. Performance standards for antimicrobial susceptibility testing. Eighteenth Informational Supplement. Clinical and Laboratory Standards Institute; Wayne, PA 2008.
49. Whitman MS, Tunkel AR. Azithromycin and clarithromycin: overview and comparison with erythromycin. Infect Control Hosp Epidemiol 1992;13(6): 357–68.
50. Goldstein EJ, Citron DM, Merriam CV, et al. In vitro activities of telithromycin and 10 oral agents against aerobic and anaerobic pathogens isolated from antral puncture specimens from patients with sinusitis. Antimicrob Agents Chemother 2003;47(6):1963–7.

51. Nagai K, Davies TA, Ednie LM, et al. Activities of a new fluoroketolide, HMR 3787, and its (des)-fluor derivative RU 64399 compared to those of telithromycin, erythromycin A, azithromycin, clarithromycin, and clindamycin against macrolide-susceptible or -resistant *Streptococcus pneumoniae* and *S. pyogenes*. Antimicrob Agents Chemother 2001;45(11):3242–5.

52. Shortridge VD, Zhong P, Cao Z, et al. Comparison of in vitro activities of ABT-773 and telithromycin against macrolide-susceptible and -resistant streptococci and staphylococci. Antimicrob Agents Chemother 2002;46(3):783–6.

53. Retsema J, Girard A, Schelkly W, et al. Spectrum and mode of action of azithromycin (CP-62,993), a new 15-membered-ring macrolide with improved potency against gram-negative organisms. Antimicrob Agents Chemother 1987;31(12): 1939–47.

54. Barry AL, Fuchs PC, Brown SD. Antipneumococcal activities of a ketolide (HMR 3647), a streptogramin (quinupristin-dalfopristin), a macrolide (erythromycin), and a lincosamide (clindamycin). Antimicrob Agents Chemother 1998;42(4):945–6.

55. Ubukata K, Iwata S, Sunakawa K. In vitro activities of new ketolide, telithromycin, and eight other macrolide antibiotics against *Streptococcus pneumoniae* having mefA and ermB genes that mediate macrolide resistance. J Infect Chemother 2003;9(3):221–6.

56. Doern GV, Heilmann KP, Huynh HK, et al. Antimicrobial resistance among clinical isolates of *Streptococcus pneumoniae* in the United States during 1999–2000, including a comparison of resistance rates since 1994–1995. Antimicrob Agents Chemother 2001;45(6):1721–9.

57. Clark JP, Langston E. Ketolides: a new class of antibacterial agents for treatment of community-acquired respiratory tract infections in a primary care setting. Mayo Clin Proc 2003;78(9):1113–24.

58. Hardy DJ, Swanson RN, Rode RA, et al. Enhancement of the in vitro and in vivo activities of clarithromycin against *Haemophilus influenzae* by 14-hydroxy-clarithromycin, its major metabolite in humans. Antimicrob Agents Chemother 1990; 34(7):1407–13.

59. Barry AL, Fuchs PC, Brown SD. In vitro activities of the ketolide HMR 3647 against recent gram-positive clinical isolates and *Haemophilus influenzae*. Antimicrob Agents Chemother 1998;42(8):2138–40.

60. Fernandes PB, Bailer R, Swanson R, et al. In vitro and in vivo evaluation of A-56268 (TE-031), a new macrolide. Antimicrob Agents Chemother 1986; 30(6):865–73.

61. Peters DH, Clissold SP. Clarithromycin: a review of its antimicrobial activity, pharmacokinetic properties and therapeutic potential. Drugs 1992;44(1):117–64.

62. Peters DH, Friedel HA, McTavish D. Azithromycin: a review of its antimicrobial activity, pharmacokinetic properties and clinical efficacy. Drugs 1992;44(5): 750–99.

63. Slover CM, Rodvold KA, Danziger LH. Tigecycline: a novel broad-spectrum antimicrobial. Ann Pharmacother 2007;41(6):965–72.

64. Hoban DJ, Bouchillon SK, Johnson BM, et al. In vitro activity of tigecycline against 6792 Gram-negative and Gram-positive clinical isolates from the global Tigecycline Evaluation and Surveillance Trial (TEST Program, 2004). Diagn Microbiol Infect Dis 2005;52(3):215–27.

65. Bouchillon SK, Hoban DJ, Johnson BM, et al. In vitro activity of tigecycline against 3989 Gram-negative and Gram-positive clinical isolates from the United States Tigecycline Evaluation and Surveillance Trial (TEST Program; 2004). Diagn Microbiol Infect Dis 2005;52(3):173–9.

66. Castanheira M, Sader HS, Deshpande LM, et al. Antimicrobial activities of tige-cycline and other broad-spectrum antimicrobials tested against serine carbape-nemase- and metallo-beta-lactamase-producing Enterobacteriaceae: report from the SENTRY Antimicrobial Surveillance Program. Antimicrob Agents Chemother 2008;52(2):570–3.

67. Hoban DJ, Bouchillon SK, Dowzicky MJ. Antimicrobial susceptibility of extended-spectrum beta-lactamase producers and multidrug-resistant *Acinetobacter baumannii* throughout the United States and comparative in vitro activity of tigecycline, a new glycylcycline antimicrobial. Diagn Microbiol Infect Dis 2007;57(4):423–8.

68. Zhanel GG, DeCorby M, Nichol KA, et al. Antimicrobial susceptibility of 3931 organisms isolated from intensive care units in Canada: Canadian National Intensive Care Unit Study, 2005/2006. Diagn Microbiol Infect Dis 2008;62(1):67–80.

69. Gales AC, Sader HS, Fritsche TR. Tigecycline activity tested against 11808 bacterial pathogens recently collected from US medical centers. Diagn Microbiol Infect Dis 2008;60(4):421–7.

70. Fritsche TR, Sader HS, Stilwell MG, et al. Antimicrobial activity of tigecycline tested against organisms causing community-acquired respiratory tract infection and nosocomial pneumonia. Diagn Microbiol Infect Dis 2005;52(3):187–93.

71. Portier H, Filipecki J, Weber P, et al. Five day clarithromycin modified release versus 10 day penicillin V for group A streptococcal pharyngitis: a multi-centre, open-label, randomized study. J Antimicrob Chemother 2002;49(2):337–44.

72. Norrby SR, Quinn J, Rangaraju M, et al. Evaluation of 5-day therapy with telithromycin, a novel ketolide antibacterial, for the treatment of tonsillopharyngitis. Clin Microbiol Infect 2004;10(7):615–23.

73. Quinn J, Ruoff GE, Ziter PS. Efficacy and tolerability of 5-day, once-daily telithromycin compared with 10-day, twice-daily clarithromycin for the treatment of group A beta-hemolytic streptococcal tonsillitis/pharyngitis: a multicenter, randomized, double-blind, parallel-group study. Clin Ther 2003;25(2):422–43.

74. McCarty JM, Phillips A, Wiisanen R. Comparative safety and efficacy of clarithromycin and amoxicillin/clavulanate in the treatment of acute otitis media in children. Pediatr Infect Dis J 1993;12(12):S122–7.

75. Block SL, Cifaldi M, Gu Y, et al. A comparison of 5 days of therapy with cefdinir or azithromycin in children with acute otitis media: a multicenter, prospective, single-blind study. Clin Ther 2005;27(6):786–94.

76. Ioannidis JP, Contopoulos-Ioannidis DG, Chew P, et al. Meta-analysis of randomized controlled trials on the comparative efficacy and safety of azithromycin against other antibiotics for upper respiratory tract infections. J Antimicrob Chemother 2001;48(5):677–89.

77. Hoberman A, Dagan R, Leibovitz E, et al. Large dosage amoxicillin/clavulanate, compared with azithromycin, for the treatment of bacterial acute otitis media in children. Pediatr Infect Dis J 2005;24(6):525–32.

78. Arguedas A, Emparanza P, Schwartz RH, et al. A randomized, multicenter, double blind, double dummy trial of single dose azithromycin versus high dose amoxicillin for treatment of uncomplicated acute otitis media. Pediatr Infect Dis J 2005;24(2):153–61.

79. Adelglass J, Jones TM, Ruoff G, et al. A multicenter, investigator-blinded, randomized comparison of oral levofloxacin and oral clarithromycin in the treatment of acute bacterial sinusitis. Pharmacotherapy 1998;18(6):1255–63.

80. Clifford K, Huck W, Shan M, et al. Double-blind comparative trial of ciprofloxacin versus clarithromycin in the treatment of acute bacterial sinusitis: Sinusitis Infection Study Group. Ann Otol Rhinol Laryngol 1999;108(4):360–7.

81. Stefansson P, Jacovides A, Jablonicky P, et al. Cefuroxime axetil versus clarithromycin in the treatment of acute maxillary sinusitis. Rhinology 1998;36(4):173–8.

82. Riffer E, Spiller J, Palmer R, et al. Once daily clarithromycin extended-release vs twice-daily amoxicillin/clavulanate in patients with acute bacterial sinusitis: a randomized, investigator-blinded study. Curr Med Res Opin 2005;21(1):61–70.

83. Murray JJ, Emparanza P, Lesinskas E, et al. Efficacy and safety of a novel, single-dose azithromycin microsphere formulation versus 10 days of levofloxacin for the treatment of acute bacterial sinusitis in adults. Otolaryngol Head Neck Surg 2005;133(2):194–200.

84. Henry DC, Riffer E, Sokol WN, et al. Randomized double-blind study comparing 3- and 6-day regimens of azithromycin with a 10-day amoxicillin-clavulanate regimen for treatment of acute bacterial sinusitis. Antimicrob Agents Chemother 2003;47(9):2770–4.

85. Desrosiers M, Ferguson B, Klossek JM, et al. Clinical efficacy and time to symptom resolution of 5-day telithromycin versus 10-day amoxicillin-clavulanate in the treatment of acute bacterial sinusitis. Curr Med Res Opin 2008;24(6):1691–702.

86. Roos K, Tellier G, Baz M, et al. Clinical and bacteriological efficacy of 5-day telithromycin in acute maxillary sinusitis: a pooled analysis. J Infect 2005;50(3):210–20.

87. Ferguson BJ, Guzzetta RV, Spector SL, et al. Efficacy and safety of oral telithromycin once daily for 5 days versus moxifloxacin once daily for 10 days in the treatment of acute bacterial rhinosinusitis. Otolaryngol Head Neck Surg 2004;131(3):207–14.

88. Langtry HD, Brogden RN. Clarithromycin. A review of its efficacy in the treatment of respiratory tract infections in immunocompetent patients. Drugs 1997;53(6):973–1004.

89. Weiss K, Vanjaka A. An open-label, randomized, multicenter, comparative study of the efficacy and safety of 7 days of treatment with clarithromycin extended-release tablets versus clarithromycin immediate-release tablets for the treatment of patients with acute bacterial exacerbation of chronic bronchitis. Clin Ther 2002;24(12):2105–22.

90. Adler JL, Jannetti W, Schneider D, et al. Phase III, randomized, double-blind study of clarithromycin extended-release and immediate-release formulations in the treatment of patients with acute exacerbation of chronic bronchitis. Clin Ther 2000;22(12):1410–20.

91. Martinot JB, Carr WD, Cullen S, et al. A comparative study of clarithromycin modified release and amoxicillin/clavulanic acid in the treatment of acute exacerbation of chronic bronchitis. Adv Ther 2001;18(1):1–11.

92. Anzueto A, Fisher CL Jr, Busman T, et al. Comparison of the efficacy of extended-release clarithromycin tablets and amoxicillin/clavulanate tablets in the treatment of acute exacerbation of chronic bronchitis. Clin Ther 2001;23(1):72–86.

93. Gotfried M, Busman TA, Norris S, et al. Role for 5-day, once-daily extended-release clarithromycin in acute bacterial exacerbation of chronic bronchitis. Curr Med Res Opin 2007;23(2):459–66.

94. Weiss LR. Open-label, randomized comparison of the efficacy and tolerability of clarithromycin, levofloxacin, and cefuroxime axetil in the treatment of adults with acute bacterial exacerbations of chronic bronchitis. Clin Ther 2002;24(9):1414–25.

95. Wilson R, Schentag JJ, Ball P, et al. A comparison of gemifloxacin and clarithromycin in acute exacerbations of chronic bronchitis and long-term clinical outcomes. Clin Ther 2002;24(4):639–52.

96. Hoeffken G, Meyer HP, Winter J, et al. The efficacy and safety of two oral moxifloxacin regimens compared to oral clarithromycin in the treatment of community-acquired pneumonia. Respir Med 2001;95(7):553–64.

97. Gotfried MH, Dattani D, Riffer E, et al. A controlled, double-blind, multicenter study comparing clarithromycin extended-release tablets and levofloxacin tablets in the treatment of community-acquired pneumonia. Clin Ther 2002; 24(5):736–51.

98. Sokol WN Jr, Sullivan JG, Acampora MD, et al. A prospective, double-blind, multicenter study comparing clarithromycin extended-release with trovafloxacin in patients with community-acquired pneumonia. Clin Ther 2002;24(4):605–15.

99. Lode H, Aronkyto T, Chuchalin AG, et al. A randomised, double-blind, double-dummy comparative study of gatifloxacin with clarithromycin in the treatment of community-acquired pneumonia. Clin Microbiol Infect 2004;10(5):403–8.

100. Kinasewitz G, Wood RG. Azithromycin versus cefaclor in the treatment of acute bacterial pneumonia. Eur J Clin Microbiol Infect Dis 1991;10(10):872–7.

101. Paris R, Confalonieri M, Dal Negro R, et al. Efficacy and safety of azithromycin 1 g once daily for 3 days in the treatment of community-acquired pneumonia: an open-label randomised comparison with amoxicillin-clavulanate 875/125 mg twice daily for 7 days. J Chemother 2008;20(1):77–86.

102. Drehobl MA, De Salvo MC, Lewis DE, et al. Single-dose azithromycin microspheres vs clarithromycin extended release for the treatment of mild-to-moderate community-acquired pneumonia in adults. Chest 2005;128(4):2230–7.

103. D'Ignazio J, Camere MA, Lewis DE, et al. Novel, single-dose microsphere formulation of azithromycin versus 7-day levofloxacin therapy for treatment of mild to moderate community-acquired pneumonia in adults. Antimicrob Agents Chemother 2005;49(10):4035–41.

104. Contopoulos-Ioannidis DG, Ioannidis JP, Chew P, et al. Meta-analysis of randomized controlled trials on the comparative efficacy and safety of azithromycin against other antibiotics for lower respiratory tract infections. J Antimicrob Chemother 2001;48(5):691–703.

105. Panpanich R, Lerttrakarnnon P, Laopaiboon M. Azithromycin for acute lower respiratory tract infections. Cochrane Database Syst Rev 2008;(1):CD001954.

106. Swanson RN, Lainez-Ventosilla A, De Salvo MC, et al. Once-daily azithromycin for 3 days compared with clarithromycin for 10 days for acute exacerbation of chronic bronchitis: a multicenter, double-blind, randomized study. Treat Respir Med 2005;4(1):31–9.

107. Amsden GW, Baird IM, Simon S, et al. Efficacy and safety of azithromycin vs levofloxacin in the outpatient treatment of acute bacterial exacerbations of chronic bronchitis. Chest 2003;123(3):772–7.

108. Zervos M, Martinez FJ, Amsden GW, et al. Efficacy and safety of 3-day azithromycin versus 5-day moxifloxacin for the treatment of acute bacterial exacerbations of chronic bronchitis. Int J Antimicrob Agents 2007;29(1):56–61.

109. Hagberg L, Carbon C, van Rensburg DJ, et al. Telithromycin in the treatment of community-acquired pneumonia: a pooled analysis. Respir Med 2003;97(6): 625–33.

110. Pullman J, Champlin J, Vrooman PS Jr. Efficacy and tolerability of once-daily oral therapy with telithromycin compared with trovafloxacin for the treatment of community-acquired pneumonia in adults. Int J Clin Pract 2003;57(5):377–84.

111. Mathers Dunbar L, Hassman J, Tellier G. Efficacy and tolerability of once-daily oral telithromycin compared with clarithromycin for the treatment of community-acquired pneumonia in adults. Clin Ther 2004;26(1):48–62.

112. Tellier G, Niederman MS, Nusrat R, et al. Clinical and bacteriological efficacy and safety of 5 and 7 day regimens of telithromycin once daily compared with a 10 day regimen of clarithromycin twice daily in patients with mild to moderate community-acquired pneumonia. J Antimicrob Chemother 2004;54(2):515–23.

113. van Rensburg DJ, Fogarty C, Kohno S, et al. Efficacy of telithromycin in community-acquired pneumonia caused by pneumococci with reduced susceptibility to penicillin and/or erythromycin. Chemotherapy 2005;51(4):186–92.

114. Carbon C, van Rensburg D, Hagberg L, et al. Clinical and bacteriologic efficacy of telithromycin in patients with bacteremic community-acquired pneumonia. Respir Med 2006;100(4):577–85.

115. Fogarty C, de Wet R, Mandell L, et al. Five-day telithromycin once daily is as effective as 10-day clarithromycin twice daily for the treatment of acute exacerbations of chronic bronchitis and is associated with reduced health-care resource utilization. Chest 2005;128(4):1980–8.

116. Aubier M, Aldons PM, Leak A, et al. Telithromycin is as effective as amoxicillin/clavulanate in acute exacerbations of chronic bronchitis. Respir Med 2002; 96(11):862–71.

117. Carbon C. A pooled analysis of telithromycin in the treatment of community-acquired respiratory tract infections in adults. Infection 2003;31(5):308–17.

118. Vergis EN, Indorf A, File TM Jr, et al. Azithromycin vs cefuroxime plus erythromycin for empirical treatment of community-acquired pneumonia in hospitalized patients: a prospective, randomized, multicenter trial. Arch Intern Med 2000; 160(9):1294–300.

119. Plouffe J, Schwartz DB, Kolokathis A, et al. Clinical efficacy of intravenous followed by oral azithromycin monotherapy in hospitalized patients with community-acquired pneumonia: the Azithromycin Intravenous Clinical Trials Group. Antimicrob Agents Chemother 2000;44(7):1796–802.

120. Feldman RB, Rhew DC, Wong JY, et al. Azithromycin monotherapy for patients hospitalized with community-acquired pneumonia: a 31/2-year experience from a veterans affairs hospital. Arch Intern Med 2003;163(14):1718–26.

121. Zervos M, Mandell LA, Vrooman PS, et al. Comparative efficacies and tolerabilities of intravenous azithromycin plus ceftriaxone and intravenous levofloxacin with step-down oral therapy for hospitalized patients with moderate to severe community-acquired pneumonia. Treat Respir Med 2004;3(5):329–36.

122. Frank E, Liu J, Kinasewitz G, et al. A multicenter, open-label, randomized comparison of levofloxacin and azithromycin plus ceftriaxone in hospitalized adults with moderate to severe community-acquired pneumonia. Clin Ther 2002;24(8):1292–308.

123. Correa JC, Badaro R, Bumroongkit C, et al. Randomized, open-label, parallel-group, multicenter study of the efficacy and tolerability of IV gatifloxacin with the option for oral stepdown gatifloxacin versus IV ceftriaxone (with or without erythromycin or clarithromycin) with the option for oral stepdown clarithromycin for treatment of patients with mild to moderate community-acquired pneumonia requiring hospitalization. Clin Ther 2003;25(5):1453–68.

124. Weiss K, Low DE, Cortes L, et al. Clinical characteristics at initial presentation and impact of dual therapy on the outcome of bacteremic *Streptococcus pneumoniae* pneumonia in adults. Can Respir J 2004;11(8):589–93.

125. Garcia Vazquez E, Mensa J, Martinez JA, et al. Lower mortality among patients with community-acquired pneumonia treated with a macrolide plus a beta-lactam agent versus a beta-lactam agent alone. Eur J Clin Microbiol Infect Dis 2005;24(3):190–5.

126. Martinez JA, Horcajada JP, Almela M, et al. Addition of a macrolide to a beta-lactam-based empirical antibiotic regimen is associated with lower in-hospital mortality for patients with bacteremic pneumococcal pneumonia. Clin Infect Dis 2003;36(4):389–95.

127. Plouffe JF, Breiman RF, Fields BS, et al. Azithromycin in the treatment of *Legionella pneumonia* requiring hospitalization. Clin Infect Dis 2003;37(11):1475–80.

128. Sahm DF, Brown NP, Draghi DC, et al. Tracking resistance among bacterial respiratory tract pathogens: summary of findings of the TRUST Surveillance Initiative, 2001–2005. Postgrad Med 2008;120(3 Suppl 1):8–15.

129. Jenkins SG, Brown SD, Farrell DJ. Trends in antibacterial resistance among *Streptococcus pneumoniae* isolated in the USA: update from PROTEKT US Years 1–4. Ann Clin Microbiol Antimicrob 2008;7:1.

130. Critchley IA, Brown SD, Traczewski MM, et al. National and regional assessment of antimicrobial resistance among community-acquired respiratory tract pathogens identified in a 2005–2006 U.S. Faropenem surveillance study. Antimicrob Agents Chemother 2007;51(12):4382–9.

131. Farrell DJ, File TM, Jenkins SG. Prevalence and antibacterial susceptibility of mef(A)-positive macrolide-resistant *Streptococcus pneumoniae* over 4 years (2000 to 2004) of the PROTEKT US Study. J Clin Microbiol 2007;45(2):290–3.

132. Sahm DF, Brown NP, Thornsberry C, et al. Antimicrobial susceptibility profiles among common respiratory tract pathogens: a GLOBAL perspective. Postgrad Med 2008;120(3 Suppl 1):16–24.

133. Rantala M, Haanpera-Heikkinen M, Lindgren M, et al. *Streptococcus pneumoniae* isolates resistant to telithromycin. Antimicrob Agents Chemother 2006; 50(5):1855–8.

134. Lau YJ, Hsueh PR, Liu YC, et al. Comparison of in vitro activities of tigecycline with other antimicrobial agents against *Streptococcus pneumoniae, Haemophilus influenzae*, and *Moraxella catarrhalis* in Taiwan. Microb Drug Resist 2006; 12(2):130–5.

135. Rowe BH, Campbell SG, Boudreaux ED, et al. Community-acquired pneumonia in North American emergency departments: drug resistance and treatment success with clarithromycin. Acad Emerg Med 2007;14(7):607–15.

136. Lonks JR, Garau J, Gomez L, et al. Failure of macrolide antibiotic treatment in patients with bacteremia due to erythromycin-resistant *Streptococcus pneumoniae*. Clin Infect Dis 2002;35(5):556–64.

137. Mandell LA, Wunderink RG, Anzueto A, et al. Infectious Diseases Society of America/American Thoracic Society consensus guidelines on the management of community-acquired pneumonia in adults. Clin Infect Dis 2007;44(Suppl 2):S27–72.

138. Lau CY, Qureshi AK. Azithromycin versus doxycycline for genital chlamydial infections: a meta-analysis of randomized clinical trials. Sex Transm Dis 2002; 29(9):497–502.

139. Pitsouni E, Iavazzo C, Athanasiou S, et al. Single-dose azithromycin versus erythromycin or amoxicillin for *Chlamydia trachomatis* infection during pregnancy: a meta-analysis of randomised controlled trials. Int J Antimicrob Agents 2007;30(3):213–21.

140. Workowski KA, Berman SM. Centers for Disease Control and Prevention. Sexually transmitted diseases treatment guidelines, 2006. MMWR Recomm Rep 2006;55(RR-11):1–94.

141. Skerk V, Schonwald S, Krhen I, et al. Comparative analysis of azithromycin and ciprofloxacin in the treatment of chronic prostatitis caused by *Chlamydia trachomatis*. Int J Antimicrob Agents 2003;21(5):457–62.

142. Skerk V, Krhen I, Lisic M, et al. Comparative randomized pilot study of azithromycin and doxycycline efficacy in the treatment of prostate infection caused by *Chlamydia trachomatis*. Int J Antimicrob Agents 2004;24(2):188–91.

143. Handsfield HH, Dalu ZA, Martin DH, et al. Multicenter trial of single-dose azithromycin vs. ceftriaxone in the treatment of uncomplicated gonorrhea: Azithromycin Gonorrhea Study Group. Sex Transm Dis 1994;21(2):107–11.

144. Bevan CD, Ridgway GL, Rothermel CD. Efficacy and safety of azithromycin as monotherapy or combined with metronidazole compared with two standard multidrug regimens for the treatment of acute pelvic inflammatory disease. J Int Med Res 2003;31(1):45–54.

145. Palmer HM, Young H, Winter A, et al. Emergence and spread of azithromycin-resistant *Neisseria gonorrhoeae* in Scotland. J Antimicrob Chemother 2008;62(3):490–4.

146. Wang SA, Harvey AB, Conner SM, et al. Antimicrobial resistance for *Neisseria gonorrhoeae* in the United States, 1988 to 2003: the spread of fluoroquinolone resistance. Ann Intern Med 2007;147(2):81–8.

147. Bai ZG, Yang KH, Liu YL, et al. Azithromycin vs. benzathine penicillin G for early syphilis: a meta-analysis of randomized clinical trials. Int J STD AIDS 2008; 19(4):217–21.

148. Riedner G, Rusizoka M, Todd J, et al. Single-dose azithromycin versus penicillin G benzathine for the treatment of early syphilis. N Engl J Med 2005;353(12):1236–44.

149. Chey WD, Wong BC, Practice Parameters Committee of the American College of Gastroenterology. American College of Gastroenterology guideline on the management of *Helicobacter pylori* infection. Am J Gastroenterol 2007;102(8):1808–25.

150. Suerbaum S, Michetti P. *Helicobacter pylori* infection. N Engl J Med 2002; 347(15):1175–86.

151. Vergara M, Vallve M, Gisbert JP, et al. Meta-analysis: comparative efficacy of different proton-pump inhibitors in triple therapy for *Helicobacter pylori* eradication. Aliment Pharmacol Ther 2003;18(6):647–54.

152. Gene E, Calvet X, Azagra R, et al. Triple vs. quadruple therapy for treating *Helicobacter pylori* infection: a meta-analysis. Aliment Pharmacol Ther 2003;17(9): 1137–43.

153. Laheij RJ, Rossum LG, Jansen JB, et al. Evaluation of treatment regimens to cure *Helicobacter pylori* infection: a meta-analysis. Aliment Pharmacol Ther 1999;13(7):857–64.

154. Calvet X, Garcia N, Lopez T, et al. A meta-analysis of short versus long therapy with a proton pump inhibitor, clarithromycin and either metronidazole or amoxycillin for treating *Helicobacter pylori* infection. Aliment Pharmacol Ther 2000;14(5):603–9.

155. Paoluzi P, Iacopini F, Crispino P, et al. 2-week triple therapy for *Helicobacter pylori* infection is better than 1-week in clinical practice: a large prospective single-center randomized study. Helicobacter 2006;11(6):562–8.

156. Vaira D, Zullo A, Vakil N, et al. Sequential therapy versus standard triple-drug therapy for *Helicobacter pylori* eradication: a randomized trial. Ann Intern Med 2007;146(8):556–63.

157. Zullo A, De Francesco V, Hassan C, et al. The sequential therapy regimen for *Helicobacter pylori* eradication: a pooled-data analysis. Gut 2007;56(10):1353–7.

158. Jafri NS, Hornung CA, Howden CW. Meta-analysis: sequential therapy appears superior to standard therapy for *Helicobacter pylori* infection in patients naive to treatment. Ann Intern Med 2008;148(12):923–31.

159. Meyer JM, Silliman NP, Wang W, et al. Risk factors for *Helicobacter pylori* resistance in the United States: the surveillance of *H. pylori* antimicrobial resistance partnership (SHARP) study, 1993–1999. Ann Intern Med 2002;136(1):13–24.

160. Duck WM, Sobel J, Pruckler JM, et al. Antimicrobial resistance incidence and risk factors among *Helicobacter pylori*-infected persons, United States. Emerg Infect Dis 2004;10(6):1088–94.

161. De Francesco V, Margiotta M, Zullo A, et al. Prevalence of primary clarithromycin resistance in *Helicobacter pylori* strains over a 15 year period in Italy. J Antimicrob Chemother 2007;59(4):783–5.

162. McMahon BJ, Hennessy TW, Bensler JM, et al. The relationship among previous antimicrobial use, antimicrobial resistance, and treatment outcomes for *Helicobacter pylori* infections. Ann Intern Med 2003;139(6):463–9.

163. Lee JH, Shin JH, Roe IH, et al. Impact of clarithromycin resistance on eradication of *Helicobacter pylori* in infected adults. Antimicrob Agents Chemother 2005;49(4):1600–3.

164. Dore MP, Leandro G, Realdi G, et al. Effect of pretreatment antibiotic resistance to metronidazole and clarithromycin on outcome of *Helicobacter pylori* therapy: a meta-analytical approach. Dig Dis Sci 2000;45(1):68–76.

165. Havlir DV, Dube MP, Sattler FR, et al. Prophylaxis against disseminated *Mycobacterium avium* complex with weekly azithromycin, daily rifabutin, or both: California Collaborative Treatment Group. N Engl J Med 1996;335(6):392–8.

166. Benson CA, Williams PL, Cohn DL, et al. Clarithromycin or rifabutin alone or in combination for primary prophylaxis of *Mycobacterium avium* complex disease in patients with AIDS: a randomized, double-blind, placebo-controlled trial. The AIDS Clinical Trials Group 196/Terry Beirn Community Programs for Clinical Research on AIDS 009 Protocol Team. J Infect Dis 2000;181(4):1289–97.

167. Kaplan JE, Masur H, Holmes KK. Guidelines for preventing opportunistic infections among HIV-infected persons–2002. Recommendations of the U.S. Public Health Service and the Infectious Diseases Society of America. MMWR Recomm Rep 2002;51(RR-8):1–52.

168. Shafran SD, Singer J, Zarowny DP, et al. A comparison of two regimens for the treatment of *Mycobacterium avium* complex bacteremia in AIDS: rifabutin, ethambutol, and clarithromycin versus rifampin, ethambutol, clofazimine, and ciprofloxacin. Canadian HIV Trials Network Protocol 010 Study Group. N Engl J Med 1996;335(6):377–83.

169. Cohn DL, Fisher EJ, Peng GT, et al. A prospective randomized trial of four three-drug regimens in the treatment of disseminated *Mycobacterium avium* complex disease in AIDS patients: excess mortality associated with high-dose clarithromycin. Terry Beirn Community Programs for Clinical Research on AIDS. Clin Infect Dis 1999;29(1):125–33.

170. Benson CA, Williams PL, Currier JS, et al. A prospective, randomized trial examining the efficacy and safety of clarithromycin in combination with ethambutol, rifabutin, or both for the treatment of disseminated *Mycobacterium avium* complex disease in persons with acquired immunodeficiency syndrome. Clin Infect Dis 2003;37(9):1234–43.

171. Dunne M, Fessel J, Kumar P, et al. A randomized, double-blind trial comparing azithromycin and clarithromycin in the treatment of disseminated *Mycobacterium avium* infection in patients with human immunodeficiency virus. Clin Infect Dis 2000;31(5):1245–52.

172. Ward TT, Rimland D, Kauffman C, et al. Randomized, open-label trial of azithromycin plus ethambutol vs. clarithromycin plus ethambutol as therapy for *Mycobacterium avium* complex bacteremia in patients with human immunodeficiency virus infection. Veterans Affairs HIV Research Consortium. Clin Infect Dis 1998;27(5):1278–85.

173. Wallace RJ Jr, Brown BA, Griffith DE, et al. Initial clarithromycin monotherapy for Mycobacterium avium-intracellulare complex lung disease. Am J Respir Crit Care Med 1994;149(5):1335–41.
174. Griffith DE, Brown BA, Girard WM, et al. Azithromycin activity against *Mycobacterium avium* complex lung disease in patients who were not infected with human immunodeficiency virus. Clin Infect Dis 1996;23(5):983–9.
175. Griffith DE, Brown BA, Murphy DT, et al. Initial (6-month) results of three-times-weekly azithromycin in treatment regimens for *Mycobacterium avium* complex lung disease in human immunodeficiency virus-negative patients. J Infect Dis 1998;178(1):121–6.
176. Griffith DE, Brown BA, Cegielski P, et al. Early results (at 6 months) with intermittent clarithromycin-including regimens for lung disease due to *Mycobacterium avium* complex. Clin Infect Dis 2000;30(2):288–92.
177. Lam PK, Griffith DE, Aksamit TR, et al. Factors related to response to intermittent treatment of *Mycobacterium avium* complex lung disease. Am J Respir Crit Care Med 2006;173(11):1283–9.
178. Griffith DE, Aksamit T, Brown-Elliott BA, et al. An official ATS/IDSA statement: diagnosis, treatment, and prevention of nontuberculous mycobacterial diseases. Am J Respir Crit Care Med 2007;175(4):367–416.
179. Sacchidanand S, Penn RL, Embil JM, et al. Efficacy and safety of tigecycline monotherapy compared with vancomycin plus aztreonam in patients with complicated skin and skin structure infections: results from a phase 3, randomized, double-blind trial. Int J Infect Dis 2005;9(5):251–61.
180. Breedt J, Teras J, Gardovskis J, et al. Safety and efficacy of tigecycline in treatment of skin and skin structure infections: results of a double-blind phase 3 comparison study with vancomycin-aztreonam. Antimicrob Agents Chemother 2005;49(11):4658–66.
181. Ellis-Grosse EJ, Babinchak T, Dartois N, et al. The efficacy and safety of tigecycline in the treatment of skin and skin-structure infections: results of 2 double-blind phase 3 comparison studies with vancomycin-aztreonam. Clin Infect Dis 2005;41(Suppl 5):S341–53.
182. Florescu I, Beuran M, Dimov R, et al. Efficacy and safety of tigecycline compared with vancomycin or linezolid for treatment of serious infections with methicillin-resistant *Staphylococcus aureus* or vancomycin-resistant enterococci: a phase 3, multicentre, double-blind, randomized study. J Antimicrob Chemother 2008;62(Suppl 1):i17–28.
183. Fomin P, Beuran M, Gradauskas A, et al. Tigecycline is efficacious in the treatment of complicated intra-abdominal infections. Int J Surg 2005;3(1):35–47.
184. Oliva ME, Rekha A, Yellin A, et al. A multicenter trial of the efficacy and safety of tigecycline versus imipenem/cilastatin in patients with complicated intra-abdominal infections [Study ID Numbers: 3074A1-301-WW; ClinicalTrials.gov Identifier: NCT00081744]. BMC Infect Dis 2005;5:88.
185. Babinchak T, Ellis-Grosse E, Dartois N, et al. The efficacy and safety of tigecycline for the treatment of complicated intra-abdominal infections: analysis of pooled clinical trial data. Clin Infect Dis 2005;41(Suppl 5):S354–67.
186. Bergallo C, Jasovich A, Teglia O, et al. Safety and efficacy of intravenous tigecycline in treatment of community-acquired pneumonia: results from a double-blind randomized phase 3 comparison study with levofloxacin. Diagn Microbiol Infect Dis 2009;63(1):52–61.
187. Tanaseanu C, Bergallo C, Teglia O, et al. Integrated results of 2 phase 3 studies comparing tigecycline and levofloxacin in community-acquired pneumonia. Diagn Microbiol Infect Dis 2008;61(3):329–38.

188. Kelesidis T, Karageorgopoulos DE, Kelesidis I, et al. Tigecycline for the treatment of multidrug-resistant Enterobacteriaceae: a systematic review of the evidence from microbiological and clinical studies. J Antimicrob Chemother 2008;62(5):895–904.

189. Vasilev K, Reshedko G, Orasan R, et al. A phase 3, open-label, non-comparative study of tigecycline in the treatment of patients with selected serious infections due to resistant Gram-negative organisms including *Enterobacter* species, *Acinetobacter baumannii* and *Klebsiella pneumoniae.* J Antimicrob Chemother 2008;62(Suppl 1):i29–40.

190. Gallagher JC, Rouse HM. Tigecycline for the treatment of *Acinetobacter* infections: a case series. Ann Pharmacother 2008;42(9):1188–94.

191. Nieman RB, Sharma K, Edelberg H, et al. Telithromycin and myasthenia gravis. Clin Infect Dis 2003;37(11):1579.

192. Anthony KB, Fishman NO, Linkin DR, et al. Clinical and microbiological outcomes of serious infections with multidrug-resistant gram-negative organisms treated with tigecycline. Clin Infect Dis 2008;46(4):567–70.

193. Hopkins S. Clinical toleration and safety of azithromycin. Am J Med 1991;91(3):40S–5S.

194. Garey KW, Amsden GW. Intravenous azithromycin. Ann Pharmacother 1999;33(2):218–28.

195. Guay DR, Patterson DR, Seipman N, et al. Overview of the tolerability profile of clarithromycin in preclinical and clinical trials. Drug Saf 1993;8(5):350–64.

196. Ketek (telithromycin) tablets: prescribing information. 2007;2008(November, 28).

197. Demolis JL, Vacheron F, Cardus S, et al. Effect of single and repeated oral doses of telithromycin on cardiac QT interval in healthy subjects. Clin Pharmacol Ther 2003;73(3):242–52.

198. Ross DB. The FDA and the case of Ketek. N Engl J Med 2007;356(16):1601–4.

199. Clay KD, Hanson JS, Pope SD, et al. Brief communication: severe hepatotoxicity of telithromycin: three case reports and literature review. Ann Intern Med 2006;144(6):415–20.

200. Perrot X, Bernard N, Vial C, et al. Myasthenia gravis exacerbation or unmasking associated with telithromycin treatment. Neurology 2006;67(12):2256–8.

201. U.S. Food and Drug Administration. Telithromycin (marketed as Ketek) Information. 2007;2008(12/22).

202. Gilson M, Moachon L, Jeanne L, et al. Acute pancreatitis related to tigecycline: case report and review of the literature. Scand J Infect Dis 2008;40(3):1–3.

203. Rubinstein E. Comparative safety of the different macrolides. Int J Antimicrob Agents 2001;18(Suppl 1):S71–6.

204. Amsden GW. Macrolides versus azalides: a drug interaction update. Ann Pharmacother 1995;29(9):906–17.

205. Rengelshausen J, Goggelmann C, Burhenne J, et al. Contribution of increased oral bioavailability and reduced nonglomerular renal clearance of digoxin to the digoxin-clarithromycin interaction. Br J Clin Pharmacol 2003;56(1):32–8.

206. Zimmerman JJ, Harper DM, Matschke K, et al. Absence of an interaction between tigecycline and digoxin in healthy men. Pharmacotherapy 2007;27(6):835–44.

207. Zimmerman JJ, Raible DG, Harper DM, et al. Evaluation of a potential tigecycline-warfarin drug interaction. Pharmacotherapy 2008;28(7):895–905.

The Newer Fluoroquinolones

Maureen K. Bolon, MD, MS

KEYWORDS

- Fluoroquinolones • Antiinfective agents • Pharmacology
- Pharmacokinetics • Microbial drug resistance
- Therapeutic use

Quinolones are unusual among antimicrobials in that they were not isolated from living organisms, but rather synthesized by chemists. The first quinolone, nalidixic acid, was derived from the antimalarial drug chloroquine.[1] Subsequent agents were derived through side chain and nuclear manipulation.[2] The development of the fluoroquinolone class may be described in generational terms, with each generation sharing similar features or antimicrobial spectra (**Table 1**).[1-3] First-generation agents possess activity against aerobic gram-negative bacteria, but little activity against aerobic gram-positive bacteria or anaerobes. Second-generation agents are the original fluoroquinolones, named for the addition of a fluorine atom at position C-6 (**Fig. 1**). These agents offer improved coverage against gram-negative bacteria and moderately improved gram-positive coverage. Third-generation agents achieve greater potency against gram-positive bacteria, particularly pneumococci, in combination with good activity against anaerobes. Fourth-generation fluoroquinolones have superior coverage against pneumococci and anaerobes. This article focuses on the fluoroquinolone agents most commonly used in clinical practice: ciprofloxacin, levofloxacin, and moxifloxacin.

CHEMISTRY
Basic Antimicrobial Activity

Fluoroquinolones interfere with bacterial cell replication, transcription, and DNA repair by disabling two bacterial enzymes crucial to these processes, DNA gyrase (formerly topoisomerase II) and topoisomerase IV. These enzymes are necessary for bacteria to manage the topological challenge of containing their genetic material. Using _Escherichia coli_ as an example, a bacterial cell that is 1 to 3 μm long must accommodate a chromosome that is a double-stranded DNA circle longer than 1000 μm. Chromosomal volume is reduced via tertiary folding and compaction. These processes must be reversed in order for bacterial replication to occur; DNA topoisomerases facilitate this.[4]

Department of Medicine, Division of Infectious Diseases, Northwestern University Feinberg School of Medicine, 645 N. Michigan Avenue, Suite 900, Chicago, IL 60611, USA
E-mail address: m-bolon@northwestern.edu

Infect Dis Clin N Am 23 (2009) 1027–1051
doi:10.1016/j.idc.2009.06.003
0891-5520/09/$ – see front matter

id.theclinics.com

Table 1
Evolution of the fluoroquinolone class of antimicrobials

Generation	Agent	Comment
First generation	Nalidixic acid	Generic form available
	Cinoxacin	Discontinued
Second generation	Norfloxacin	Available as Noroxin
	Ciprofloxacin	Available as Cipro and generic form
	Lomefloxacin	Discontinued
	Ofloxacin	Available as Floxin and generic form
	Levofloxacin	Available as Levaquin
Third generation	Sparfloxacin	Discontinued
	Gatifloxacin	Discontinued
	Grepafloxacin	Discontinued
Fourth generation	Trovafloxacin	Discontinued
	Moxifloxacin	Available as Avelox
	Gemifloxacin	Available as Factive
	Garenoxacin	Not approved

Data from Andriole VT. The quinolones: past, present, and future. Clinical Infectious Diseases 2005;41 Suppl 2(S113–9); Ball P. Adverse drug reactions: Implications for the development of fluoroquinolones. Journal of Antimicrobial Chemotherapy 2003;51 Suppl 1(21–7); and Drugs@FDA page. Available at: http://www.accessdata.fda.gov/scripts/cder/drugsatfda/index.cfm. Accessed November 25, 2008.

DNA gyrase is a tetramer of two A and two B subunits, encoded by *gyrA* and *gyrB*.[4] DNA gyrase introduces negative DNA supercoils, removes positive and negative supercoils, and catenates and decatenates (links and unlinks) chromosomal material.[5] Topoisomerase IV is a homologue of DNA gyrase and possesses two C and two E subunits, encoded by *parC* and *parE*.[4] It too can remove positive and negative supercoils, but is primarily involved in the separation of the daughter chromosome.[5,6]

Fluoroquinolones bind to the enzyme–DNA complex, causing a conformational change in the enzyme. This leads to DNA cleavage by the enzyme while the continued presence of the fluoroquinolone prevents ligation of broken DNA strands. The fluoroquinolone traps the enzyme on the DNA as a fluoroquinolone–enzyme–DNA complex, inhibiting further DNA replication. The process of complex formation inhibits bacterial cell growth and is thus believed to be bacteriostatic in nature. The bactericidal action of fluoroquinolones is attributed to DNA cleavage.[4,5]

Structure–activity Relationships

Decades of fluoroquinolone development provide considerable insight into the effects of structural modification upon the antimicrobial activity and pharmacologic properties of these agents. **Fig. 1** depicts the core quinolone nucleus. Position 1 affects drug

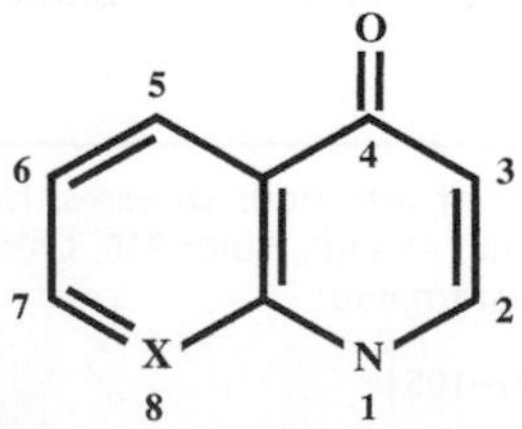

Fig. 1. The core quinolone nucleus.

potency, pharmacokinetics, and the potential for interaction with theophylline. Positions 2, 3, and 4 determine antibacterial activity by influencing the affinity for bacterial enzymes. Additionally, positions 3 and 4 are involved in metal chelation and the resulting interaction with di- and trivalent cations. The presence of a methoxy side chain at position 5 enhances gram-positive activity and phototoxicity. The addition of a fluorine atom to position 6 transforms a quinolone into a fluoroquinolone, enhancing drug penetration into the bacterial cell and activity against gram-negative bacteria. Position 7, like position 1, is instrumental in drug potency, pharmacokinetics, and the interaction with theophylline. This position is also implicated in the central nervous system toxicity of some fluoroquinolones owing to their proclivity to bind to gamma-aminobutyric acid (GABA). The addition of a piperazine moiety at position 7 augments activity against *Pseudomonas aeruginosa*, whereas a pyrrolidine group improves gram-positive activity. The presence of any halogen at position 8 can increase a drug's half-life, absorption, and antianaerobic activity; however, the resulting phototoxicity of di-halogenated compounds renders them unacceptable for clinical use. In contrast, superior pneumococcal activity is achieved by the addition of a methoxy group at position 8 without attendant phototoxicity.[6,7]

Pharmacologic Considerations

Fluoroquinolones have favorable pharmacokinetic properties that have encouraged their widespread use (**Table 2**). They are well absorbed and have good tissue penetration, which facilitates their use for many clinical syndromes.[6,8] While ciprofloxacin must be dosed more frequently, the longer half-lives of the later generation fluoroquinolones allow them to be dosed daily. Most fluoroquinolones are eliminated via the kidney. Moxifloxacin, which is eliminated via the hepatic route, is unusual among fluoroquinolones in lacking efficacy for the treatment of genitourinary infections.

In general, because fluoroquinolones are not highly protein-bound and inhibition of the cytochrome P450 system is limited to the CYP1A2 enzyme, concerns for drug–drug interactions are somewhat minimized.[6,8,9] Fluoroquinolones are known to interact with xanthines, including theophylline and caffeine; however, this is primarily a concern for the older agents.[10] Concomitant use of fluoroquinolones and warfarin can result in supratherapeutic anticoagulation.[11] Perhaps the most common fluoroquinolone interaction involves di- and trivalent cations. Coadministration with antacids may result in subtherapeutic levels of fluoroquinolone agents and, potentially, clinical failure. This issue may be particularly relevant in the inpatient setting given the prevalent use of both fluoroquinolones and antacids; coadministration of fluoroquinolones

Table 2
Pharmacokinetic properties of fluoroquinolones

Agent	Dose (mg)	Bioavailability (%)	Protein Binding (%)	Half-life (Hours)	Elimination	Formulation
Ciprofloxacin	500	60–80	20–40	3–5	Renal/other	IV and PO
Gemifloxacin	320	71	60	7	Renal/other	PO only
Levofloxacin	500	99	40	7	Renal	IV and PO
Moxifloxacin	400	90	50	13	Hepatic	IV and PO

Abbreviations: IV, intravenous; PO, by mouth.
Data from Ball P. The quinolones: history and overview. In: Andriole VT, editor. The quinolones, Third edition. San Diego: Academic Press; 2000. p. 1–33; and O'Donnell JA, Gelone SP. The newer fluoroquinolones. Infect Disease Clinics of North America 2004;18(3):691–716.

and antacids has been implicated by some authors in the emergence of resistance to fluoroquinolones.[12,13]

Pharmacodynamics

Decisions regarding the choice and dosing of an agent are greatly enhanced by considering the pharmacokinetic and pharmacodynamic properties of that agent. Using the minimal inhibitory concentration (MIC) of a bacterial isolate as the sole criterion for choosing an agent fails to take into account the likely concentration of the agent at the site of the infection, individual variation in drug metabolism and clearance, and the mechanism of antimicrobial killing. The pharmacodynamic parameters typically used to predict antimicrobial efficacy are: the time over MIC (T>MIC), the ratio of peak concentration to the MIC (C_{max}/MIC), and the ratio of the area under the concentration-versus-time curve to the MIC (AUC/MIC).[14] Consistent with the characterization of fluoroquinolones as concentration-dependent killers, the parameters regarded as most useful for predicting fluoroquinolone efficacy are C_{max}/MIC and AUC/MIC. These parameters may also be useful to guide therapy in order to prevent the development of resistance to fluoroquinolone agents.

One of the earliest studies to correlate pharmacodynamic parameters with bacteriologic and clinical outcomes evaluated several regimens of intravenous ciprofloxacin administered to acutely ill subjects.[15] Although subjects were treated for a variety of infectious syndromes, the majority were receiving therapy for gram-negative pneumonia. An AUC/MIC ratio greater than 125 was associated with a superior likelihood of clinical and microbiologic cure. Additionally, the time to bacterial eradication was significantly shorter if the AUC/MIC exceeded 125. Subsequent studies have not validated the AUC/MIC threshold value of 125 for all infectious processes, but rather suggest that this value varies by disease state and target pathogen.[16,17] As an example, an AUC/MIC ratio of greater than 33.7 was necessary for a superior microbiologic response when treating pneumococcal pneumonia using levofloxacin or gatifloxacin.[18] Another study in subjects who had nosocomial pneumonia determined that an AUC/MIC threshold of 87 was required for bacterial eradication when treating with levofloxacin.[19] The usefulness of the C_{max}/MIC parameter was established by modeling the pharmacodynamic data from phase 3 trials for levofloxacin.[20] Favorable clinical and microbiologic outcomes were associated with a C_{max}/MIC ratio of at least 12.2. In this particular study, the C_{max}/MIC was highly correlated with the AUC/MIC.

One of the earliest studies to examine whether pharmacodynamic parameters correlate with the emergence of resistance analyzed retrospective data from four nosocomial pneumonia trials.[21] The AUC/MIC ratio was a significant predictor of resistance: resistance was significantly more likely to occur when the AUC/MIC was below 100. Although dosing antimicrobials aggressively in order to achieve adequate pharmacodynamic parameters is fairly well accepted, subsequent studies have not conclusively established that this approach prevents the emergence of resistance. Falagas and colleagues[22] reviewed 12 studies that compared different dosing regimens of fluoroquinolones and reported the development of resistance. Only five of the studies identified fluoroquinolone-resistant isolates following treatment. There was no statistical difference in the emergence of resistance between the high- and low-dose arms, highlighting the need for more studies in this area.

Given trends of worsening antimicrobial resistance, the feasibility of achieving desirable pharmacodynamic thresholds has become an issue of great concern. Pharmacodynamic modeling using antimicrobial susceptibility data from gram-negative organisms collected in the United States for the 2004 Meropenem Yearly Susceptibility Test Information Collection (MYSTIC) surveillance program substantiates this concern.[23] Ciprofloxacin and levofloxacin could be anticipated to be active against only 78% of *E coli*, 40.4%–65.5% of *P aeruginosa* and 43.6%–48.2% of *Acinetobacter baumannii*. These are findings that call into question whether these agents can continue to be used empirically for nonfermenters and Enterobacteriaceae. Finally, altered pharmacokinetics may impact the likelihood of achieving desirable pharmacodynamic thresholds on an individual level. Target AUC/MIC ratios for ciprofloxacin in critically ill individuals are attainable for organisms with the lowest levels of resistance.[24] However, standard doses of ciprofloxacin do not achieve AUC/MIC ratios above 125 for organisms with higher MICs in this population. Higher doses of ciprofloxacin should be considered in critically ill patients to accommodate the MICs of bacteria likely to be encountered.

MECHANISMS OF RESISTANCE

Resistance to fluoroquinolones was traditionally believed to be caused by one of two possible mechanisms: mutation of the target enzymes or reduction of intracellular drug concentrations by way of efflux pumps or alterations in porin channels. The discovery of transferable resistance due to plasmids has uncovered additional mechanisms.[5] A complete understanding of resistance mechanisms continues to evolve— one contemporary appraisal in *E coli* estimated that 50–70% of resistance was explained by known mechanisms.[25]

Target Mutations

Mutations in DNA gyrase or topoisomerase IV are due to amino acid substitutions in the corresponding genes (*gyrA* or *gyrB* for DNA gyrase and *parC* or *parE* for topoisomerase IV) at a site known as the quinolone resistance determining region (QRDR). This location corresponds to a region on the DNA-binding surface of the enzyme and influences drug affinity at the DNA–enzyme complex.[5] Resistance to fluoroquinolones occurs in a stepwise fashion, with accumulation of additional mutations resulting in a greater degree of resistance. The primary target enzyme for an organism is generally the first affected by mutation. Thus, *gyrA* mutations are the first to occur in *E coli*, because DNA gyrase is the primary target of fluoroquinolones in gram-negative organisms.[4,26] Additional mutations in *gyrA* and *parC* lead to higher levels of resistance in gram-negative organisms.[27] The fact that relatively more mutations are required for high-level resistance in *E coli* may account for the superior activity of fluoroquinolones in *E coli* compared to that of other gram-negatives with intrinsic resistance to fluoroquinolones.[28,29]

Topoisomerase IV is believed to be the primary target of fluoroquinolones in the gram-positive organisms. Typically, *parC* mutations are first to occur in *Staphylococcus aureus* or *Streptococcus pneumoniae* and are associated with low-level resistance. Progressive resistance in gram-positives also occurs in a stepwise fashion, with accumulation of subsequent mutations in *gyrA* leading to higher levels of fluoroquinolone resistance.[30,31] Many of the older studies in the gram-positives were performed using older agents, such as ciprofloxacin. Studies of the newer generations of fluoroquinolones demonstrate some divergence from the previously held understanding. For instance, gatifloxacin and moxifloxacin bind strongly to both DNA gyrase and topoisomerase IV.[32] Thus, the primary mutations leading to resistance to these agents occur in *gyrA*, rather than *parC*.[33,34] This feature may explain the preserved activity of later generation fluoroquinolones against *S pneumoniae* strains that are resistant to ciprofloxacin.

One continuing challenge for clinicians is the failure of standard susceptibility testing methods to identify isolates with low-level resistance caused by single-step mutations. These isolates may develop high-level resistance upon exposure to fluoro-quinolone therapy. Studies indicate a high prevalence of single-step mutants exists among pneumococcal isolates.[35] The clinical relevance of this issue has been under-scored by a report of treatment failure and death due to the emergence of high-level resistance in a single-step mutant following levofloxacin therapy.[36] This phenomenon has led to calls advocating for use of a more sensitive screening test for single-step mutants, similar to what is done for *Salmonella* isolates.[37]

Efflux Pumps

Efflux pumps are intrinsic components of the bacterial cell membrane that expel waste and other harmful substances from cells. In general, efflux pumps are responsible for lower levels of resistance to fluoroquinolones than target enzyme mutations.[38] However, by allowing short-term survival of the organism in the presence of the drug, efflux pumps encourage the development of mutations in the QRDR.[16]

The efflux transport mechanism is seen in wild-type *E coli*[39] and may explain the intrinsic fluoroquinolone resistance among *P aeruginosa*.[40] This mechanism has also been described in gram-positive organisms, including *S aureus* and *S pneumo-niae*,[38,41] although agents with a bulky side chain at position 7 such as moxifloxacin are less susceptible to efflux pumps.[32] Because efflux pumps may expel multiple anti-microbial agents, the phenomenon of efflux pump overexpression may contribute to the selection of multidrug-resistant organisms.[42]

Plasmid-mediated Resistance Mechanisms

Transferable fluoroquinolone resistance was conclusively established by the inadver-tent discovery of a plasmid from *Klebsiella pneumoniae* that conferred resistance to ciprofloxacin.[43] The plasmid-mediated locus was initially termed *qnr*. Although the impact upon the MIC for ciprofloxacin was fairly minimal in wild-type strains, clinically significant resistance was achieved in strains with deficient porin channels. It was theorized that the low levels of resistance conferred by this mechanism could facilitate the development of secondary mutations that would produce greater resistance. The implication of this discovery was the understanding that Enterobacteriaceae were vulnerable to the rapid development and dissemination of fluoroquinolone and multi-drug resistance.

Since the initial discovery of plasmid-mediated fluoroquinolone resistance, several additional plasmid-mediated resistance determinants have been described. Qnr-type determinants, which are now thought to produce proteins that protect DNA gyrase and topoisomerase IV from fluoroquinolone inhibition, are geographically widespread and have been identified in many species of Enterobacteriaceae.[44,45] Another plasmid-mediated resistance determinant is an aminoglycoside acetyltransferase, AAC(6')-Ib-cr, which acts in Enterobacteriaceae by acetylating the piperazinyl substit-uent of ciprofloxacin and norfloxacin and is frequently found in association with extended-spectrum β-lactamases.[44,45] The latest plasmid-mediated fluoroquinolone resistance determinant to be described is QepA, an efflux pump that has been iden-tified in *E coli* isolates.[44,45]

EPIDEMIOLOGY OF RESISTANCE
Surveillance Studies

Large surveillance studies report fluoroquinolone resistance rates among a variety of pathogens (**Table 3**).[46-56] Data for gram-negative pathogens predominantly come from intensive care units, where one would expect to see the highest rates of resistance. Indeed, the rates of ciprofloxacin resistance are quite high for *P aeruginosa* and other nosocomial pathogens. Notably, fluoroquinolone resistance among Enterobacteriaceae approaches that of nonfermenters in some settings. Data from the National Nosocomial Infections Surveillance (NNIS) system demonstrate that resistance to ciprofloxacin is also being observed in the outpatient setting.[46]

Emerging fluoroquinolone resistance in *S pneumoniae* has been monitored very closely following a report of very high rates of levofloxacin resistance in Hong Kong (13.3% and 27.3% among penicillin-susceptible and penicillin-resistant pneumococci, respectively).[57] As of this writing, pneumococcal resistance to the newer fluoroquinolone agents does not appear to be prevalent outside of Asia.

Correlation with Use

Fluoroquinolone use has been correlated with the development of resistance in gram-negative organisms on an individual level and on an ecologic level.[58–60] These studies are consistent with the understanding that fluoroquinolone use encourages resistance in gram-negatives by selecting organisms whose survival is favored because of target enzyme mutations or other resistance determinants. The association of fluoroquinolone use with methicillin-resistanct *S aureus* (MRSA) is also fairly well established,[61–64] but the explanation for this association is not akin to that for gram-negative organisms. De novo resistance to methicillin in *S aureus* is not believed to explain the development of MRSA colonization or infection. Rather, MRSA strains are acquired from contact with colonized individuals or the environment. Fluoroquinolones may increase the likelihood of acquisition of MRSA colonization or amplify the resistant population following colonization.[63]

Clostridium Difficile Infection

The association between fluoroquinolone use and the epidemic of *Clostridium difficile* infection (CDI) noted in Quebec and other regions of North America deserves mention. The responsible strain of *C difficile*, referred to as BI/NAP/027, is a fluoroquinolone-resistant, binary toxin-producing strain that also produces high levels of toxins A and B.[65,66] Numerous studies have demonstrated a relationship between fluoroquinolone use and this epidemic strain of *C difficile*.[65,67,68] Some investigators have proposed that the risk for CDI may be higher in association with the newer generations of respiratory fluoroquinolones, possibly because of their greater anaerobic activity.[69] Other investigators have failed to correlate a differential risk among individual fluoroquinolone agents.[7,70]

Resistance in Gonococcal Infections

Although ciprofloxacin received an indication from the US Food and Drug Administration (FDA) for treatment of gonococcal infections, the utility of this drug has been steadily decreasing secondary to the advance of resistance among vulnerable populations. Resistance in *Neisseria gonorrhoeae* is tracked by the Gonococcal Isolate Surveillance Project (GISP), a surveillance program sponsored by the Centers for Disease Control and Prevention (CDC).[71] In 2007, the CDC recommended that fluoroquinolones no longer be used in the United States to treat gonococcal infections and associated conditions. This was based on GISP data that demonstrated that 8.6% of *N gonorrhoeae* isolates outside of Hawaii and California were fluoroquinolone resistant. Of 26 GISP sites, fluoroquinolone resistance was identified in 25.

Table 3
Summary data of fluoroquinolone resistance from selected large surveillance studies

Author or Name of Study	Patient Population	Details of Microbiologic Isolate Collection	Time Period of Study	Summary of Findings
Gram-negative pathogens				
Meropenem Yearly Susceptibility Test Information Collection (MYSTIC) Program[53]	15 United States medical centers	Up to 200 consecutive clinical isolates submitted by each center; 2894 total isolates	2007	Ciprofloxacin resistance in 18.3% of Enterobacteriaceae Ciprofloxacin resistance in 3.4% of *Citrobacter* spp Ciprofloxacin resistance in 8.8% of *Enterobacter* spp Ciprofloxacin resistance in 29% of *E coli* Ciprofloxacin resistance in 20.8% of *Klebsiella* spp Ciprofloxacin resistance in 20.3% of *P mirabilis* Ciprofloxacin resistance in 4.3% of *Serratia* spp Ciprofloxacin resistance in 19.6% of *P aeruginosa* Ciprofloxacin resistance in 60.9% of *Acinetobacter* spp
International Nosocomial Infection Control Consortium (INICC) surveillance study[55]	ICU patients from 98 ICUs in Latin America, Asia, Africa, and Europe	Bacterial susceptibilities provided from patients with device-associated infections	2002–2007	Ciprofloxacin or ofloxacin resistance in 52.4% of *P aeruginosa* Ciprofloxacin or ofloxacin resistance in 42.9% of *E coli*

Lockhart et al[54]	ICU patients from multiple US hospitals	74,000 gram-negative clinical isolates	1993–2004	Ciprofloxacin resistance in *Acinetobacter* spp increased from 38.5% to 64.8% Ciprofloxacin resistance in *P aeruginosa* increased from 16.8% to 33.7% Ciprofloxacin resistance in *E coli* increased from 1.1% to 17.5% Ciprofloxacin resistance in *C freundii* increased from 12% to 26.1% Ciprofloxacin resistance in *P mirabilis* increased from 3.6% to 17.1% Ciprofloxacin resistance in *E cloacae* increased from 6.5% to 14.1% Ciprofloxacin resistance in *K pneumoniae* increased from 11% to 18.2% Multidrug resistance (resistance to one or more of extended-spectrum cephalosporins, one aminoglycoside and ciprofloxacin) increased fourfold in *Acinetobacter* spp and more than fivefold in *P aeruginosa*.
National Nosocomial Infections Surveillance (NNIS) system[46]	United States patients in ICU, non-ICU inpatient areas, and outpatient areas	Bacterial susceptibilities reported by participating centers	1992–2004	In the ICU: ciprofloxacin or ofloxacin resistance in 34.8% of *P aeruginosa* In the ICU: ciprofloxacin or ofloxacin resistance in 7.3% of *E coli* In non-ICU inpatient areas: ciprofloxacin or ofloxacin resistance in 27.7% of *P aeruginosa* In non-ICU inpatient areas: ciprofloxacin or ofloxacin resistance in 8.2% of *E coli* In outpatient areas: ciprofloxacin or ofloxacin resistance in 23.4% of *P aeruginosa* In outpatient areas: ciprofloxacin or ofloxacin resistance in 3.6% of *E coli*

(continued on next page)

Table 3
(continued)

S pneumoniae and other respiratory pathogens

Author or Name of Study	Patient Population	Details of Microbiologic Isolate Collection	Time Period of Study	Summary of Findings
MOXIAKTIV Study[51]	Patients admitted to one of 29 hospitals in Germany	Laboratories submitted respiratory or bloodstream isolates: 426 S pneumoniae isolates; 398 H influenzae isolates; 112 M catarrhalis isolates	Not specified	Moxifloxacin resistance in 0.7% of S pneumoniae isolates Moxifloxacin resistance in 0.8% of H influenzae isolates Moxifloxacin resistance in 0.9% of M catarrhalis isolates
Ip et al[50]	Patients admitted to a 1350-bed teaching hospital in Hong Kong	1388 nonduplicate S pneumoniae isolates from respiratory tract or blood	2000–2005	Ciprofloxacin resistance in 10.5% Levofloxacin resistance in 1.6% In penicillin-nonsusceptible isolates, ciprofloxacin resistance was 11.2% In penicillin nonsusceptible isolates, levofloxacin resistance was 2.2%
Prospective Resistant Organism Tracking and Epidemiology for the Ketolide Telithromycin (PROTEKT)[48]	151 centers from 40 countries worldwide	20,142 respiratory tract isolates of S pneumoniae from outpatients with community-acquired respiratory tract infections and from hospitalized patients within 48 hours of admission	2001–2004	Levofloxacin resistance in 0.8% to 1.1%
SENTRY Antimicrobial Surveillance Program[52]	Medical centers in North America, Latin America, and Europe	2379 strains of S pneumoniae from patients diagnosed with community-acquired respiratory tract infections	1999–2003	Ciprofloxacin resistance in 4.9%–8.0% Levofloxacin resistance in 0–1.1% Gatifloxacin resistance in 0–1%

Prospective Resistant Organism Tracking and Epidemiology for the Ketolide Telithromycin (PROTEKT)[49]	Six centers from Japan, two centers from South Korea, and one center from Hong Kong	515 isolates of S pneumoniae, 373 isolates of H influenzae, 165 isolates of M catarrhalis from blood and respiratory samples	1999–2000	Levofloxacin resistance in 4.7% of S pneumoniae Moxifloxacin resistance in 3.3% of S pneumoniae In Hong Kong, 14% of S pneumoniae isolates were resistant to fluoroquinolones No fluoroquinolone resistance in H influenzae or M catarrhalis isolates
Other organisms				
Canadian National Intensive Care Unit (CAN-ICU)[56]	19 medical centers from all regions of Canada	Consecutive isolates from clinical specimens: 687 MSSA isolates, 197 MRSA isolates	2005–2006	Ciprofloxacin resistance in 9.2% of MSSA Levofloxacin resistance in 7.5% of MSSA Moxifloxacin resistance in 7.3% of MSSA Ciprofloxacin resistance in 91.8% of MRSA Levofloxacin resistance in 91.8% of MRSA Moxifloxacin resistance in 91.1% of MRSA
Bozeman et al[47]	United States and Canadian patients enrolled in Tuberculosis Trials Consortium (TBTC) studies	1373 M tuberculosis isolates from the TBTC studies	1995–2001	Ciprofloxacin resistance in 0.15%
	Isolates from state health departments submitted to the CDC microbiology lab for additional testing	1852 M tuberculosis isolates referred to CDC	1996–2000	Ciprofloxacin resistance in 1.8% 75.8% of ciprofloxacin-resistant isolates were multidrug resistant

Abbreviations: ICU, intensive care unit; MSSA, methicillin-susceptible Staphylococcus aureus; MRSA, methicillin-resistant Staphylococcus aureus; CDC, Centers for Disease Control and Prevention.

TOXICITY

Although generally considered safe and well tolerated, a number of fluoroquinolones have been removed from the United States market for reasons of toxicity. Reported toxicities may be class-wide or limited to single agents or to agents that share a particular structural characteristic. The discussion below is divided into a general account of adverse effects, followed by mention of toxicities that are fairly unique to the fluoroquinolone class, and concludes with a description of the idiosyncratic and typically most severe toxicities that have been associated with individual agents.

Adverse Effects

As with many other antimicrobials, patients may experience gastrointestinal distress when taking fluoroquinolones. In clinical trials, nausea and diarrhea were the most commonly reported adverse effects.[7] There is no particular structural component of fluoroquinolones known to correlate with gastrointestinal toxicity.[72]

A range of adverse effects of the central nervous system can accompany fluoroquinolone administration. Symptoms can range from relatively mild, such as headache or drowsiness, to more severe, such as dizziness or confusion. Seizures have been reported, but are quite rare and are most likely to occur in patients who have a predisposition.[2,72] As mentioned above, fluoroquinolones with certain substituents at position 7 can cause CNS stimulation through one of several hypothesized mechanisms: displacement of GABA, competition with GABA at the receptor site, or interaction with glutamate receptors.[7]

Rash due to fluoroquinolones is fairly uncommon and should be distinguished from phototoxicity, which is specific to certain agents and is discussed in more detail below. Gemifloxacin had an increased rate of rash in clinical trials that appeared to be associated with prolonged use (longer than 5 days) and with use in younger women.[72,73]

Apart from the severe, immune-mediated idiosyncratic reactions leading to hepatitis and renal failure that are discussed below, hepatotoxicity and nephrotoxicity are uncommon following administration of available fluoroquinolones. Liver enzyme abnormalities are reported in 2% to 3% of patients.[74] These have generally been limited to mild, reversible elevations in serum transaminases and alkaline phosphatase.

Anaphylactoid reactions and anaphylaxis can occur following fluoroquinolone administration, but are fairly infrequent, occurring in 0.46 to1.2 cases per 100,000.[74] Unfortunately, there is substantial crossreactivity among the fluoroquinolones, and skin testing is believed to be unreliable due to the frequency of false-positive results.[72]

Class-wide Toxicities

Arthropathy

Tendinopathy was reported in association with the earliest quinolones, and subsequent study established it as a class-wide effect. In 2008, the FDA added a "black box" warning to all fluoroquinolone agents cautioning of the risk of tendonitis and tendon rupture that may be increased in certain populations.[75–79] Although the Achilles tendon is most frequently involved, other tendons of weight-bearing joints may also be affected. Patients typically complain of pain, stiffness, and joint swelling within the first few days of therapy.[80] Symptoms typically resolve within several weeks after discontinuation, although recovery can be prolonged. Achilles tendon rupture may occur in up to half of those with involvement at this site.[80] Fluoroquinolones should be discontinued in patients who have symptoms of tendonitis and exercise should be avoided until recovery.

The mechanism for fluoroquinolone-induced tendinopathy has not been fully elucidated. Fluoroquinolones may be directly toxic to collagen fibers or may cause defective proteoglycan and procollagen synthesis.[7,72] Yet another possibility is that magnesium deficiency caused by fluoroquinolone chelation of ions alters the functionality of chondrocyte surface integrin receptors.[72,81]

QT prolongation

QT interval prolongation is a potentially serious class effect of fluoroquinolones that may provoke torsades de pointes or other ventricular arrhythmias. Grepafloxacin and sparfloxacin were removed from the market for increased risk of arrhythmia.[7] There are certain patient populations who are at increased risk for developing arrhythmia in association with fluoroquinolone use. Fluoroquinolones should be used cautiously in elderly female patients, those who have electrolyte abnormalities (particularly hypokalemia or hypomagnesemia), those who have significant cardiac disease or pre-existing arrhythmia or QTc prolongation, and those receiving coadministration of other drugs likely to prolong the QT interval (particularly class Ia or class III antiarrhythmics).[2,7] The package inserts for levofloxacin, moxifloxacin, and gemifloxacin recommend that these drugs be avoided in patients who have known QTc interval prolongation, uncorrected hypokalemia, and in patients receiving class Ia or class III antiarrhythmics.[7]

The structural moiety responsible for QT interval prolongation by fluoroquinolones has not been identified. The mechanism, however, is known to be blockade of the delayed rectifier potassium current, which regulates the outward flow of potassium ions from the myocyte.[82] The resultant accumulation of intracellular potassium ions within the myocyte delays ventricular repolarization. Because the degree of the effect upon repolarization is influenced by fluoroquinolone concentration, factors that increase drug concentration or reduce clearance increase the risk for arrhythmia.[82]

QT interval prolongation should be considered to be a possibility for all available fluoroquinolone agents, although there is some variation in the reported risk. A review of case reports of torsades de pointes from 1996 to 2001 demonstrated an extremely low risk for ciprofloxacin and moxifloxacin, whereas that for levofloxacin and gatifloxacin was 10- to 100-fold higher, respectively.[83] However, no case reports of torsades de pointes caused by moxifloxacin existed at the time of this review. Data that were submitted to the FDA confirm that moxifloxacin may prolong the QT interval.[7] Several case reports documenting torsades de pointes following moxifloxacin administration have since been published.[84,85] Although there is certainly more accumulated clinical experience with ciprofloxacin, it is difficult to compare older and new agents for the risk of torsades de pointes. Agents that have been approved since 2002 undergo much more rigorous testing for QT interval prolongation as directed by the FDA's International Conference on Harmonization S7B document.[72]

Dysglycemia

Fluoroquinolones may cause both hypoglycemia and hyperglycemia. Although a number of fluoroquinolones may have this effect, there is clearly a greater risk associated with gatifloxacin, which was consequently removed from the market in 2006.[7] Development of the agent clinafloxacin was also halted for this reason. Park-Wyllie and colleagues'[86] influential study established that gatifloxacin administration was associated with an increased risk of both hypoglycemia and hyperglycemia. Levofloxacin use was noted to slightly increase the risk for hypoglycemia.

The structural moiety responsible for dysglycemia is not known at this time. Fluoroquinolones are believed to increase pancreatic insulin secretion by inhibiting adenosine triphosphate–sensitive potassium channels in the beta cells.[7] The mechanism of hyperglycemia is unknown, but, according to one theory, gatifloxacin may reduce insulin levels by triggering the vacuolation of pancreatic beta cells.[86]

Phototoxicity

Fluoroquinolone-induced phototoxicity typically manifests as an intense sunburn that occurs within hours of exposure to UV light.[72] Reactions can be severe, however, particularly in association with multifluorinated agents or agents with halogen atoms at position 8, such as clinafloxacin and sitafloxacin, which are no longer available.[2] Patients should be cautioned to avoid excessive UV exposure during fluoroquinolone administration.[7] Phototoxicity following fluoroquinolone use is believed to be secondary to the generation of reactive oxygen species and free radicals following exposure of these agents to UV light.[7]

Idiosyncratic Toxicities

Several fluoroquinolone agents are known to cause severe, idiosyncratic reactions that are believed to be immune-mediated. Two such agents, temofloxacin and trovafloxacin, are both trifluorinated compounds and possess a 1-2,4-difluorophenyl substituent.[2,72] Temafloxacin was withdrawn from the market after reports of an association with immune hemolytic anemia. The original report by the FDA detailed 95 cases of fevers, rigors, and jaundice that developed within a week of therapy and was associated with hemolysis, hepatitis, and new renal insufficiency.[87] Trovafloxacin was also removed from the market following reports of the development of severe hepatotoxicity, in some cases progressing to hepatic failure, liver transplant, and death.[2]

INDICATIONS
FDA-approved Indications

Table 4 lists complete details regarding indications for the most commonly prescribed fluoroquinolone agents: ciprofloxacin, gemifloxacin, levofloxacin, and moxifloxacin.[76–79]

Ciprofloxacin is the only fluoroquinolone agent approved for gram-negative bone and joint infections. It is also the primary fluoroquinolone approved for gastrointestinal infections, including infectious diarrhea (when therapy is warranted) and typhoid fever. Ciprofloxacin is approved for treatment of uncomplicated and complicated urinary tract infections and chronic bacterial prostatitis. It is also approved for treatment of urethral and cervical gonococcal infections, although it should be noted that the CDC no longer recommends fluoroquinolones for this indication.[71] Ciprofloxacin may be used to treat a range of respiratory tract infections, but is not the agent of choice for *S pneumoniae*. The intravenous formulation of ciprofloxacin may be used for nosocomial pneumonia. Ciprofloxacin is approved for the management of skin and skin structure infections. Ciprofloxacin is approved for postexposure prophylaxis following anthrax exposure. It is the only fluoroquinolone approved for empiric therapy for neutropenic fever, although combination with piperacillin–sodium is recommended. Finally, ciprofloxacin has approval for two pediatric indications: complicated urinary tract infections and pyelonephritis due to *E coli* and postexposure prophylaxis to anthrax.

Gemifloxacin is approved only for respiratory indications: acute bacterial exacerbation of chronic bronchitis and community-acquired pneumonia, including that caused by known or suspected multidrug resistant strains of *S pneumoniae*.

Levofloxacin is approved for uncomplicated and complicated urinary tract infections and prostatitis. It is unique in that it has an indication for short-course regimens (5 days) for complicated urinary tract infections and pyelonephritis. Levofloxacin is approved for the treatment of respiratory tract infections, including community-acquired pneumonia caused by multidrug resistant strains of *S pneumoniae*. A short-course regimen of 5 days may be used to treat community-acquired pneumonia due to sensitive strains of *S pneumoniae*. Levofloxacin is the only fluoroquinolone agent specifically approved for treatment of *Legionella pneumophila* using the longer course of therapy (7–14 days). Levofloxacin may be used for the treatment of nosocomial pneumonia; it is suggested that combination therapy with an antipseudomonal β-lactam be used for *P aeruginosa*. Levofloxacin is approved for the treatment of uncomplicated and complicated skin and skin structure infections due to gram-positive organisms. Lastly, levofloxacin is approved in both adult and pediatric patients for postexposure prophylaxis for inhalation anthrax.

Moxifloxacin is approved for the treatment of complicated intra-abdominal infections, including polymicrobial infections and abscesses. Moxifloxacin is approved for respiratory tract infections, including community-acquired pneumonia caused by multidrug resistant strains of *S pneumoniae*. Finally, moxifloxacin is approved for the treatment of uncomplicated and complicated skin and skin structure infections caused by gram-positive organisms.

Special Indications

There are several special uses for fluoroquinolones that do not specifically have FDA approval, but nonetheless deserve mention.

Tuberculosis

There are a number of arguments for including a fluoroquinolone agent in a treatment regimen for *Mycobacterium tuberculosis* (MTB). These agents act by a mechanism that is unique among antituberculous agents, achieve good penetration into many tissues, and their good safety profile and convenient dosing schedule is likely to improve adherence to therapy. However, these agents are not without toxicity and may interact with other antituberculous and antiretroviral agents. A Cochrane review of 11 trials assessed the use of fluoroquinolones as additional or substitute components in antituberculous regimens for both sensitive and resistant strains.[88] There were no significant differences observed in trials substituting ciprofloxacin, ofloxacin, or moxifloxacin for first-line drugs in relation to cure, treatment failure, or clinical or radiologic improvement. However, substituting ciprofloxacin into first-line regimens for cases of drug-sensitive MTB led to a higher incidence of relapse and longer time to sputum culture conversion for HIV-positive subjects. Adding or substituting levofloxacin to basic regimens in drug-resistant areas did not result in adverse outcomes. The sole conclusion of the review was that ciprofloxacin should not be used to treat MTB.

Legionella

Although levofloxacin does have FDA approval for the treatment of pneumonia due to *L pneumophila*, all agents in the class have become workhorses for lower respiratory tract infections. Thus, it is instructive to examine the evidence supporting the use of fluoroquinolones for this indication. Although fluoroquinolones have been shown to have superior efficacy compared with macrolides in animal and in vitro models, clinical evidence favoring fluoroquinolone use primarily comes from observational studies.[89] It should be noted that no prospective studies or randomized trials have directly

Table 4
FDA-approved indications for the most commonly prescribed fluoroquinolone agents[a]

Type and/or Severity of Infection	Agent	Target Organisms	Dose, Frequency, Route	Duration
Bone and joint infections				
Mild/moderate	Ciprofloxacin	E cloacae, S marcescens, P aeruginosa	500 mg q 12 h PO or 400 mg q 12 h IV	≥4–6 wk
Severe/complicated	Ciprofloxacin	See mild/moderate infections above	750 mg q 12 h PO or 400mg q 8 h IV	≥4–6 wk
Gastrointestinal infections				
Complicated intra-abdominal infections	Ciprofloxacin[b]	E coli, P aeruginosa, P mirabilis, K pneumoniae, B fragilis	500 mg q 12 h PO or 400 mg q 12 h IV	7–14 d
	Moxifloxacin	E coli, B fragilis, S anginosus, S constellatus, E faecalis, P mirabilis, C perfringens, B thetaiotamicron, Peptostreptococcus spp	400 mg q 24 h PO or 400 mg q 24 h IV	5–14 d
Infectious diarrhea, mild/moderate/severe	Ciprofloxacin	E coli (enterotoxigenic strains), C jejuni, S boydii, S dysenteriae, S flexneri, S sonnei	500 mg q 12 h PO	5–7 d
Typhoid fever, mild/moderate	Ciprofloxacin[c]	S typhi	500 mg q 12 h PO	10 d
Genitourinary Infections				
Urinary tract infection, acute/uncomplicated	Ciprofloxacin	E coli, K pneumoniae, E cloacae, S marcescens, P mirabilis, P rettgeri, M morganii, C diversus, C freundii, P aeruginosa, methicillin-susceptible S epidermidis, S saprophyticus, E faecalis	250 mg q 12 h PO	3 d
	Levofloxacin	E coli, K pneumoniae, S saprophyticus	250 mg q 24 h PO or 250 mg q 24 h IV	3 d
Urinary tract infection, mild/moderate	Ciprofloxacin	See acute/uncomplicated infections above	250 mg q 12 h PO or 200 mg q 12 h IV	7–14 d
Urinary tract infection, severe/complicated	Ciprofloxacin	See acute/uncomplicated infections above	500 mg q 12 h PO or 400 mg q 12 h IV	7–14 d

Complicated urinary tract infection	Levofloxacin	E coli, K pneumoniae, P mirabilis	750 mg q 24 h PO	5 d
		E faecalis, E cloacae, E coli, K pneumoniae, P mirabilis, P aeruginosa	250 mg q 24 h PO or 250 mg q 24 h IV	10 d
Acute pyelonephritis	Levofloxacin	E coli	750 mg q 24 h PO	5 d
			250 mg q 24 h PO or 250 mg q 24 h IV	10 d
Chronic bacterial prostatitis	Ciprofloxacin	E coli, P mirabilis	500 mg q 12 h PO or 400 mg q 12 IV	28 d
	Levofloxacin	E coli, E faecalis, methicillin-susceptible S epidermidis	500 mg q 24 h PO	28 d
Urethral and cervical gonococcal infections[d]	Ciprofloxacin	N gonorrhoeae	250 mg PO	Single dose
Respiratory infections				
Acute bacterial sinusitis	Ciprofloxacin	H influenzae, penicillin-susceptible S pneumoniae, M catarrhalis	500 mg q 12 h PO or 400 mg q 12 h IV	10 d
	Levofloxacin	S pneumoniae, H influenzae, M catarrhalis	750 mg q 24 h PO	5 d
			500 mg q 24 h PO or 500 mg q 24 h IV	10-14 d
	Moxifloxacin	S pneumoniae, H influenzae, M catarrhalis	400 mg q 24 h PO or 400 mg q 24 h IV	10 d
Lower respiratory tract, mild/moderate	Ciprofloxacin	E coli, K pneumoniae, E cloacae, P mirabilis, P aeruginosa, H influenzae, H parainfluenzae, penicillin-susceptible S pneumoniae,[e] M catarrhalis[f]	500 mg q 12 h PO or 400 mg q 12 h IV	7–14 d
Lower respiratory tract, severe/complicated	Ciprofloxacin	See mild/moderate infections above	750 mg q 12 h PO or 400 mg q 8 h IV	7–14 d
Acute bacterial exacerbation of chronic bronchitis	Gemifloxacin	S pneumoniae, H influenzae, H parainfluenzae, M catarrhalis	320 mg q 24 h PO	5 d
	Levofloxacin	MSSA, S pneumoniae, H influenzae, H parainfluenzae, M catarrhalis	500 mg q 24 h PO or 500 mg q 24 h IV	7 d
	Moxifloxacin	S pneumoniae, H influenzae, H parainfluenzae, K pneumoniae, MSSA, M catarrhalis	400 mg q 24 h PO or 400 mg q 24 h IV	5 d

(continued on next page)

Table 4
(continued)

Type and/or Severity of Infection	Agent	Target Organisms	Dose, Frequency, Route	Duration
Community-acquired pneumonia	Gemifloxacin	S pneumoniae, H influenzae, M pneumoniae, C pneumoniae	320 mg q 24 h PO	5 d
	Gemifloxacin	Known or suspected multidrug resistant strains of S pneumoniae, K pneumoniae, or M catarrhalis	320 mg q 24 h PO	7 d
	Levofloxacin	S pneumoniae (not multidrug resistant strains), H influenzae, H parainfluenzae, M pneumoniae, C pneumoniae	750 mg q 24 h PO	5 d
	Levofloxacin	MSSA, S pneumoniae (including multidrug resistant strains), H influenzae, H parainfluenzae, K pneumoniae, M catarrhalis, C pneumoniae, L pneumophila, M pneumoniae	500 mg q 24 h PO or 500 mg q 24 h IV	7–14 d
	Moxifloxacin	S pneumoniae (including multidrug resistant strains), H influenzae, M catarrhalis, MSSA, K pneumoniae, M pneumoniae, C pneumoniae	400 mg q 24 h PO or 400 mg q 24 h IV	7–14 d
Nosocomial pneumonia	Ciprofloxacin	H influenzae, K pneumoniae	400 mg q 8 h IV	10–14 d
	Levofloxacin	MSSA, P aeruginosa,[9] S marcescens, E coli, K pneumoniae, H influenzae, S pneumoniae	750 mg q 24 h PO	7–14 d
Skin and skin structure infections				
Mild/moderate	Ciprofloxacin	E coli, K pneumoniae, E cloacae, P mirabilis, P vulgaris, P stuartii, M morganni, C freundii, P aeruginosa, MSSA, methicillin-susceptible S epidermidis, S pyogenes	500 mg q 12 h PO or 400 mg q 12 h IV	7–14 d
Uncomplicated	Levofloxacin	MSSA, S pyogenes	500 mg q 24 h PO or 500 mg q 24 h IV	7–10 d
	Moxifloxacin	MSSA, S pyogenes	400 mg q 24 h PO or 400 mg q 24 h IV	7 d
Severe/complicated	Ciprofloxacin	See mild/moderate infections above	750 mg q 12 h PO or 400 mg q 8 h IV	7–14 d
Complicated	Levofloxacin	MSSA, E faecalis, S pyogenes, P mirabilis	750 mg q 24 h PO	7–14 d
	Moxifloxacin	MSSA, E coli, K pneumoniae, E cloacae	400 mg q 24 h PO or 400 mg q 24 h IV	7–21 d
Other				
Inhalation anthrax (postexposure)	Ciprofloxacin	B anthracis	500 mg q 12 h PO or 400 mg q 12 h IV	60 d
	Levofloxacin	B anthracis	500 mg q 24 h PO	60 d

Empirical therapy in febrile neutropenia	Ciprofloxacin[h]		400 mg q 8 h IV	7–14 d
Indications approved for use in pediatric patients (1–17 years of age)				
Complicated urinary tract infections and pyelonephritis	Ciprofloxacin	E coli	10–20 mg/kg q 12 h PO (not to exceed 750 mg dose) or 6–10 mg/kg q 8 h IV (not to exceed 400 mg dose)	10–21 d
Inhalation anthrax (postexposure)	Ciprofloxacin	B anthracis	15 mg/kg q 12 h PO (not to exceed 500 mg dose) or 10 mg/kg q 12 h IV (not to exceed 400 mg dose)	60 d
	Levofloxacin	B anthracis	For patients <50 kg: 8 mg/kg q 12 h PO (not to exceed 250 mg dose) For patients >50 kg: 500 mg q 24 h PO	60 d

Abbreviations: PO, by mouth; IV, intravenous; MSSA, methicillin-susceptible *Staphylococcus aureus.*

[a] Please note that the indications, target organisms, dosing, and durations listed below are based on FDA labeling information, but are not consistent with best practices in all cases.

[b] Use in combination with metronidazole.

[c] The efficacy of ciprofloxacin in eradication of the chronic typhoid carrier state has not been demonstrated.

[d] Fluoroquinolones no longer recommended by the CDC for treatment of gonococcal infections.

[e] Ciprofloxacin is not a drug of first choice in the treatment of presumed or confirmed pneumonia secondary to *S pneumonia.*

[f] For acute exacerbations of chronic bronchitis.

[g] Combination therapy with an antipseudomonal β-lactam is recommended.

[h] Use in combination with piperacillin–sodium.

Data from Cipro labeling information, October 2008. Available at: http://www.fda.gov/cder/foi/label/2008/019537s68,19847s42,19857s49,20780s26,21473s24lbl. pdf; Factive labeling information, October 2008. Available at: http://www.fda.gov/cder/foi/label/2008/021158s012lbl.pdf; Levaquin labeling information, October 2008. Available at: http://www.fda.gov/cder/foi/label/2008/021721s020_020635s57_020634s52_lbl.pdf; Avelox labeling information, October 2008. Available at: http://www.fda.gov/cder/foi/label/2008/021085s040,021277s034lbl.pdf. All accessed on November 14, 2008.

compared the clinical efficacy of fluoroquinolones with that of newer macrolides such as azithromycin.

Antibacterial prophylaxis after chemotherapy

Clinical trials have evaluated the practice of administering fluoroquinolone prophylaxis during periods of chemotherapy-induced neutropenia. Two studies of note, one of which included subjects who had solid tumors and lymphoma[90] and another that enrolled subjects who had solid tumors, lymphoma, and acute leukemia,[91] found a benefit of levofloxacin compared to placebo for the outcomes of fever and documented infection. The study in subjects who had solid tumors and lymphoma also demonstrated a reduction in hospitalization for infection following levofloxacin prophylaxis. Neither study demonstrated a reduction in mortality attributable to the prophylaxis. A follow-up meta-analysis of randomized, blinded, placebo-controlled trials of fluoroquinolone prophylaxis for neutropenic subjects similarly failed to establish a significant reduction in mortality associated with prophylaxis.[92]

Prevention of meningococcal infections following exposure

Ciprofloxacin may be used for the prevention of meningococcal disease following exposure to an infected individual. A Cochrane review has examined the outcomes associated with the common antimicrobial agents used for this indication.[93] Because no meningococcal disease occurred among secondary contacts in any of the trials, the efficacy of different agents for the prevention of future disease could not be assessed. Ciprofloxacin proved effective at eradicating pharyngeal carriage of *Neisseria meningitidis* for up to 2 weeks following treatment in healthy carriers. The authors concluded that ciprofloxacin could be considered as an alternative to rifampin.

SUMMARY

Fluoroquinolones have gained widespread use owing to their favorable pharmacokinetics and broad antimicrobial spectra. Although a number of agents have been withdrawn from the market for serious safety concerns, the remaining agents have proved quite safe. Worrisome levels of fluoroquinolone resistance have developed as a consequence of heavy use. Resistance in gram-negative organisms, in particular, threatens to jeopardize the continued empiric use of fluoroquinolones. However, recent advances in fluoroquinolone development have primarily resulted in improved pneumococcal coverage, with the consequence that the treatment of respiratory tract infections may become the main use for this class. Appropriate choice of agent and dose while keeping pharmacodynamic principles in mind will, we hope, preserve these very useful agents.

REFERENCES

1. Andriole VT. The quinolones: past, present, and future. Clin Infect Dis 2005; 41(Suppl 2):S113–9.
2. Ball P. Adverse drug reactions: implications for the development of fluoroquinolones. J Antimicrob Chemother 2003;51(Suppl 1):21–7.
3. Drugs@FDA page. Available at: http://www.accessdata.fda.gov/scripts/cder/drugsatfda/index.cfm. Accessed November 25, 2008.
4. Hawkey PM. Mechanisms of quinolone action and microbial response. J Antimicrob Chemother 2003;51(Suppl 1):29–35.
5. Jacoby GA. Mechanisms of resistance to quinolones. Clin Infect Dis 2005; 41(Suppl 2):S120–6.

6. O'Donnell JA, Gelone SP. The newer fluoroquinolones. Infect Dis Clin North Am 2004;18(3):691–716, x.

7. Mehlhorn AJ, Brown DA. Safety concerns with fluoroquinolones. Ann Pharmacother 2007;41(11):1859–66.

8. Ball P. The quinolones: history and overview. In: Andriole VT, editor. The quinolones. 3rd edition. San Diego (CA): Academic Press; 2000. p. 1–33.

9. Stahlman R, Lode H. Safety overview: toxicity, adverse effects, and drug interactions. In: Andriole VT, editor. The quinolones. 3rd edition. San Diego (CA): Academic Press; 2000. p. 397–453.

10. Niki Y, Hashiguchi K, Okimoto N, et al. Quinolone antimicrobial agents and theophylline [letter]. Chest 1992;101(3):881.

11. Carroll DN, Carroll DG. Interactions between warfarin and three commonly prescribed fluoroquinolones. Ann Pharmacother 2008;42(5):680–5.

12. Barton TD, Fishman NO, Weiner MG, et al. High rate of coadministration of di- or trivalent cation-containing compounds with oral fluoroquinolones: risk factors and potential implications. Infect Control Hosp Epidemiol 2005;26(1):93–9.

13. Cohen KA, Lautenbach E, Weiner MG, et al. Coadministration of oral levofloxacin with agents that impair absorption: impact on antibiotic resistance. Infect Control Hosp Epidemiol 2008;29(10):975–7.

14. Rybak MJ. Pharmacodynamics: relation to antimicrobial resistance. Am J Med 2006;119(6 Suppl 1):S37–44 [discussion: S62–70].

15. Forrest A, Nix DE, Ballow CH, et al. Pharmacodynamics of intravenous ciprofloxacin in seriously ill patients. Antimicrob Agents Chemother 1993;37(5):1073–81.

16. Dalhoff A, Schmitz FJ. In vitro antibacterial activity and pharmacodynamics of new quinolones. Eur J Clin Microbiol Infect Dis 2003;22(4):203–21.

17. Wispelwey B. Clinical implications of pharmacokinetics and pharmacodynamics of fluoroquinolones. Clin Infect Dis 2005;41(Suppl 2):S127–35.

18. Ambrose PG, Grasela DM, Grasela TH, et al. Pharmacodynamics of fluoroquinolones against Streptococcus pneumoniae in patients with community-acquired respiratory tract infections. Antimicrob Agents Chemother 2001; 45(10):2793–7.

19. Drusano GL, Preston SL, Fowler C, et al. Relationship between fluoroquinolone area under the curve: minimum inhibitory concentration ratio and the probability of eradication of the infecting pathogen, in patients with nosocomial pneumonia. J Infect Dis 2004;189(9):1590–7.

20. Preston SL, Drusano GL, Berman AL, et al. Pharmacodynamics of levofloxacin: a new paradigm for early clinical trials. JAMA 1998;279(2):125–9.

21. Thomas JK, Forrest A, Bhavnani SM, et al. Pharmacodynamic evaluation of factors associated with the development of bacterial resistance in acutely ill patients during therapy. Antimicrob Agents Chemother 1998;42(3):521–7.

22. Falagas ME, Bliziotis IA, Rafailidis PI. Do high doses of quinolones decrease the emergence of antibacterial resistance? A systematic review of data from comparative clinical trials. J Infect 2007;55(2):97–105.

23. DeRyke CA, Kuti JL, Nicolau DP. Pharmacodynamic target attainment of six beta-lactams and two fluoroquinolones against Pseudomonas aeruginosa, Acinetobacter baumannii, Escherichia coli, and Klebsiella species collected from United States intensive care units in 2004. Pharmacotherapy 2007;27(3): 333–42.

24. van Zanten AR, Polderman KH, van Geijlswijk IM, et al. Ciprofloxacin pharmacokinetics in critically ill patients: a prospective cohort study. J Crit Care 2008;23(3): 422–30.

25. Morgan-Linnell SK, Becnel Boyd L, Steffen D, et al. Mechanisms accounting for fluoroquinolone resistance in *Escherichia coli* clinical isolates. Antimicrob Agents Chemother 2009;53(1):235–41.

26. Oram M, Fisher LM. 4-quinolone resistance mutations in the DNA gyrase of *Escherichia coli* clinical isolates identified by using the polymerase chain reaction. Antimicrob Agents Chemother 1991;35(2):387–9.

27. Khodursky AB, Zechiedrich EL, Cozzarelli NR. Topoisomerase IV is a target of quinolones in *Escherichia coli*. Proc Natl Acad Sci U S A 1995;92(25):11801–5.

28. Vila J, Ruiz J, Goni P, et al. Detection of mutations in *parC* in quinolone-resistant clinical isolates of *Escherichia coli*. Antimicrob Agents Chemother 1996;40(2): 491–3.

29. Vila J, Ruiz J, Goni P, et al. Quinolone-resistance mutations in the topoisomerase IV *parC* gene of *Acinetobacter baumannii*. J Antimicrob Chemother 1997;39(6): 757–62.

30. Ferrero L, Cameron B, Crouzet J. Analysis of *gyrA* and *grlA* mutations in step-wise-selected ciprofloxacin-resistant mutants of *Staphylococcus aureus*. Antimicrob Agents Chemother 1995;39(7):1554–8.

31. Pan XS, Ambler J, Mehtar S, et al. Involvement of topoisomerase IV and DNA gyrase as ciprofloxacin targets in *Streptococcus pneumoniae*. Antimicrob Agents Chemother 1996;40(10):2321–6.

32. Scheld WM. Maintaining fluoroquinolone class efficacy: review of influencing factors. Emerg Infect Dis 2003;9(1):1–9.

33. Fukuda H, Hiramatsu K. Primary targets of fluoroquinolones in *Streptococcus pneumoniae*. Antimicrob Agents Chemother 1999;43(2):410–2.

34. Pestova E, Millichap JJ, Noskin GA, et al. Intracellular targets of moxifloxacin: a comparison with other fluoroquinolones. J Antimicrob Chemother 2000;45(5): 583–90.

35. Pletz MW, Shergill AP, McGee L, et al. Prevalence of first-step mutants among levofloxacin-susceptible invasive isolates of *Streptococcus pneumoniae* in the United States. Antimicrob Agents Chemother 2006;50(4):1561–3.

36. de Cueto M, Rodriguez JM, Soriano MJ, et al. Fatal levofloxacin failure in treatment of a bacteremic patient infected with *Streptococcus pneumoniae* with a pre-existing *parC* mutation. J Clin Microbiol 2008;46(4):1558–60.

37. Hakanen A, Kotilainen P, Jalava J, et al. Detection of decreased fluoroquinolone susceptibility in *Salmonella*s and validation of nalidixic acid screening test. J Clin Microbiol 1999;37(11):3572–7.

38. Kaatz GW, Seo SM, Ruble CA. Efflux-mediated fluoroquinolone resistance in *Staphylococcus aureus*. Antimicrob Agents Chemother 1993;37(5):1086–94.

39. Cohen SP, Hooper DC, Wolfson JS, et al. Endogenous active efflux of norfloxacin in susceptible *Escherichia coli*. Antimicrob Agents Chemother 1988;32(8): 1187–91.

40. Li XZ, Livermore DM, Nikaido H. Role of efflux pump(s) in intrinsic resistance of *Pseudomonas aeruginosa*: resistance to tetracycline, chloramphenicol, and nor-floxacin. Antimicrob Agents Chemother 1994;38(8):1732–41.

41. Brenwald NP, Gill MJ, Wise R. Prevalence of a putative efflux mechanism among fluoroquinolone-resistant clinical isolates of *Streptococcus pneumoniae*. Antimicrob Agents Chemother 1998;42(8):2032–5.

42. Kriengkauykiat J, Porter E, Lomovskaya O, et al. Use of an efflux pump inhibitor to determine the prevalence of efflux pump-mediated fluoroquinolone resistance and multidrug resistance in *Pseudomonas aeruginosa*. Antimicrob Agents Chemother 2005;49(2):565–70.

43. Martinez-Martinez L, Pascual A, Jacoby GA. Quinolone resistance from a transferable plasmid. Lancet 1998;351(9105):797–9.

44. Poirel L, Cattoir V, Nordmann P. Is plasmid-mediated quinolone resistance a clinically significant problem? Clin Microbiol Infect 2008;14(4):295–7.

45. Yamane K, Wachino J, Suzuki S, et al. New plasmid-mediated fluoroquinolone efflux pump, QepA, found in an *Escherichia coli* clinical isolate. Antimicrob Agents Chemother 2007;51(9):3354–60.

46. National Nosocomial Infections Surveillance System. National nosocomial infections surveillance (NNIS) system report, data summary from January 1992 through June 2004, issued October 2004. Am J Infect Control 2004;32(8):470–85.

47. Bozeman L, Burman W, Metchock B, et al. Fluoroquinolone susceptibility among *Mycobacterium tuberculosis* isolates from the United States and Canada. Clin Infect Dis 2005;40(3):386–91.

48. Felmingham D, Canton R, Jenkins SG. Regional trends in beta-lactam, macrolide, fluoroquinolone and telithromycin resistance among *Streptococcus pneumoniae* isolates 2001–2004. J Infect 2007;55(2):111–8.

49. Inoue M, Lee NY, Hong SW, et al. Protekt 1999–2000: a multicentre study of the antibiotic susceptibility of respiratory tract pathogens in Hong Kong, Japan and South Korea. Int J Antimicrob Agents 2004;23(1):44–51.

50. Ip M, Chau SS, Chi F, et al. Longitudinally tracking fluoroquinolone resistance and its determinants in penicillin-susceptible and -nonsusceptible *Streptococcus pneumoniae* isolates in Hong Kong, 2000 to 2005. Antimicrob Agents Chemother 2007;51(6):2192–4.

51. Jacobs E, Dalhoff A, Korfmann G. Susceptibility patterns of bacterial isolates from hospitalised patients with respiratory tract infections (MOXIAKTIV study). Int J Antimicrob Agents 2009;33(1):52–7.

52. Johnson DM, Stilwell MG, Fritsche TR, et al. Emergence of multidrug-resistant *Streptococcus pneumoniae*: report from the SENTRY antimicrobial surveillance program (1999–2003). Diagn Microbiol Infect Dis 2006;56(1):69–74.

53. Jones RN, Kirby JT, Rhomberg PR. Comparative activity of meropenem in US medical centers (2007): initiating the 2nd decade of MYSTIC program surveillance. Diagn Microbiol Infect Dis 2008;61(2):203–13.

54. Lockhart SR, Abramson MA, Beekmann SE, et al. Antimicrobial resistance among gram-negative bacilli causing infections in intensive care unit patients in the United States between 1993 and 2004. J Clin Microbiol 2007;45(10):3352–9.

55. Rosenthal VD, Maki DG, Mehta A, et al. International nosocomial infection control consortium report, data summary for 2002–2007, issued January 2008. Am J Infect Control 2008;36(9):627–37.

56. Zhanel GG, DeCorby M, Laing N, et al. Antimicrobial-resistant pathogens in intensive care units in Canada: results of the Canadian National Intensive Care Unit (CAN-ICU) study, 2005–2006. Antimicrob Agents Chemother 2008;52(4):1430–7.

57. Ho PL, Yung RW, Tsang DN, et al. Increasing resistance of *Streptococcus pneumoniae* to fluoroquinolones: results of a Hong Kong multicentre study in 2000. J Antimicrob Chemother 2001;48(5):659–65.

58. Gagliotti C, Nobilio L, Moro ML. Emergence of ciprofloxacin resistance in *Escherichia coli* isolates from outpatient urine samples. Clin Microbiol Infect 2007;13(3):328–31.

59. Kaye KS, Kanafani ZA, Dodds AE, et al. Differential effects of levofloxacin and ciprofloxacin on the risk for isolation of quinolone-resistant *Pseudomonas aeruginosa*. Antimicrob Agents Chemother 2006;50(6):2192–6.

60. Ray GT, Baxter R, DeLorenze GN. Hospital-level rates of fluoroquinolone use and the risk of hospital-acquired infection with ciprofloxacin-nonsusceptible *Pseudomonas aeruginosa*. Clin Infect Dis 2005;41(4):441–9.

61. Weber SG, Gold HS, Hooper DC, et al. Fluoroquinolones and the risk for methicillin-resistant *Staphylococcus aureus* in hospitalized patients. Emerg Infect Dis 2003;9(11):1415–22.

62. LeBlanc L, Pepin J, Toulouse K, et al. Fluoroquinolones and risk for methicillin-resistant *Staphylococcus aureus*, Canada. Emerg Infect Dis 2006;12(9):1398–405.

63. MacDougall C, Harpe SE, Powell JP, et al. *Pseudomonas aeruginosa, Staphylococcus aureus*, and fluoroquinolone use. Emerg Infect Dis 2005;11(8):1197–204.

64. MacDougall C, Powell JP, Johnson CK, et al. Hospital and community fluoroquinolone use and resistance in *Staphylococcus aureus* and *Escherichia coli* in 17 US hospitals. Clin Infect Dis 2005;41(4):435–40.

65. Labbe AC, Poirier L, Maccannell D, et al. *Clostridium difficile* infections in a Canadian tertiary care hospital before and during a regional epidemic associated with the bi/nap1/027 strain. Antimicrob Agents Chemother 2008;52(9):3180–7.

66. Razavi B, Apisarnthanarak A, Mundy LM. *Clostridium difficile*: emergence of hypervirulence and fluoroquinolone resistance. Infection 2007;35(5):300–7.

67. Pepin J, Saheb N, Coulombe MA, et al. Emergence of fluoroquinolones as the predominant risk factor for *Clostridium difficile*-associated diarrhea: a cohort study during an epidemic in Quebec. Clin Infect Dis 2005;41(9):1254–60.

68. Loo VG, Poirier L, Miller MA, et al. A predominantly clonal multi-institutional outbreak of *Clostridium difficile*-associated diarrhea with high morbidity and mortality. N Engl J Med 2005;353(23):2442–9.

69. Gaynes R, Rimland D, Killum E, et al. Outbreak of *Clostridium difficile* infection in a long-term care facility: association with gatifloxacin use. Clin Infect Dis 2004;38(5):640–5.

70. McFarland LV, Clarridge JE, Beneda HW, et al. Fluoroquinolone use and risk factors for *Clostridium difficile*-associated disease within a Veterans Administration health care system. Clin Infect Dis 2007;45(9):1141–51.

71. del Rio C, Hall G, Hook EW, et al. Update to CDC's sexually transmitted diseases treatment guidelines, 2006: Fluoroquinolones no longer recommended for treatment of gonococcal infections. MMWR Morb Mortal Wkly Rep 2007;56(14):332–6.

72. Owens RC Jr, Ambrose PG. Antimicrobial safety: focus on fluoroquinolones. Clin Infect Dis 2005;41(Suppl 2):S144–57.

73. Iannini P, Mandell L, Patou G, et al. Cutaneous adverse events and gemifloxacin: observations from the clinical trial program. J Chemother 2006;18(1):3–11.

74. Lipsky BA, Baker CA. Fluoroquinolone toxicity profiles: a review focusing on newer agents. Clin Infect Dis 1999;28(2):352–64.

75. Tanne JH. FDA adds "black box" warning label to fluoroquinolone antibiotics [comment]. BMJ 2008;337:a816.

76. Cipro. [label information October 2008]. Available at: http://www.fda.gov/cder/foi/label/2008/019537s68, 19847s42, 19857s49, 20780s26, 21473s24lbl.pdf. Accessed November 14, 2008.

77. Factive. [label information October 2008]. Available at: http://www.fda.gov/cder/foi/label/2008/021158s012lbl.pdf. Accessed November 14, 2008.

78. Levaquin. [label information October 2008]. Available at: http://www.fda.gov/cder/foi/label/2008/021721s020_020635s57_020634s52_lbl.pdf. Accessed November 14, 2008.

79. Avelox. [label information October 2008]. Available at: http://www.fda.gov/cder/foi/label/2008/021085s040, 021277s034lbl.pdf. Accessed November 14, 2008.

80. Khaliq Y, Zhanel GG. Fluoroquinolone-associated tendinopathy: a critical review of the literature. Clin Infect Dis 2003;36(11):1404–10.
81. Stahlmann R, Forster C, Shakibaei M, et al. Magnesium deficiency induces joint cartilage lesions in juvenile rats which are identical to quinolone-induced arthropathy. Antimicrob Agents Chemother 1995;39(9):2013–8.
82. Owens RC Jr, Nolin TD. Antimicrobial-associated QT interval prolongation: pointes of interest. Clin Infect Dis 2006;43(12):1603–11.
83. Frothingham R. Rates of torsades de pointes associated with ciprofloxacin, ofloxacin, levofloxacin, gatifloxacin, and moxifloxacin. Pharmacotherapy 2001;21(12):1468–72.
84. Dale KM, Lertsburapa K, Kluger J, et al. Moxifloxacin and torsades de pointes. Ann Pharmacother 2007;41(2):336–40.
85. Altin T, Ozcan O, Turhan S, et al. Torsades de pointes associated with moxifloxacin: a rare but potentially fatal adverse event. Can J Cardiol 2007;23(11):907–8.
86. Park-Wyllie LY, Juurlink DN, Kopp A, et al. Outpatient gatifloxacin therapy and dysglycemia in older adults. N Engl J Med 2006;354(13):1352–61.
87. Blum MD, Graham DJ, McCloskey CA. Temafloxacin syndrome: review of 95 cases. Clin Infect Dis 1994;18(6):946–50.
88. Ziganshina LE, Squire SB. Fluoroquinolones for treating tuberculosis. Cochrane Database Syst Rev 2008;(1):CD004795.
89. Pedro-Botet L, Yu VL. Legionella: macrolides or quinolones? Clin Microbiol Infect 2006;12(Suppl 3):25–30.
90. Cullen M, Steven N, Billingham L, et al. Antibacterial prophylaxis after chemotherapy for solid tumors and lymphomas. N Engl J Med 2005;353(10):988–98.
91. Bucaneve G, Micozzi A, Menichetti F, et al. Levofloxacin to prevent bacterial infection in patients with cancer and neutropenia. N Engl J Med 2005;353(10):977–87.
92. Imran H, Tleyjeh IM, Arndt CA, et al. Fluoroquinolone prophylaxis in patients with neutropenia: a meta-analysis of randomized placebo-controlled trials. Eur J Clin Microbiol Infect Dis 2008;27(1):53–63.
93. Fraser A, Gafter-Gvili A, Paul M, et al. Antibiotics for preventing meningococcal infections. Cochrane Database Syst Rev 2006;(4):CD004785.

Current Use for Old Antibacterial Agents: Polymyxins, Rifamycins, and Aminoglycosides

Luke F. Chen, MBBS (Hons), CIC, FRACP[a],*, Donald Kaye, MD[b,c]

KEYWORDS

• Rifaximin • Pharmacokinetics • Pharmacodynamics
• Toxicity • Polymyxins • Aminoglycoside • Rifampin

The polymyxins, rifamycins, and the aminoglycosides may be considered special use antibacterial agents. They are all old agents and are rarely considered the drugs of choice for common bacterial infections.

The polymyxins are increasingly important because of the continued emergence of multidrug resistant (MDR) gram-negative organisms, such as strains of *Pseudomonas aeruginosa* or carbapenemase-producing Enterobacteriaceae that are susceptible to few remaining drugs. Rifampin is only considered in nonmycobacterial infections where its role is limited and sometimes controversial. Rifaximin is a new enteric rifamycin that is increasingly used for gastrointestinal infections such as traveler's diarrhea and *Clostridium difficile* infections (CDIs). This article will also review the current role of aminoglycosides in nonmycobacterial systemic infections, with an emphasis on the use of single daily administration.

POLYMYXINS

The polymyxins were discovered in 1947. Although there are five known polymyxin molecules, sequentially named polymyxin A through polymyxin E, only two polymyxins are available for therapeutic use: polymyxin B and polymyxin E (colistin) (Table 1). Both polymyxin B and polymyxin E are large cyclic cationic polypeptide detergents with molecular weights of 1000 or more. Polymyxin B was initially isolated from *Bacillus polymyxa*, and colistin was isolated from *Bacillus colistinus*. There are two

[a] Department of Medicine, Division of Infectious Diseases and International Health, Duke University Medical Center, Box 102359, Hanes House, Durham, NC 27710, USA
[b] Drexel University, College of Medicine, Philadelphia, PA 19035, USA
[c] Department of Medicine, 1535 Sweet Briar Road, Gladwyne, PA 19035, USA
* Corresponding author.
E-mail address: luke.chen@duke.edu (L.F. Chen).

Infect Dis Clin N Am 23 (2009) 1053–1075
doi:10.1016/j.idc.2009.06.004
0891-5520/09/$ – see front matter © 2009 Elsevier Inc. All rights reserved.

Table 1			
Routes of administration of different forms of polymyxins			
	Alternate Name	**Available Preparations**	**Routes of Administration**
Polymyxin B	—	Polymyxin B	Parenteral/topical intrathecal/intraventricular
Polymyxin E	Colistin	Colistin sulfate Colistimethate sodium (Colistin methanesulfonate)	Oral Parenteral/nebulization intrathecal/intraventricular

preparations of colistin: colistin sulfate and colistimethate sodium. Colistimethate sodium is inactive until hydrolyzed and such hydrolysis occurs in both in vivo and in vitro testing systems. Notably, colistimethate sodium is the least active polymyxin in vitro (as much as fourfold to eightfold less active)[1] but also is the least nephrotoxic compound compared with polymyxin B and colistin sulfate.[2,3]

The polymyxins were used to treat serious infections caused by gram-negative bacilli in the early 1960s until aminoglycosides active against P aeruginosa (eg, gentamicin) came into common use. The polymyxins fell into further disuse by 1980 because of their nephrotoxicity and subsequently they became mainly reserved for topical and oral administration.[4,5] The recent emergence of P aeruginosa, Acinetobacter baumannii, and MDR gram-negative bacilli resistant to all other antimicrobial agents has resulted in the increasing need for an injectable polymyxin.[6,7]

In recent years, colistimethate sodium has been the most commonly used form of polymyxin for parenteral therapy. Colistimethate has also been used for nebulization therapy in patients with cystic fibrosis and for intrathecal and intraventricular injection. Colistin, on the other hand, has been available as colistin sulfate for use topically and orally, except in the United States, where only colistimethate and polymyxin B are available commercially.

Polymyxin B sulfate can be given intramuscularly and intravenously and is available for topical use (see article by Lio & Kaye on topical antibacterial agents elsewhere in this issue). Polymyxin B has also been used intrathecally and intraventricularly for central nervous system infections.

Mechanism of Action and Antimicrobial Activity

The polymyxins act on the cell wall of gram-negative bacteria by way of three known mechanisms of action. (1) Polymyxins are cationic molecules that electrostatically disrupt bacterial surface membranes by displacing Ca^{2+} and Mg^{2+} ions that stabilize lipopolysaccharide (LPS) molecules. (2) Polymyxins are surface-active amphipathic agents containing both lipophilic and lipophobic groups. They penetrate into cell membranes and interact with phospholipids in the membranes, leading to permeability changes that quickly disrupt cell membranes leading to cell death. (3) Polymyxins also bind to the lipid A portion of endotoxin or LPS molecules and, in animal studies, block many of the biologic effects of endotoxins.[8]

The polymyxins are active against commonly isolated gram-negative aerobic bacilli with the exception of Proteus spp, which are generally very resistant to the polymyxins. In addition, the polymyxins have poor activity against Serratia, Providencia, Burkholderia, Vibrio, Brucella, Helicobacter, Moraxella, Aeromonas, Morganella, and Edwardsiella.[5,9] Fortunately, the polymyxins have retained activity against many drug-resistant gram-negative bacilli, such as P aeruginosa and A baumannii. When tested against colistin sulfate, most gram-negative bacilli are inhibited by 1.0 μg/mL; P aeruginosa strains are more resistant, but most strains are inhibited by 2.0 μg/mL.[9] *Pseudomonas* strains with a minimal inhibitory concentration (MIC) greater than 4.0 μg/mL and *Acinetobacter* strains with a colistin MIC of 2 μg/mL or greater are defined as resistant.[10]

Polymyxins are not active against gram-positive organisms and most anaerobes. Fortunately, resistance of gram-negative bacteria to the polymyxins is uncommon. When resistance is present however, there is complete cross-resistance between the polymyxins. Such resistance of gram-negative bacteria to the polymyxins is usually related to changes in the architecture of LPS molecules in the cell wall that interfere with the interaction between peptides of the polymyxin (which are positively charged) and the LPS molecules (which are negatively charged).[5] Studies have shown less common mechanisms of resistance to polymyxins. For example, one study of colistin-resistant *Pseudomonas* isolates revealed alterations in bacterial cell membrane, including reduced density of LPS molecules, and reduced concentration of Ca^{2+} and Mg^{2+} ions.[1] Interestingly, the emergence of polymyxin-resistant *P aeruginosa* has been linked to the use of nebulized colistimethate in patients who have cystic fibrosis.[2,11] Another recent report showed that efflux pump/potassium channels may mediate resistance in isolates of polymyxin-resistant *Yersinia* spp.[12] The activity of the polymyxins is diminished in the presence of high concentrations of divalent cations such as calcium and magnesium.[1]

Pharmacokinetics

The basic and clinical evaluation of the polymyxins took place many years ago, and reliable pharmacokinetic data are lacking. Furthermore, review articles often do not differentiate forms of polymyxin and often have internally inconsistent data concerning pharmacokinetics, especially blood levels.[13]

When administered orally, none of the polymyxins are absorbed. According to old literature, following intramuscular injection of 2–4 mg/kg polymyxin B, peak serum levels of 1–8 μg/mL were achieved. There is little reliable data on serum levels after IV administration of polymyxin B. A very recent study using 0.5–1.25 mg/kg polymyxin B, given by IV infusions over an hour to critically ill subjects, reported peak plasma concentrations of 2.4–14 μg/mL drawn after at least 2 days of therapy. Serum protein binding was 79%–92%.[14]

When colistimethate was given intramuscularly to adults at a dose of 2.5 mg/kg, a peak serum level of 5–7 μg/mL was achieved. In old reports, the peak serum level following intravenous administration of colistimethate was about 20 μg/mL. The package insert for colistimethate shows peak levels of about 8 μg/mL and 20 μg/mL, respectively, following intramuscular and intravenous administration of 150 mg.

In very limited recent studies, however, following 2 to 3 mg/kg intravenous administration of colistimethate, the peak level of colistin, the active metabolite was only about 2μg/ml (which is much lower than the peak of colistimethate).[15] Because serum protein binding of colistin is about 50%, the peak antibacterial activity in serum of active colistin following administration of recommended doses is borderline at best.[15]

According to past literature, the excretion of polymyxin B and colistin is primarily by glomerular filtration. After the initial dose of polymyxin B (but not colistimethate) there is a 12- to 24-hour lag period before significant amounts of drug are found in the urine. After administration of subsequent doses, the urine levels of both polymyxin B and colistimethate exceed 15 μg/mL for at least 6 hours. In a recent study, less than 1% of infused polymyxin B was recovered unchanged in the urine.[14]

The half-life of polymyxin B in serum is about 4.5 to 6 hours.[16] There is relatively little information available on the serum half-life of colistin (the active antibiotic) following injection of colistimethate. In subjects who have cystic fibrosis, the serum half-lives of colistimethate and colistin were 2 hours and 4 hours, respectively.[15] Half-lives of these agents are prolonged when given to patients who have renal insufficiency. Distribution to the cerebrospinal fluid (CSF), biliary tract, pleural fluid, and joint fluid is poor. However, in one report, the peak CSF levels following the intravenous administration of colistimethate were 25% of the peak serum levels.[17]

Serum levels of the polymyxins are very low following inhalation therapy.[18] The polymyxins are poorly dialyzed and there is minimal hepatic metabolism or biliary excretion.

Pharmacodynamics

Polymyxin B and colistin have rapid bactericidal effect in vitro in a concentration-dependent manner. There is well-described postantibiotic effect (PAE) for *P aeruginosa* with delayed regrowth, as compared with rapid regrowth of MDR *A baumannii* with no PAE because of heteroresistance.[5,19] Because of the potential lack of PAE, three times a day dosing has been suggested by in vitro studies.[20] It has also been suggested that the polymyxins be used in combination with another active drug if there is one. Studies of in vitro synergy have been limited to relatively few organisms. Using colistin-susceptible strains of MDR bacteria, synergism has been demonstrated between a polymyxin and ceftazidime, rifampin, trimethoprim-sulfamethoxazole, imipenem, cefepime, and azithromycin.[21–27]

Toxicity

Dose-related nephrotoxicity is the most common and the most important adverse effect associated with polymyxins. The nephrotoxicity is attributed to direct damage of the cells in the distal convoluted tubules,[28] and is usually reversible after the drug is discontinued.[13,29] Early literature suggested that 10%–30% of subjects who received polymyxins developed reversible renal impairment. However, recent reports indicate that the nephrotoxicity with polymyxins may be less than aminoglycosides.[15] In addition, studies that adjusted for severity of illness and pre-existing renal impairment have found that subjects receiving colistimethate experienced similar rates of nephrotoxicity compared with cohorts receiving carbapenems and other agents for infections caused by *P aeruginosa* and *A baumanii*.[7,30,31] Nephrotoxic effects are enhanced, however, when the polymyxins are used in subjects receiving other nephrotoxic agents.

Dose-related neurotoxicity occurs in approximately 5% of subjects receiving polymyxins, according to more recent literature. There are several manifestations of neurotoxicity: (1) Neuromuscular blockade, which can involve the respiratory musculature and cause apnea and can be potentiated by aminoglycosides;[13,29] (2) Sensory disturbance with perioral paresthesias, parethesias of the tongue, and parethesias of the extremities; and (3) Polyneuropathy, including cranial nerve palsies (diplopia, nystagmus).

Neuromuscular blockade is most likely to occur when the drug is used in excessive doses in patients who have renal failure, or in those who are receiving curariform drugs. When respiratory paralysis occurs, it is necessary to support respiratory function until the effects of the drug wear off. Intravenous calcium may help reverse the respiratory paralysis. Aminoglycosides may potentiate the neurotoxic effects. Other neurotoxic side effects, such as perioral paresthesias, parethesias of the tongue and extremities, and peripheral neuropathy are not uncommon.[4] Toxicity is less likely to occur with colistimethate than with polymyxin B.

Hypersensitivity to polymyxins is unusual, but up to 2% of patients receiving parenteral polymyxins can develop allergic manifestations, including fever, eosinophilia, and rashes.

In general, toxicity is less likely to occur with colistimethate than with polymyxin B. Intraventricular and intrathecal administration of the polymyxins are generally well tolerated.[32] Nebulization may result in bronchoconstriction. A warning has been issued by the FDA against premixing colistimethate too far in advance of nebulization because of one possible drug-related death.[33]

Clinical Indications

In the United States, polymyxin B and colistimethate are approved only for use intravenously (which is preferred) and intramuscularly. However, aerosols and the intrathecal and intraventricular routes have become relatively common.[17,32,34–37]

Polymyxin B is very painful when given intramuscularly, and this route of administration should be avoided. The dosage of polymyxins below are expressed in terms of the polymyxin base. If IM injection is necessary, the usual IM dose is 2.5–3 mg/kg/day in divided doses every 4 to 6 hours. The IV dose is 1.5–2.5 mg/kg/day by continuous IV infusion or in divided doses every 12 hours over a period of 60 to 90 minutes.

For treatment of gram-negative bacillary central nervous system infection, the Infectious Diseases Society of America guidelines recommend a daily dose of 5 mg polymyxin B intraventricularly.[38] Polymyxin B has been given intrathecally in doses of 5–10 mg/day for the initial 3 days of therapy and then every other day until cultures are negative.

The recommended dosage of colistimethate in adults who have normal renal function is 2.5–5 mg/kg (depending on the severity of infection) each day intramuscularly or intravenously in two to four divided doses. The dose should be based on ideal body weight and should not exceed 300 mg/day. Doses must be decreased in patients who have impaired renal function to avoid drug accumulation and toxicity. When given intravenously, colistimethate is administered over 3 to 5 minutes. Administration of doses as high as 8 mg/kg/day has been reported recently.[39] The question has been raised about the use of colistimethate as a single daily dose to theoretically lower the risk of toxicity, but clinical validation is lacking and, for reasons stated above, is probably not a good idea.

For treatment of central nervous system infection, the Infectious Diseases Society of America guidelines suggest an intraventricular dose of 10 mg of colistimethate.[38] The same dose would presumably be used intrathecally.

Colistin sulfate has been used orally for intestinal decontamination. The oral preparation is not available in the United States.

Inhalation therapy with aerosolized colistimethate has been used with varying success to treat colonization or infection of the bronchial system, especially with MDR *P aeruginosa*, in patients who have cystic fibrosis.[36,37] Systemic blood levels are not achieved with inhalation therapy. The usual dose in adults is 80 mg every 12 hours. Up to 160 mg every 8 hours has been used.

Most of the literature on the use of the polymyxins for parenteral therapy is old. In recent years, colistimethate has been used parenterally to treat systemic infections caused by MDR gram-negative bacilli, mainly ventilator-associated pneumonia.[1,5,13,17,29,30,32,34–37,39,40] In contrast with past experience, recent reports claim little in the way of nephrotoxicity or neurotoxicity.[1,4,5,13,17,29,30,32,34–37,39,40] However, more modern-day experience is necessary before colistimethate can be considered a relatively nontoxic systemic agent. Reports of use of polymyxin B in modern medicine have been sparse.

Recent observations have indicated that emergence of polymyxin resistance in *P aeruginosa, K pneumoniae*, and *A baumannii* is associated with the use of this class of agents.[2,11,41]

Until more clinical data become available, parenteral polymyxin B and colistimethate should be reserved for use only when no other less toxic or potentially more effective drug can be used.

RIFAMPIN AND RIFAXIMIN

Rifamycins are a group of broad-spectrum antibiotics that interfere with bacterial DNA-dependent RNA polymerase and are active against mycobacteria and various gram-positive and gram-negative organisms. This section focuses on the use of rifampin against nonmycobacterial organisms, and is followed by a discussion of rifaximin, a novel rifamycin derivative that is increasingly used as an enteric antibiotic against traveler's diarrhea[42] and is being evaluated for CDIs.[43]

Rifampin

Rifampin, or rifampicin, the prototypical rifamycin, was first synthesized in 1965 from a fermentation product of *Streptomyces mediterranei*. It kills proliferating extracellular organisms, intracellular mycobacteria, and semidormant subpopulations of mycobacteria that reside in tissues.[44]

Although rifampin is best known for its antimycobacterial activity, the drug is highly active against both coagulase-positive and -negative staphylococci and other gram-positive cocci, such as *S pyogenes* and *S pneumoniae*. Enterococci are only moderately susceptible. Among gram-negative organisms, *N meningitidis, N gonorrhoeae,* and *Hemophilus influenzae* are the most susceptible.

In addition to its broad spectrum of activity, rifampin has interesting pharmacokinetic properties and has the unusual ability to enter cells and mediate antibacterial activity at intracellular sites.[45]

Mechanism of action and antimicrobial activity

Rifampin acts by inhibiting DNA-dependent RNA polymerase after binding to the beta subunit of the enzyme.[46] This interaction interferes with protein synthesis by preventing chain initiation. Rifampin is usually bactericidal, but may be bacteriostatic depending on the organism and the drug concentration. Hence, rifampin demonstrates concentration-dependent killing and has a very long PAE.[47] Those organisms inhibited by 1.0 μg/mL or less are considered to be susceptible to rifampin, those inhibited by 2.0 μg/mL are intermediate, and those with a MIC of 4.0 μg/mL or more are resistant.[10]

Most gram-positive cocci (staphylococci and streptococci) are highly susceptible to rifampin (MICs <1 μg/mL); enterococci, which are only moderately sensitive, are an important exception.[48,49]

Meningococci, gonococci, and *H influenzae* are susceptible to rifampin. In contrast, most gram-negative bacilli are intrinsically resistant to rifampin.

Acquired resistance to rifampin occurs rapidly when it is inappropriately used as monotherapy and often develops by mutations in the gene (*rpoB*) encoding the beta subunit of DNA-dependent RNA polymerase. Additionally, resistance can be mediated by alterations in membrane permeability.[50]

The effects of combining rifampin with other antibiotics remain a confusing area due to conflicting in vitro and in vivo data. When rifampin is added to other bactericidal agents, the effect may be synergistic, additive, indifferent, or antagonistic depending on the drugs, their concentrations, the organisms being studied, and the model. Examples of some of the results follow.

Addition of rifampin to penicillinase-resistant penicillins in vitro inhibited the bactericidal activity of the penicillins against S aureus.[51] In a rabbit model of S aureus endocarditis, the combination of a penicillinase-resistant penicillin and rifampin was synergistic for some strains and indifferent or antagonistic for other strains.[52] The addition of rifampin to vancomycin or to vancomycin-plus-gentamicin improved the effectiveness of therapy in a rabbit model of Staphylococcus epidermidis endocarditis.[53] Similarly, substantial improvements in cure rates for S epidermidis prosthetic valve endocarditis were achieved by adding rifampin, gentamicin, or both, to vancomycin.[54]

Experimental meningitis studies with limited number of strains of pneumococci have demonstrated that addition of rifampin to vancomycin or ceftriaxone may have differing effects on the rate of killing of pneumococci in CSF. One study showed a beneficial effect.[55] In contrast, another study demonstrated no increase in killing rate against pneumococci when rifampin was added to vancomycin.[56] Interestingly, an in vitro study showed that the addition of rifampin to ceftriaxone resulted in a marked decrease in killing rates of ceftriaxone-susceptible pneumococci, compared with ceftriaxone alone.[57]

Synergism has been demonstrated between colistin and rifampin in vitro and in vivo against certain MDR strains of bacteria.[22,24,26,58]

Pharmacokinetics

Rifampin is well absorbed when given orally with peak serum concentrations of 7 to 10 µg/mL following a dose of 600 mg. Food interferes with enteric absorption and rifampin should therefore be administered on an empty stomach. An intravenous preparation is available when the oral route cannot be used. Dosing is identical for the oral and intravenous preparations.

Rifampin is widely distributed into tissues and different compartments despite being 80% protein-bound. It penetrates well into body fluids, achieving therapeutic levels in saliva, bile, bone, pleural fluid, prostate, and CSF. Moreover, rifampin readily enters phagocytic cells and can kill microorganisms in the cells.

Rifampin undergoes a multistep process of elimination. It is first de-acetylated in the liver and then cleared by hepatic metabolism and biliary excretion. The half-life of rifampin is 2 to 5 hours, which can be prolonged by hepatic disease and shortened by repeated dosing due to rifampin's propensity to induce its own metabolism by way of the P450 enzymes. Rifampin does not need dose-adjustment in the setting of renal insufficiency.

Toxicity

With administration of rifampin, urine and sweat often develop an orange tinge and soft contact lenses may be stained. This adverse effect of discoloring body fluids is almost universal and may be used as a surrogate marker of adherence. A flulike syndrome can occur in up to 5% of patients who have had prolonged intermittent use of rifampin. Rash and gastrointestinal adverse effects (eg, nausea, vomiting, diarrhea, heartburn) may occur in up to 5% of patients. Abnormal liver function tests are common but frank hepatitis is uncommon (<1%), especially with short courses used for nonmycobacterial infections.

The potential for rifampin to induce hepatic microsomal enzymes can cause multiple drug–drug interactions;[59] such interactions can occur with oral contraceptives, cyclosporine, digoxin, fluconazole, sulfonylureas, theophylline, thyroxine, warfarin, antipsychotics[60] and antiretroviral agents.[61]

Clinical indications

Rifampin should always be coupled with another bacterioactive agent and should never be used as monotherapy, except when used for chemoprophylaxis of meningococcal and *H influenzae* infections.[62,63] The course of chemoprophylaxis is always short and is designed to eradicate the organism from the nasopharynx. Furthermore, rifampin is now seldom used to prevent *H influenzae* infections because of decreased rates of the infection due to widespread use of the *H influenzae* vaccine.

Rifampin is administered in a dose of 10 mg/kg (not to exceed 600 mg) in patients at least 1 month of age, twice a day for 2 days for prevention of meningococcal disease; this generally has had an efficacy of more than 90%. However, rifampin has several shortcomings, including nasopharyngeal eradication rates of only about 70%–80% in some studies, adverse effects, and the necessity for multiple doses over 2 days. Moreover, resistance to rifampin in isolates of *N meningitidis* in the United States is increasingly detected (up to 10%–27% of *N meningitidis* isolates).[64,65] Ciprofloxacin may be more effective in eradicating meningococci.[66] To protect children under 4 years of age who have been incompletely immunized against *H influenzae* type B, all household contacts who have been in contact with a case of severe infection should receive rifampin prophylaxis. The dose in adults is 600 mg twice daily for 2 days.

Rifampin has been used in combination with other nonmycobacterial agents in some limited situations, including (1) Staphylococcal infections, especially on foreign bodies (eg, prosthetic valve endocarditis);[67] (2) Pneumococcal meningitis in which corticosteroids are being given in addition to vancomycin and a third generation cephalosporin; and (3) As combination therapy for certain zoonoses, such as Brucellosis, Q fever, Bartonellosis and Rhodococcus infections.[68]

Staphylococcal infection In an attempt to achieve higher rates of cure, rifampin has been increasingly used by some in combination with standard antistaphylococcal therapy for severe infections caused by staphylococci. Rifampin has several properties that are theoretically advantageous in the treatment of complicated staphylococcal infections: (1) Rifampin is bactericidal against *S aureus*, (2) Rifampin achieves high intracellular levels, and (3) Rifampin can penetrate biofilms.[69]

Even though rifampin has these desirable characteristics, data to support the practice of combining rifampin and another antistaphylococcal agent are limited and are typically based on small clinical studies or animal and in vitro investigations. A recent meta-analysis concluded that many animal studies showed a microbiologic benefit of adjunctive rifampin use, particularly in osteomyelitis and infected foreign body infection models.[67] Few human studies have adequately addressed the role of adjunctive rifampin therapy. Adjunctive therapy seems most promising for the treatment of osteomyelitis and prosthetic device-related infections, although studies typically have been underpowered and benefits were not always seen.[67]

A substantial improvement in cure rates for *S epidermidis* prosthetic valve endocarditis was reported in a noncontrolled study by adding rifampin, gentamicin, or both, to vancomycin.[54] As a result of this study and in vitro and animal studies, the American Heart Association recommends the addition of 300 mg rifampin orally every 8 hours for treatment of *S epidermidis* prosthetic valve endocarditis.[70]

Because of the excellent penetration of rifampin into tissues and organ spaces, there is a general enthusiasm for including rifampin in regimens when treating staphylococcal infections in the presence of abscesses or foreign bodies.

Despite the benefit of adding rifampin to the regimen in animal models of *S aureus* osteomyelitis,[71] clinical studies have not been convincing.[72] However, in the presence of a foreign body, it is reasonable to add rifampin.

Rifampin alone or in combination with another drug (eg, trimethoprim-sulfamethoxazole) has been used to eradicate nasal carriage of *S aureus*, including methicillin-resistant strains (MRSA).[73,74] These combinations have also been used for oral treatment of non–life-threatening MRSA infections.

Pneumococcal meningitis Despite high in vitro susceptibility against *S pneumoniae*, rifampin should never be used alone to treat pneumococcal meningitis. When the infecting organism is highly resistant to ceftriaxone and cefotaxime but is rifampin-susceptible, combination therapy with vancomycin plus ceftriaxone plus rifampin might be effective.[55] In these circumstances, vancomycin concentrations should be maximized to ensure adequate CNS penetration. Steroid therapy can reduce antimicrobial penetration into CSF by decreasing inflammation; in animal models, steroid therapy has been associated with failure of cephalosporin or vancomycin monotherapy, although this has not been observed in all experimental studies. For these reasons the Infectious Disease Society of America recommends addition of rifampin to the vancomycin, third generation cephalosporin, and dexamethasone regimen used for pneumococcal meningitis.[38]

Despite these recommendations, there are no reliable clinical data concerning results of the addition of rifampin to vancomycin and/or a third-generation cephalosporin in subjects who have pneumococcal meningitis. Because there are conflicting results of the benefits of rifampin in animal model and in vitro studies, it has been suggested that rifampin be used for patients in whom the pneumococcal isolate is sensitive to rifampin in vitro and who are not responding appropriately to standard therapy.

Brucellosis Rifampin in combination with doxycycline plus and minus an aminoglycoside has been shown to have better cure rates for brucellosis than other antibiotic combinations in recent meta-analyses.[75,76]

Rifaximin

Rifaximin is a new enteric antibiotic that is only available as an oral preparation. Like other rifamycins, rifaximin binds the beta subunit of the DNA-dependent RNA polymerase, and inhibits RNA synthesis.[77] Unlike rifampicin, however, rifaximin acts exclusively in the gastrointestinal tract and is poorly absorbed due to the presence of a pyridoimidazole moiety.

Spectrum of activity

Rifaximin is active against most gram-positive organisms, including *C difficile* and essentially all enteric gram-negative pathogens, including *E coli, H pylori, Y enterocolitica,* and *Shigella* spp.[78]

Despite its broad antibiotic spectrum, rifaximin appears to have little impact on normal gastrointestinal flora.[79] In one study, there was an initial decrease in the gastrointestinal flora following rifaximin administration, followed by rapid normalization of enteric flora within the month.[80] Development of resistance to rifaximin appears to occur with low frequency.[81]

Adverse effects

Rifaximin is generally well tolerated, with similar rates of adverse effects in subjects receiving comparator drugs and placebos.[82–84] Headache was more common in one study. Rifaximin is not expected to have drug–drug interactions via the CYP 450 system because it is not systemically absorbed.[85]

Clinical indications

Rifaximin is currently approved for the treatment of traveler's diarrhea caused by noninvasive strains of E coli. Three studies showed rifaximin to be effective in shortening the duration of diarrhea. The approved dosage is 200 mg three times per day for 3 days.

Rifaximin is also being considered in the therapy for C difficile infections.[43,86,87] One study in the hamster model showed oral rifaximin to be as effective, if not more effective, than oral vancomycin for two standard strains of C difficile.[88] Several treatment strategies with rifaximin have shown positive outcomes in refractory C difficile infections, including combination therapy of vancomycin and rifaximin,[89] drug-cycling regimen of vancomycin and rifaximin,and even a strategy of sequential monotherapy of vancomycin and rifaximin.[90]

In one small case series, eight subjects who had recurrent symptoms of C difficile infection received sequential therapy of oral vancomycin and then rifaximin.[90] At the end of the study, all but one subject remained symptom free. Unfortunately, the study also reported that the rifaximin MIC for C difficile isolates recovered after therapy (>256 µg/mL) was much higher than the MIC for isolates recovered before therapy (0.0078 µg/mL). The use of rifaximin for C difficile infections remains off-label and caution should be exercised because drug resistance was clearly demonstrated after rifaximin use in the study.

AMINOGLYCOSIDES

The aminoglycosides are a class of bactericidal antibiotics characterized by the presence of a six-carbon aminocyclitol ring, covalently bonded to multiple amino sugar groups. Aminoglycosides were once widely used as primary agents in the therapy of gram-negative bacillary infections. However, because of their toxicity and the availability of newer effective agents, systemic aminoglycosides have been primarily relegated to a role as companion drugs either to broaden coverage against gram-negative aerobic bacilli or to provide synergistic killing against gram-positive cocci or certain gram-negative bacilli. Now, because of the emergence of MDR gram-negative bacilli, the aminoglycosides, along with the polymyxins, may become antibiotics of last resort.[91]

The major change in the use of aminoglycosides has been a trend toward single daily dosage, even though this is not an FDA-approved dosing regimen. Gentamicin, the most widely administered and the most studied of the aminoglycosides, is the prototype for our discussion.

Mechanism of Action and Antimicrobial Activity

The aminoglycosides act in part by impairing bacterial protein synthesis through irreversible binding to the 30S subunit of the bacterial ribosome. They are rapidly bactericidal against a broad range of aerobic gram-negative bacilli (including P aeruginosa), but lack activity against anaerobes. Although there is activity against some gram-positive aerobic cocci, it is unreliable. The aminoglycosides are generally used against gram-positive cocci such as enterococci and staphylococci in combination with beta-lactam antibiotics and vancomycin to achieve synergistic bactericidal activity.

This clinical application of drug synergy is based primarily on in vitro and animal studies because there are no comparative trials showing better cure rates with addition of an aminoglycoside.[92] Synergy is lacking or variable when aminoglycosides are combined with newer drugs such as daptomycin, quinupristin-dalfopristin, or linezolid.[93]

Acquired resistance to the aminoglycosides is usually mediated by bacterial elaboration of aminoglycoside-inactivating enzymes. These enzymes are widely distributed in both gram-positive and gram-negative bacteria, and usually are plasmid-mediated.[94] Amikacin is the most likely of all aminoglycosides to be effective against MDR gram-negative bacilli because amikacin only has one locus that is susceptible to aminoglycoside-inactivating enzymes compared with six susceptible loci on gentamicin and tobramycin.[95,96]

Among gram-positive cocci, the most clinically significant resistance occurs in enterococci, where the synergistic killing activity of aminoglycosides is required for a high cure rate of endocarditis. Although all enterococci are intrinsically resistant to low concentrations of aminoglycosides, the clinical problem arises with high level gentamicin resistant (HLGR) enterococci.[70] HLGR enterococci are resistant to all other aminoglycosides in clinical use in the United States, with the possible exception of streptomycin, and do not demonstrate synergistic killing of enterococci when aminoglycosides are combined with penicillin or vancomycin.[70] Detection of HLGR requires either special susceptibility wells or screening plates with high concentrations of gentamicin or streptomycin (eg, ≥ 500 µg/mL gentamicin; ≥ 1000µg/ml streptomycin).

The synergistic killing effect of beta-lactam antibiotics and aminoglycosides has been demonstrated with multiple aerobic gram-negative bacilli and gram-positive cocci and in multiple animal models. In uncontrolled clinical studies, synergistic activity has been demonstrated to be important in the treatment of native valve endocarditis caused by enterococci and in prosthetic valve endocarditis due to S epidermidis.[70] There is a lack of clinical studies to clearly demonstrate benefits of drug synergy with aminoglycosides in serious P aeruginosa infections, and in infections caused by gram-negative bacilli in neutropenic patients. The aminoglycosides remain among the most active antibiotics against P aeruginosa.[94]

Pharmacokinetics

Aminoglycosides are poorly absorbed orally. After intravenous infusion of 1.7 mg/kg gentamicin (every 8 hour dosage), peak serum levels (C_{max}) are 4 to10 µg/mL. After infusion of 5 mg/kg (once daily dosage), peak levels are about 20 µg/mL serum. The half-life of all of the aminoglycosides is about 2 to 3 hours. Protein binding is low (<10%) and, because the agents are water soluble, they are distributed in the intravascular space and into interstitial fluid. The drugs diffuse into synovial, pleural, and peritoneal fluids, but penetration into CSF and bile is poor.

In general, in the absence of large effusions and edema, the volume of distribution is low. Increases in the volume of distribution tend to decrease the C_{max} and area under the serum-concentration-time curve (AUC), and increases in clearance tend to decrease the AUC. For example, the volume of distribution tends to be elevated and peak serum levels decreased in patients who have large effusions, fever, burns, or congestive heart failure and in critically ill patients.[97] Excretion of aminoglycosides is primarily by glomerular filtration; clearance is decreased with renal insufficiency and increased in children, in pregnancy and in patients who have cystic fibrosis.

Pharmacodynamics

The aminoglycosides show the following well-studied pharmacodynamic properties: (1) Concentration-dependent killing, (2) PAE, and (3) Postantibiotic leucocyte enhancement.

Concentration-dependent killing

Bacterial killing by aminoglycosides in vitro is concentration-dependent.[94] In vivo, higher doses of the drug not only increase the rate of reduction of bacteria, but also the length of time of drug exposure to bactericidal concentrations as measured by the AUC. In animal studies, aminoglycoside efficacy is correlated with the ratio of C_{max} to MIC of the infecting organism and also with the AUC. In animal studies, effective dosing regimens for concentration-dependent antibiotics require that either the 24-hour AUC/MIC be 80 to100 against gram-negative bacilli or the C_{max}/MIC of the causative pathogen be 8 to10.[98]

Some clinical studies have demonstrated a relationship between peak aminoglycoside concentrations and response to therapy. For concentration-dependent drugs, such as aminoglycosides, giving the total daily dose once every 24 hours rather than smaller divided doses would maximize the C_{max} and possibly allow for comparable or better efficacy at greater convenience and lower cost. A C_{max}/MIC of 10 to 12 appears to be the optimal ratio to ensure clinical response.[94] To achieve this ratio with single daily dose gentamicin, the MIC must be 2μg/ml or less and preferably 1μg/ml or less.

PAE

Aminoglycoside antibiotics have a PAE for both staphylococci and gram-negative bacilli, meaning that suppression of bacterial growth persists despite concentrations of antibiotic below the MIC.[94,99,100] This permits longer intervals before another dose of aminoglycoside is given.

Postantibiotic leucocyte enhancement

Enhanced phagocytosis of aminoglycoside-exposed bacteria by host leukocytes has also been observed in vitro.[101] This phenomenon has been referred to as postantibiotic leukocyte enhancement (PALE). The absence of PALE may help explain the decreased efficacy of once-daily dosing that has been described in neutropenic animals as compared with nonneutropenic animals.[102]

The antibacterial effects of aminoglycosides can be impaired in a couple of settings. First, an acidic or an anaerobic environment is known to impair the activity of aminoglycosides.[103–105] Second, adaptive resistance refers to the phenomenon of transient reduction in rate of bacterial killing by an antibiotic following pre-exposure to that drug.[106] Adaptive resistance to aminoglycoside agents has been observed principally in *P aeruginosa*, but also in other gram-negative bacilli and more recently in staphylococci.[107,108] Once-daily dosing may circumvent the possibility of adaptive resistance through the provision of a drug-free interval.[94]

Toxicity

The major adverse effects of the aminoglycosides are nephrotoxicity and oto-vestibular toxicity. The aminoglycosides mediate toxic damage to the proximal convoluted tubules in the kidneys, and to the cochlear and vestibular bodies of the inner ear.[91,94] In addition, aminoglycosides can cause neuromuscular blockade due to interference of neurotransmission at neuromuscular junctions.[94] The uptake of aminoglycosides by renal cortical cells appears to be a saturable process.[91,94,109] Once proximal tubular cells are saturated with aminoglycoside, the higher peak serum concentrations seen with once-daily dosing should not cause greater intracellular accumulation of drug than is seen with multiple lower doses. In fact, renal cortical accumulation of gentamicin in rodents is lower following once-daily dosing regimens than after multiple daily doses, and greater increases in serum creatinine are seen with multiple-daily dosing regimens.[110]

Correlation of increased renal cortical accumulation of aminoglycosides with dosing frequency rather than with peak serum concentrations has been demonstrated in a cohort of human subjects undergoing nephrectomy for cancer.[109] There have been many clinical studies of nephrotoxicity of aminoglycosides. A recent review compiled a summary of the results of meta-analyses of once-daily dosing of aminoglycosides versus multiple-daily dosing.[98] Although some of these reported a decrease in nephrotoxicity with once-daily dosing, most of the meta-analyses demonstrated no significant decrease in nephrotoxicity. However, once-daily administration of aminoglycoside was less likely to result in nephrotoxicity than twice-daily administration in the only randomized double-blind study of aminoglycoside use.[111]

Increased nephrotoxicity has been observed in the elderly; in patients who have elevated trough levels; with prolonged use; in patients who have diabetes mellitus; with concurrent use of vancomycin, loop diuretics, cyclosporine, and cisplatin; and when the drug is administered at time of rest as opposed to activity.[111–114]

Aminoglycoside therapy may result in both vestibular and cochlear toxicity.[115] In rats (but not in guinea pigs), gentamicin uptake into perilymph, endolymph, and inner ear tissues appears to be a saturable process, as in the kidney.[116] It is unknown whether gentamicin uptake is a saturable process in humans and it is unclear whether aminoglycoside accumulation in the inner ear predicts ototoxicity.[116]

Risk of ototoxicity has been associated with elevated trough levels of aminoglycoside, although some investigators have found no association between drug levels and ototoxicity after controlling for age.[117,118] Nonetheless, the suggestion that aminoglycoside uptake into inner ear fluids is saturable has raised the possibility that once-daily dosing of aminoglycosides may decrease ototoxicity. However, most published meta-analyses have reported no difference in ototoxicity between once- and multiple-daily dosing.[98]

Clinical Indications

The most common indication for aminoglycosides is combination therapy with other antimicrobial agents for serious gram-negative bacillary infections. In addition, the aminoglycosides are important drugs in the treatment of mycobacterial infections and in infections caused by less common pathogens, such as *Yersinia pestis*, *Brucella* spp, and *Francisella tularensis*.

The aminoglycosides are also used in combination with cell-wall–active antibiotics to provide synergistic bactericidal activity in treatment of serious gram-positive coccal infections such as staphylococcal, enterococcal, and streptococcal endocarditis.[70]

The major change in therapy with aminoglycosides has been the increasing use of single daily dosage for treatment of gram-negative bacillary infections versus divided daily doses. For example, the daily dose of gentamicin is usually 5 mg/kg. It can be given as 5 mg/kg in one single daily IV dose over 30 to 60 minutes or as 1.7 mg/kg IM or IV every 8 hours in gram-negative meningitis (FDA approved). Once-daily dosing should be performed in a manner that ensures a high C_{max}/MIC ratio for the pathogen being treated and ensures that trough levels are low enough to minimize toxicity and permit the loss of adaptive resistance. Maximizing concentrations of aminoglycosides by using single daily dosing optimizes the rate and extent of bactericidal activity and results in lower residual bacterial counts and longer intervals before significant regrowth occurs.

The potential for increased efficacy with once-daily aminoglycoside dosing has been evaluated in a multitude of randomized clinical trials. In general, these individual trials have lacked sufficient power to determine whether observed differences in efficacy between once-daily and multiple-daily dosage regimens were due to chance alone. Therefore, meta-analysis has been used to synthesize the data contained in these multiple studies. Most meta-analyses demonstrated an improvement (albeit small) in the clinical efficacy of once-daily aminoglycoside dosing.[98]

Overall, in vitro, animal, and existing clinical data suggest that once-daily administration of aminoglycosides may be more efficacious and less nephrotoxic, or at least not more nephrotoxic, than multiple-daily dosing. Giving the total 24-hour dose as a single dose, rather than in smaller divided doses, and using extended dosing intervals has now become the standard for use in gram-negative bacillary infections in many clinical settings.[98] This strategy may be especially appropriate for treatment of infections caused by borderline susceptible pathogens (eg, P aeruginosa), with MICs that are close to the breakpoint.[119]

The dosages of once-daily administration of gentamicin, netilmicin, and tobramycin have varied from 4–7 mg/kg/day in clinical trials.[119] A starting dose of 5 mg/kg has been suggested for adults 30 to 60 years of age with doses of 6 mg/kg for adults below 30 years and 4 mg/kg for those over 60.[98] Because of patient-to-patient variability, 4 mg/kg dosing does not always ensure sufficiently high peak concentrations to provide optimal activity against organisms such as P aeruginosa.[119] The use of 7 mg/kg dosing of gentamicin in 2148 adult inpatients was associated with only 27 incidents of nephrotoxicity and 3 of vestibulotoxicity; however, the median duration of therapy was only 3 days.[119] It has been suggested that the initial once-daily doses should be 7 mg/kg for gentamicin and tobramycin and 15 mg/kg for amikacin in the critically ill; the dose is then tapered to yield a C_{max}/MIC greater than or equal to 10.[94] Other investigators have suggested a dose of 5 mg/kg for gentamicin, which is more in line with the FDA-approved daily dosage.[91]

Two different approaches have been suggested to treat patients who have impaired renal function: reduction of daily drug dosage, and increase in dosing interval beyond 24 hours.[119,120] Intuitively, it seems most reasonable to give daily doses that will yield peak serum levels that result in an appropriate C_{max} and to stop administration as soon as feasible. Regardless of the approach used, vigilant monitoring of aminoglycoside serum levels is of utmost importance when renal function is decreased.

The doses of aminoglycosides used for synergistic bactericidal activity in the treatment of gram-positive coccal endocarditis have been lower than those used for serious gram-negative infections (target serum peak level of gentamicin 3 μg/mL). The most compelling data on the need for synergistic bactericidal activity requiring aminoglycosides concern enterococcal endocarditis. Although a significant PAE has been demonstrated against enterococci with aminoglycoside/beta-lactam combinations in vitro, no PAE was demonstrated in an animal model of enterococcal endocarditis.[121] Animal models of enterococcal endocarditis using single daily doses of aminoglycosides compared with 8-hour doses have yielded conflicting results.[70] The current recommendations from the American Heart Association state that until more data demonstrate that once-daily dosing of an aminoglycoside is as effective as multiple-daily dosing, gentamicin or streptomycin should be administered in multiple divided doses rather than a daily single dose to patients who have enterococcal endocarditis.[70]

Aminoglycoside antibiotics have been used in the treatment of pulmonary exacerbations in patients who have cystic fibrosis and P aeruginosa colonization.[122–125] Antibiotic treatment of such exacerbations is typically prolonged, and often occurs in the home setting. Once-daily dosing for home therapy has obvious advantages. Evidence also suggests that inhaled tobramycin can reduce infective exacerbations and other health care costs in cystic fibrosis patients.[126–128] Debate continues, however, over whether aminoglycoside therapy significantly contributes to the long-term risk of nephrotoxicity in cystic fibrosis patients.[129]

Patients who have cystic fibrosis clear aminoglycosides at an increased rate.[130] Higher doses of aminoglycosides (eg, tobramycin at doses up to 15 mg/kg/d) once daily have been used successfully with little or no increase in nephrotoxicity,[131–136] although transient ototoxicity has been associated with these doses.[132]

Several different methods of monitoring once-daily aminoglycoside dosing have been suggested. Some investigators have suggested monitoring trough concentrations only, with dose adjustments for troughs greater than 2 μg/mL.[137,138] However, this approach does not allow clinicians to appreciate underdosage of drug, and trough levels of 2 μg/mL are too high and indicate reduced clearance with once-daily dosing.

Another proposed approach to monitoring of once-daily dosage is with a drug level taken 6 to14 hours after infusion and adjusting the doses according to a nomogram.[119,139,140] Suboptimal peaks are not recognized by this method. A third approach measures two levels (at 0.5–1 h and 6–14 h) and calculates the AUC.[141–143]

It has been proposed that aminoglycoside levels need not be measured with once-daily dosing in patients who have ClCr greater than 60 mL/min who receive fewer than 5 days of therapy.[119,144] However, levels should be checked in patients at increased risk for toxicity or clinical failure, such as the elderly, those receiving other nephrotoxic drugs, those with severe infections, or those expected to require longer than 5 days of treatment. In patients on long-term therapy, aminoglycoside levels should be measured weekly as long as the serum creatinine is stable.[119,144]

SUMMARY

This article reviews three classes of antibacterial agents that are uncommonly used in bacterial infections (other than mycobacterial infections) and therefore can be thought of as special-use agents. The polymyxins are reserved for gram-negative bacilli that are resistant to virtually all other classes of drugs. Rifampin is used therapeutically, mainly as a companion drug in treatment of refractory gram-positive coccal infections, especially involving foreign bodies. Rifaximin is a new rifamycin that is a strict enteric antibiotic approved for use for treatment of traveler's diarrhea and is showing promise as a possible agent for refractory *C difficile* infections. The aminoglycosides are used mainly as companion drugs for the therapy of resistant gram-negative bacillary infection and for gram-positive coccal endocarditis. The major change in use of aminoglycosides has been a shift to once-daily dosing in many situations.

REFERENCES

1. Hermsen ED, Sullivan CJ, Rotschafer JC. Polymyxins: pharmacology, pharmacokinetics, pharmacodynamics, and clinical applications. Infect Dis Clin North Am 2003;17(3):545–62.
2. Li J, Turnidge J, Milne R, et al. In vitro pharmacodynamic properties of colistin and colistin methanesulfonate against *Pseudomonas aeruginosa* isolates from patients with cystic fibrosis. Antimicrob Agents Chemother 2001;45(3):781–5.
3. Kwa A, Kasiakou SK, Tam VH, et al. Polymyxin B: similarities to and differences from colistin (polymyxin E). Expert Rev Anti Infect Ther 2007;5(5):811–21.
4. Falagas ME, Kasiakou SK. Toxicity of polymyxins: a systematic review of the evidence from old and recent studies. Crit Care 2006;10(1):R27.
5. Zavascki AP, Goldani LZ, Li J, et al. Polymyxin B for the treatment of multidrug-resistant pathogens: a critical review. J Antimicrob Chemother 2007;60(6): 1206–15.

6. Falagas ME, Rafailidis PI. Re-emergence of colistin in today's world of multidrug-resistant organisms: personal perspectives. Expert Opin Investig Drugs 2008; 17(7):973–81.

7. Reina R, Estenssoro E, Saenz G, et al. Safety and efficacy of colistin in acinetobacter and pseudomonas infections: a prospective cohort study. Intensive Care Med 2005;31(8):1058–65.

8. From AH, Fong JS, Good RA. Polymyxin B sulfate modification of bacterial endotoxin: effects on the development of endotoxin shock in dogs. Infect Immun 1979;23(3):660–4.

9. Gales AC, Reis AO, Jones RN. Contemporary assessment of antimicrobial susceptibility testing methods for polymyxin B and colistin: review of available interpretative criteria and quality control guidelines. J Clin Microbiol 2001; 39(1):183–90.

10. Clinical and Laboratory Standards Institute. Performance standards for antimicrobial susceptibility testing. Wayne (PA): Clinical and Laboratory Standards Institute (CLSI); 2008.

11. Livermore DM. Multiple mechanisms of antimicrobial resistance in *Pseudomonas aeruginosa*: our worst nightmare? Clin Infect Dis 2002;34(5):634–40.

12. Bengoechea JA, Skurnik M. Temperature-regulated efflux pump/potassium antiporter system mediates resistance to cationic antimicrobial peptides in Yersinia. Mol Microbiol 2000;37(1):67–80.

13. Evans ME, Feola DJ, Rapp RP. Polymyxin B sulfate and colistin: old antibiotics for emerging multiresistant gram-negative bacteria. Ann Pharmacother 1999; 33(9):960–7.

14. Zavascki AP, Goldani LZ, Cao G, et al. Pharmacokinetics of intravenous polymyxin B in critically ill patients. Clin Infect Dis 2008;47(10):1298–304.

15. Nation RL, Li J. Optimizing use of colistin and polymyxin B in the critically ill. Semin Respir Crit Care Med 2007;28(6):604–14.

16. Reed MD, Stern RC, O'Riordan MA, et al. The pharmacokinetics of colistin in patients with cystic fibrosis. J Clin Pharmacol 2001;41(6):645–54.

17. Jimenez-Mejias ME, Pichardo-Guerrero C, Marquez-Rivas FJ, et al. Cerebrospinal fluid penetration and pharmacokinetic/pharmacodynamic parameters of intravenously administered colistin in a case of multidrug-resistant *Acinetobacter baumannii* meningitis. Eur J Clin Microbiol Infect Dis 2002;21(3):212–4.

18. Ratjen F, Rietschel E, Kasel D, et al. Pharmacokinetics of inhaled colistin in patients with cystic fibrosis. J Antimicrob Chemother 2006;57(2):306–11.

19. Owen RJ, Li J, Nation RL, et al. In vitro pharmacodynamics of colistin against *Acinetobacter baumannii* clinical isolates. J Antimicrob Chemother 2007;59(3):473–7.

20. Bergen PJ, Li J, Nation RL, et al. Comparison of once-, twice- and thrice-daily dosing of colistin on antibacterial effect and emergence of resistance: studies with *Pseudomonas aeruginosa* in an in vitro pharmacodynamic model. J Antimicrob Chemother 2008;61(3):636–42.

21. Gunderson BW, Ibrahim KH, Hovde LB, et al. Synergistic activity of colistin and ceftazidime against multiantibiotic-resistant *Pseudomonas aeruginosa* in an in vitro pharmacodynamic model. Antimicrob Agents Chemother 2003;47(3):905–9.

22. Giamarellos-Bourboulis EJ, Karnesis L, Giamarellou H. Synergy of colistin with rifampin and trimethoprim/sulfamethoxazole on multidrug-resistant *Stenotrophomonas maltophilia*. Diagn Microbiol Infect Dis 2002;44(3):259–63.

23. Rahal JJ. Novel antibiotic combinations against infections with almost completely resistant *Pseudomonas aeruginosa* and *Acinetobacter* species. Clin Infect Dis 2006;43(Suppl 2):S95–9.

24. Chitnis S, Chitnis V, Chitnis DS. In vitro synergistic activity of colistin with amino-glycosides, beta-lactams and rifampin against multidrug-resistant gram-negative bacteria. J Chemother 2007;19(2):226–9.

25. Petrosillo N, Ioannidou E, Falagas ME. Colistin monotherapy vs. combination therapy: evidence from microbiological, animal and clinical studies. Clin Microbiol Infect 2008;14(9):816–27.

26. Song JY, Lee J, Heo JY, et al. Colistin and rifampicin combination in the treatment of ventilator-associated pneumonia caused by carbapenem-resistant Acinetobacter baumannii. Int J Antimicrob Agents 2008;32(3):281–4.

27. Tascini C, Ferranti S, Messina F, et al. In vitro and in vivo synergistic activity of colistin, rifampin, and amikacin against a multiresistant Pseudomonas aeruginosa isolate. Clin Microbiol Infect 2000;6(12):690–1.

28. Wallace SJ, Li J, Nation RL, et al. Subacute toxicity of colistin methanesulfonate in rats: comparison of various intravenous dosage regimens. Antimicrob Agents Chemother 2008;52(3):1159–61.

29. Bosso JA, Liptak CA, Seilheimer DK, et al. Toxicity of colistin in cystic fibrosis patients. DICP 1991;25(11):1168–70.

30. Garnacho-Montero J, Ortiz-Leyba C, Jimenez-Jimenez FJ, et al. Treatment of multidrug-resistant Acinetobacter baumannii ventilator-associated pneumonia (VAP) with intravenous colistin: a comparison with imipenem-susceptible VAP. Clin Infect Dis 2003;36(9):1111–8.

31. Rios FG, Luna CM, Maskin B, et al. Ventilator-associated pneumonia due to colistin susceptible-only microorganisms. Eur Respir J 2007;30(2):307–13.

32. Falagas ME, Bliziotis IA, Tam VH. Intraventricular or intrathecal use of poly-myxins in patients with gram-negative meningitis: a systematic review of the available evidence. Int J Antimicrob Agents 2007;29(1):9–25.

33. FDA Alert [6/28/2007] Colistimethate (marketed as Coly-Mycin M and generic products) information. FDA. Available at: http://www.fda.gov/DrugsSafety/PostmarketDrugSafetyInformationforPatientsandProviders/ucm118080.htm. Accessed July 28, 2009.

34. Segal-Maurer S, Mariano N, Qavi A, et al. Successful treatment of ceftazidime-resistant Klebsiella pneumoniae ventriculitis with intravenous meropenem and intraventricular polymyxin B: case report and review. Clin Infect Dis 1999;28(5):1134–8.

35. Gump WC, Walsh JW. Intrathecal colistin for treatment of highly resistant pseudomonas ventriculitis. Case report and review of the literature. J Neurosurg 2005;102(5):915–7.

36. Linden PK, Paterson DL. Parenteral and inhaled colistin for treatment of ventilator-associated pneumonia. Clin Infect Dis 2006;43(Suppl 2):S89–94.

37. Hartzell JD, Kim AS, Kortepeter MG, et al. Acinetobacter pneumonia: a review. MedGenMed 2007;9(3):4.

38. Tunkel AR, Hartman BJ, Kaplan SL, et al. Practice guidelines for the management of bacterial meningitis. Clin Infect Dis 2004;39(9):1267–84.

39. Beringer P. The clinical use of colistin in patients with cystic fibrosis. Curr Opin Pulm Med 2001;7(6):434–40.

40. Maragakis LL, Perl TM. Acinetobacter baumannii: epidemiology, antimicrobial resistance, and treatment options. Clin Infect Dis 2008;46(8):1254–63.

41. Matthaiou DK, Michalopoulos A, Rafailidis PI, et al. Risk factors associated with the isolation of colistin-resistant gram-negative bacteria: a matched case-control study. Crit Care Med 2008;36(3):807–11.

42. Huang DB, DuPont HL. Rifaximin–a novel antimicrobial for enteric infections. J Infect 2005;50(2):97–106.

43. Nelson R. Antibiotic treatment for *Clostridium difficile*-associated diarrhea in adults. Cochrane Database Syst Rev 2007;(3):CD004610.

44. Paramasivan CN, Sulochana S, Kubendiran G, et al. Bactericidal action of gatifloxacin, rifampin, and isoniazid on logarithmic- and stationary-phase cultures of Mycobacterium tuberculosis. Antimicrob Agents Chemother 2005;49(2):627–31.

45. Cappelletty DM. Evaluation of an intracellular pharmacokinetic in vitro infection model as a tool to assess tuberculosis therapy. Int J Antimicrob Agents 2007; 29(2):212–6.

46. Wehrli W, Knusel F, Schmid K, et al. Interaction of rifamycin with bacterial RNA polymerase. Proc Natl Acad Sci U S A 1968;61(2):667–73.

47. Bundtzen RW, Gerber AU, Cohn DL, et al. Postantibiotic suppression of bacterial growth. Rev Infect Dis 1981;3(1):28–37.

48. Thornsberry C, Hill BC, Swenson JM, et al. Rifampin: spectrum of antibacterial activity. Rev Infect Dis 1983;5(Suppl 3):S412–7.

49. Pohlod DJ, Saravolatz LD, Somerville MM. In-vitro susceptibility of gram-positive cocci to LY146032 teicoplanin, sodium fusidate, vancomycin, and rifampicin. J Antimicrob Chemother 1987;20(2):197–202.

50. Klugman KP, Madhi SA. Emergence of drug resistance. Impact on bacterial meningitis. Infect Dis Clin North Am 1999;13(3):637–46, vii.

51. Watanakunakorn C, Tisone JC. Antagonism between nafcillin or oxacillin and rifampin against *Staphylococcus aureus*. Antimicrob Agents Chemother 1982; 22(5):920–2.

52. Zak O, Scheld WM, Sande MA. Rifampin in experimental endocarditis due to *Staphylococcus aureus* in rabbits. Rev Infect Dis 1983;5(Suppl 3):S481–90.

53. Kobasa WD, Kaye KL, Shapiro T, et al. Therapy for experimental endocarditis due to *Staphylococcus epidermidis*. Rev Infect Dis 1983;5(Suppl 3):S533–7.

54. Karchmer AW, Archer GL, Dismukes WE. *Staphylococcus epidermidis* causing prosthetic valve endocarditis: microbiologic and clinical observations as guides to therapy. Ann Intern Med 1983;98(4):447–55.

55. Friedland IR, Paris M, Ehrett S, et al. Evaluation of antimicrobial regimens for treatment of experimental penicillin- and cephalosporin-resistant pneumococcal meningitis. Antimicrob Agents Chemother 1993;37(8):1630–6.

56. Martinez-Lacasa J, Cabellos C, Martos A, et al. Experimental study of the efficacy of vancomycin, rifampicin and dexamethasone in the therapy of pneumococcal meningitis. J Antimicrob Chemother 2002;49(3):507–13.

57. Fitoussi F, Doit C, Geslin P, et al. Killing activities of trovafloxacin alone and in combination with beta-lactam agents, rifampin, or vancomycin against *Streptococcus pneumoniae* isolates with various susceptibilities to extended-spectrum cephalosporins at concentrations clinically achievable in cerebrospinal fluid. Antimicrob Agents Chemother 1999;43(10):2372–5.

58. Bassetti M, Repetto E, Righi E, et al. Colistin and rifampicin in the treatment of multidrug-resistant *Acinetobacter baumannii* infections. J Antimicrob Chemother 2008;61(2):417–20.

59. Baciewicz AM, Chrisman CR, Finch CK, et al. Update on rifampin and rifabutin drug interactions. Am J Med Sci 2008;335(2):126–36.

60. Mahatthanatrakul W, Nontaput T, Ridtitid W, et al. Rifampin, a cytochrome P450 3A inducer, decreases plasma concentrations of antipsychotic risperidone in healthy volunteers. J Clin Pharm Ther 2007;32(2):161–7.

61. Nijland HM, L'Homme RF, Rongen GA, et al. High incidence of adverse events in healthy volunteers receiving rifampicin and adjusted doses of lopinavir/ritonavir tablets. AIDS 2008;22(8):931–5.

62. Fraser A, Gafter-Gvili A, Paul M, et al. Antibiotics for preventing meningococcal infections. Cochrane Database Syst Rev 2006;(4):CD004785.
63. Fraser A, Gafter-Gvili A, Paul M, et al. Prophylactic use of antibiotics for prevention of meningococcal infections: systematic review and meta-analysis of randomised trials. Eur J Clin Microbiol Infect Dis 2005;24(3):172–81.
64. Rainbow J, Cebelinski E, Bartkus J, et al. Rifampin-resistant meningococcal disease. Emerg Infect Dis 2005;11(6):977–9.
65. Stefanelli P, Neri A, Carattoli A, et al. Detection of resistance to rifampicin and decreased susceptibility to penicillin in *Neisseria meningitidis* by real-time multiplex polymerase chain reaction assay. Diagn Microbiol Infect Dis 2007;58(2): 241–4.
66. Cuevas LE, Kazembe P, Mughogho GK, et al. Eradication of nasopharyngeal carriage of *Neisseria meningitidis* in children and adults in rural Africa: a comparison of ciprofloxacin and rifampicin. J Infect Dis 1995;171(3):728–31.
67. Perlroth J, Kuo M, Tan J, et al. Adjunctive use of rifampin for the treatment of *Staphylococcus aureus* infections: a systematic review of the literature. Arch Intern Med 2008;168(8):805–19.
68. Morris AB, Brown RB, Sands M. Use of rifampin in nonstaphylococcal, nonmycobacterial disease. Antimicrob Agents Chemother 1993;37(1):1–7.
69. Bayston R, Nuradeen B, Ashraf W, et al. Antibiotics for the eradication of *Propionibacterium acnes* biofilms in surgical infection. J Antimicrob Chemother 2007; 60(6):1298–301.
70. Baddour LM, Wilson WR, Bayer AS, et al. Infective endocarditis: diagnosis, antimicrobial therapy, and management of complications: a statement for healthcare professionals from the Committee on Rheumatic Fever, Endocarditis, and Kawasaki Disease, Council on Cardiovascular Disease in the Young, and the Councils on Clinical Cardiology, Stroke, and Cardiovascular Surgery and Anesthesia, American Heart Association: endorsed by the Infectious Diseases Society of America. Circulation 2005;111(23):e394–434.
71. Norden CW. Experimental chronic staphylococcal osteomyelitis in rabbits: treatment with rifampin alone and in combination with other antimicrobial agents. Rev Infect Dis 1983;5(Suppl 3):S491–4.
72. Bliziotis IA, Ntziora F, Lawrence KR, et al. Rifampin as adjuvant treatment of gram-positive bacterial infections: a systematic review of comparative clinical trials. Eur J Clin Microbiol Infect Dis 2007;26(12):849–56.
73. Falagas ME, Bliziotis IA, Fragoulis KN. Oral rifampin for eradication of *Staphylococcus aureus* carriage from healthy and sick populations: a systematic review of the evidence from comparative trials. Am J Infect Control 2007;35(2):106–14.
74. Simor AE, Phillips E, McGeer A, et al. Randomized controlled trial of chlorhexidine gluconate for washing, intranasal mupirocin, and rifampin and doxycycline versus no treatment for the eradication of methicillin-resistant *Staphylococcus aureus* colonization. Clin Infect Dis 2007;44(2):178–85.
75. Skalsky K, Yahav D, Bishara J, et al. Treatment of human brucellosis: systematic review and meta-analysis of randomised controlled trials. BMJ 2008;336(7646): 701–4.
76. Ranjbar M, Keramat F, Mamani M, et al. Comparison between doxycycline-rifampin-amikacin and doxycycline-rifampin regimens in the treatment of brucellosis. Int J Infect Dis 2007;11(2):152–6.
77. Pelosini I, Scarpignato C. Rifaximin, a peculiar rifamycin derivative: established and potential clinical use outside the gastrointestinal tract. Chemotherapy 2005; 51(Suppl 1):122–30.

78. Ripa S, Mignini F, Prenna M, et al. In vitro antibacterial activity of rifaximin against *Clostridium difficile, Campylobacter jejunii* and *Yersinia spp.* Drugs Exp Clin Res 1987;13(8):483–8.

79. DuPont HL, Jiang ZD. Influence of rifaximin treatment on the susceptibility of intestinal gram-negative flora and enterococci. Clin Microbiol Infect 2004; 10(11):1009–11.

80. Brigidi P, Swennen E, Rizzello F, et al. Effects of rifaximin administration on the intestinal microbiota in patients with ulcerative colitis. J Chemother 2002;14(3): 290–5.

81. Adachi JA, DuPont HL. Rifaximin: a novel nonabsorbed rifamycin for gastroin-testinal disorders. Clin Infect Dis 2006;42(4):541–7.

82. DuPont HL, Jiang ZD, Ericsson CD, et al. Rifaximin versus ciprofloxacin for the treatment of traveler's diarrhea: a randomized, double-blind clinical trial. Clin Infect Dis 2001;33(11):1807–15.

83. DuPont HL, Ericsson CD, Mathewson JJ, et al. Rifaximin: a nonabsorbed antimi-crobial in the therapy of travelers' diarrhea. Digestion 1998;59(6):708–14.

84. Steffen R, Sack DA, Riopel L, et al. Therapy of travelers' diarrhea with rifaximin on various continents. Am J Gastroenterol 2003;98(5):1073–8.

85. Trapnell CB, Connolly M, Pentikis H, et al. Absence of effect of oral rifaximin on the pharmacokinetics of ethinyl estradiol/norgestimate in healthy females. Ann Pharmacother 2007;41(2):222–8.

86. Garey KW, Salazar M, Shah D, et al. Rifamycin antibiotics for treatment of *Clos-tridium difficile*-associated diarrhea. Ann Pharmacother 2008;42(6):827–35.

87. Halsey J. Current and future treatment modalities for *Clostridium difficile*-associ-ated disease. Am J Health Syst Pharm 2008;65(8):705–15.

88. Kokkotou E, Moss AC, Michos A, et al. Comparative efficacies of rifaximin and vancomycin for treatment of *Clostridium difficile*-associated diarrhea and prevention of disease recurrence in hamsters. Antimicrob Agents Chemother 2008;52(3):1121–6.

89. Berman AL. Efficacy of rifaximin and vancomycin combination therapy in a patient with refractory *Clostridium difficile*-associated diarrhea. J Clin Gastro-enterol 2007;41(10):932–3.

90. Johnson S, Schriever C, Galang M, et al. Interruption of recurrent *Clostridium difficile*-associated diarrhea episodes by serial therapy with vancomycin and rifaximin. Clin Infect Dis 2007;44(6):846–8.

91. Drusano GL, Ambrose PG, Bhavnani SM, et al. Back to the future: using amino-glycosides again and how to dose them optimally. Clin Infect Dis 2007;45(6): 753–60.

92. Falagas ME, Matthaiou DK, Bliziotis IA. The role of aminoglycosides in combina-tion with a beta-lactam for the treatment of bacterial endocarditis: a meta-anal-ysis of comparative trials. J Antimicrob Chemother 2006;57(4):639–47.

93. Lentino JR, Narita M, Yu VL. New antimicrobial agents as therapy for resistant gram-positive cocci. Eur J Clin Microbiol Infect Dis 2008;27(1):3–15.

94. Rea RS, Capitano B. Optimizing use of aminoglycosides in the critically ill. Semin Respir Crit Care Med 2007;28(6):596–603.

95. Cunha BA. New uses for older antibiotics: nitrofurantoin, amikacin, colistin, poly-myxin B, doxycycline, and minocycline revisited. Med Clin North Am 2006;90(6): 1089–107.

96. Friedland I, Gallagher G, King T, et al. Antimicrobial susceptibility patterns in *Pseudomonas aeruginosa*: data from a multicenter Intensive Care Unit Surveil-lance Study (ISS) in the United States. J Chemother 2004;16(5):437–41.

97. Buijk SE, Mouton JW, Gyssens IC, et al. Experience with a once-daily dosing program of aminoglycosides in critically ill patients. Intensive Care Med 2002; 28(7):936–42.

98. Turnidge J. Pharmacodynamics and dosing of aminoglycosides. Infect Dis Clin North Am 2003;17(3):503–28, v.

99. Isaksson B, Maller R, Nilsson LE, et al. Postantibiotic effect of aminoglycosides on staphylococci. J Antimicrob Chemother 1993;32(2):215–22.

100. Isaksson B, Nilsson L, Maller R, et al. Postantibiotic effect of aminoglycosides on gram-negative bacteria evaluated by a new method. J Antimicrob Chemother 1988;22(1):23–33.

101. McDonald PJ, Wetherall BL, Pruul H. Postantibiotic leukocyte enhancement: increased susceptibility of bacteria pretreated with antibiotics to activity of leukocytes. Rev Infect Dis 1981;3(1):38–44.

102. Kapusnik JE, Hackbarth CJ, Chambers HF, et al. Single, large, daily dosing versus intermittent dosing of tobramycin for treating experimental pseudomonas pneumonia. J Infect Dis 1988;158(1):7–12.

103. Baudoux P, Bles N, Lemaire S, et al. Combined effect of pH and concentration on the activities of gentamicin and oxacillin against Staphylococcus aureus in pharmacodynamic models of extracellular and intracellular infections. J Antimicrob Chemother 2007;59(2):246–53.

104. Simmen HP, Battaglia H, Kossmann T, et al. Effect of peritoneal fluid pH on outcome of aminoglycoside treatment of intraabdominal infections. World J Surg 1993;17(3):393–7.

105. Harrell LJ, Evans JB. Anaerobic resistance of clinical isolates of Staphylococcus aureus to aminoglycosides. Antimicrob Agents Chemother 1978;14(6):927–9.

106. Barclay ML, Begg EJ. Aminoglycoside adaptive resistance: importance for effective dosage regimens. Drugs 2001;61(6):713–21.

107. Daikos GL, Lolans VT, Jackson GG. First-exposure adaptive resistance to aminoglycoside antibiotics in vivo with meaning for optimal clinical use. Antimicrob Agents Chemother 1991;35(1):117–23.

108. Chandrakanth RK, Raju S, Patil SA. Aminoglycoside-resistance mechanisms in multidrug-resistant Staphylococcus aureus clinical isolates. Curr Microbiol 2008;56(6):558–62.

109. Verpooten GA, Giuliano RA, Verbist L, et al. Once-daily dosing decreases renal accumulation of gentamicin and netilmicin. Clin Pharmacol Ther 1989;45(1):22–7.

110. Bennett WM, Plamp CE, Gilbert DN, et al. The influence of dosage regimen on experimental gentamicin nephrotoxicity: dissociation of peak serum levels from renal failure. J Infect Dis 1979;140(4):576–80.

111. Rybak MJ, Abate BJ, Kang SL, et al. Prospective evaluation of the effect of an aminoglycoside dosing regimen on rates of observed nephrotoxicity and ototoxicity. Antimicrob Agents Chemother 1999;43(7):1549–55.

112. Beauchamp D, Labrecque G. Chronobiology and chronotoxicology of antibiotics and aminoglycosides. Adv Drug Deliv Rev 2007;59(9–10):896–903.

113. Baciewicz AM, Sokos DR, Cowan RI. Aminoglycoside-associated nephrotoxicity in the elderly. Ann Pharmacother 2003;37(2):182–6.

114. Rougier F, Claude D, Maurin M, et al. Aminoglycoside nephrotoxicity. Curr Drug Targets Infect Disord 2004;4(2):153–62.

115. Rybak LP, Ramkumar V. Ototoxicity. Kidney Int 2007;72(8):931–5.

116. Tran Ba Huy P, Bernard P, Schacht J. Kinetics of gentamicin uptake and release in the rat. Comparison of inner ear tissues and fluids with other organs. J Clin Invest 1986;77(5):1492–500.

117. Gatell JM, Ferran F, Araujo V, et al. Univariate and multivariate analyses of risk factors predisposing to auditory toxicity in patients receiving aminoglycosides. Antimicrob Agents Chemother 1987;31(9):1383–7.

118. Ariano RE, Zelenitsky SA, Kassum DA. Aminoglycoside-induced vestibular injury: maintaining a sense of balance. Ann Pharmacother 2008;42(9): 1282–9.

119. Nicolau DP, Freeman CD, Belliveau PP, et al. Experience with a once-daily aminoglycoside program administered to 2,184 adult patients. Antimicrob Agents Chemother 1995;39(3):650–5.

120. Prins JM, Weverling GJ, de Blok K, et al. Validation and nephrotoxicity of a simplified once-daily aminoglycoside dosing schedule and guidelines for monitoring therapy. Antimicrob Agents Chemother 1996;40(11):2494–9.

121. Graham JC, Gould FK. Role of aminoglycosides in the treatment of bacterial endocarditis. J Antimicrob Chemother 2002;49(3):437–44.

122. Smyth AR, Tan KH. Once-daily versus multiple-daily dosing with intravenous aminoglycosides for cystic fibrosis. Cochrane Database Syst Rev 2006;3: CD002009.

123. Ratjen F. Treatment of early *Pseudomonas aeruginosa* infection in patients with cystic fibrosis. Curr Opin Pulm Med 2006;12(6):428–32.

124. Wood DM, Smyth AR. Antibiotic strategies for eradicating *Pseudomonas aeruginosa* in people with cystic fibrosis. Cochrane Database Syst Rev 2006;(1):CD004197.

125. Smyth A, Tan KH, Hyman-Taylor P, et al. Once versus three-times daily regimens of tobramycin treatment for pulmonary exacerbations of cystic fibrosis–the TOPIC study: a randomised controlled trial. Lancet 2005;365(9459):573–8.

126. Weiner JR, Toy EL, Sacco P, et al. Costs, quality of life and treatment compliance associated with antibiotic therapies in patients with cystic fibrosis: a review of the literature. Expert Opin Pharmacother 2008;9(5):751–66.

127. Dopfer R, Brand P, Mullinger B, et al. Inhalation of tobramycin in patients with cystic fibrosis: comparison of two methods. J Physiol Pharmacol 2007;58(Suppl 5 Pt 1):141–54.

128. Lenoir G, Antypkin YG, Miano A, et al. Efficacy, safety, and local pharmacokinetics of highly concentrated nebulized tobramycin in patients with cystic fibrosis colonized with *Pseudomonas aeruginosa*. Paediatr Drugs 2007;9(Suppl 1):11–20.

129. Goss CH. Should we stop using intravenous gentamicin in patients with cystic fibrosis? Thorax 2008;63(6):479–80.

130. de Groot R, Smith AL. Antibiotic pharmacokinetics in cystic fibrosis. Differences and clinical significance. Clin Pharmacokinet 1987;13(4):228–53.

131. Vic P, Ategbo S, Turck D, et al. Efficacy, tolerance, and pharmacokinetics of once daily tobramycin for pseudomonas exacerbations in cystic fibrosis. Arch Dis Child 1998;78(6):536–9.

132. Bragonier R, Brown NM. The pharmacokinetics and toxicity of once-daily tobramycin therapy in children with cystic fibrosis. J Antimicrob Chemother 1998; 42(1):103–6.

133. Banerjee D, Stableforth D. The treatment of respiratory pseudomonas infection in cystic fibrosis: what drug and which way? Drugs 2000;60(5):1053–64.

134. Beringer PM, Vinks AA, Jelliffe RW, et al. Pharmacokinetics of tobramycin in adults with cystic fibrosis: implications for once-daily administration. Antimicrob Agents Chemother 2000;44(4):809–13.

135. Byl B, Baran D, Jacobs F, et al. Serum pharmacokinetics and sputum penetration of amikacin 30 mg/kg once daily and of ceftazidime 200 mg/kg/day as

a continuous infusion in cystic fibrosis patients. J Antimicrob Chemother 2001; 48(2):325-7.

136. Touw DJ, Knox AJ, Smyth A. Population pharmacokinetics of tobramycin administered thrice daily and once daily in children and adults with cystic fibrosis. J Cyst Fibros 2007;6(5):327-33.

137. Al-Lanqawi Y, Capps P, Abdel-hamid M, et al. Therapeutic drug monitoring of gentamicin: evaluation of five nomograms for initial dosing at Al-Amiri hospital in Kuwait. Med Princ Pract 2007;16(5):348-54.

138. Barclay ML, Kirkpatrick CM, Begg EJ. Once daily aminoglycoside therapy. Is it less toxic than multiple daily doses and how should it be monitored? Clin Pharmacokinet 1999;36(2):89-98.

139. Bailey TC, Little JR, Littenberg B, et al. A meta-analysis of extended-interval dosing versus multiple daily dosing of aminoglycosides. Clin Infect Dis 1997; 24(5):786-95.

140. Tod MM, Padoin C, Petitjean O. Individualising aminoglycoside dosage regimens after therapeutic drug monitoring: simple or complex pharmacokinetic methods? Clin Pharmacokinet 2001;40(11):803-14.

141. Barclay ML, Duffull SB, Begg EJ, et al. Experience of once-daily aminoglycoside dosing using a target area under the concentration-time curve. Aust N Z J Med 1995;25(3):230-5.

142. Paterson DL, Robson JM, Wagener MM, et al. Monitoring of serum aminoglycoside levels with once-daily dosing. Pathology 1998;30(3):289-94.

143. Bartal C, Danon A, Schlaeffer F, et al. Pharmacokinetic dosing of aminoglycosides: a controlled trial. Am J Med 2003;114(3):194-8.

144. Urban AW, Craig WA. Daily dosage of aminoglycosides. Curr Clin Top Infect Dis 1997;17:236-55.

Index

Note: Page numbers of article titles are in **boldface** type.

A

Absorption, of antibacterial agents, 793

Acinetobacter spp.
   antibacterial susceptibility testing for, 775
   resistance to antibacterial agents, 830–831

Active surveillance
   in screening of high-risk patients, in antimicrobial resistance control in hospitals, 850
   universal, in antimicrobial resistance control in hospitals, 850–851

Agar dilution, in antibacterial susceptibility testing, 759

Amikacin, in renal failure patients, 904

Aminoglycoside(s), 1062–1067
   antimicrobial activity of, 1062–1063
   concentration-dependent killing by, 1064
   described, 1062
   in children, 872–873
   in renal failure patients, 904
   indications for, 1065–1067
   mechanism of action of, 1062–1063
   once-daily, for renal failure patients, 903, 912
   PAE of, 1064
   PALE of, 1064
   pharmacodynamics of, 1063–1064
   pharmacokinetics of, 1063
   toxicity of, 1064–1065

Amoxicillin, in renal failure patients, 910

AmpC, gram-negative rods producing, resistance to antibacterial agents, 829–830

Ampicillin, in renal failure patients, 910

Anaerobe(s), antibacterial susceptibility testing for, 776–777

Antiacne agents, profile of, 947

Antibacterial agents. See also specific indications and *Antimicrobial agents.*
   absorption of, 793
      food effects on, 794
   bacteriostatic activity of, 808–809
   concentration-dependent bactericidal action of, time course of, 807–808
   distribution of, 775–798
   elimination of, 798–801
   in children, **865–880**
   in renal failure, **899–924**
   in the elderly, **881–898**
   in vitro activity of, 791–793
   intravenous administration of, 793

Infect Dis Clin N Am 23 (2009) 1077–1091
doi:10.1016/S0891-5520(09)00091-9
0891-5520/09/$ – see front matter © 2009 Elsevier Inc. All rights reserved.

id.theclinics.com

United States Postal Service

Statement of Ownership, Management, and Circulation
(All Periodicals Publications Except Requestor Publications)

1. Publication Title	2. Publication Number	3. Filing Date
Infectious Disease Clinics of North America	0 0 1 - 5 5 6	9/15/09

4. Issue Frequency	5. Number of Issues Published Annually	6. Annual Subscription Price
Mar, Jun, Sep, Dec	4	$218.00

7. Complete Mailing Address of Known Office of Publication (Not printer) (Street, city, county, state, and ZIP+4®)

Elsevier Inc.
360 Park Avenue South
New York, NY 10010-1710

Contact Person
Stephen Bushing

Telephone (Include area code)
215-239-3688

8. Complete Mailing Address of Headquarters or General Business Office of Publisher (Not printer)

Elsevier Inc., 360 Park Avenue South, New York, NY 10010-1710

9. Full Names and Complete Mailing Addresses of Publisher, Editor, and Managing Editor (Do not leave blank)

Publisher (Name and complete mailing address)

John Schrefer, Elsevier, Inc., 1600 John F. Kennedy Blvd. Suite 1800, Philadelphia, PA 19103-2899

Editor (Name and complete mailing address)

Barbara Cohen-Kligerman, Elsevier, Inc., 1600 John F. Kennedy Blvd. Suite 1800, Philadelphia, PA 19103-2899

Managing Editor (Name and complete mailing address)

Catherine Bewick, Elsevier, Inc., 1600 John F. Kennedy Blvd. Suite 1800, Philadelphia, PA 19103-2899

10. Owner (Do not leave blank. If the publication is owned by a corporation, give the name and address of the corporation immediately followed by the names and addresses of all stockholders owning or holding 1 percent or more of the total amount of stock. If not owned by a corporation, give the names and addresses of the individual owners. If owned by a partnership or other unincorporated firm, give its name and address as well as those of each individual owner. If the publication is published by a nonprofit organization, give its name and address.)

Full Name	Complete Mailing Address
Wholly owned subsidiary of	4520 East-West Highway
Reed/Elsevier, US holdings	Bethesda, MD 20814

11. Known Bondholders, Mortgagees, and Other Security Holders Owning or Holding 1 Percent or More of Total Amount of Bonds, Mortgages, or Other Securities. If none, check box ☐ None

Full Name	Complete Mailing Address
N/A	

12. Tax Status (For completion by nonprofit organizations authorized to mail at nonprofit rates) (Check one)
The purpose, function, and nonprofit status of this organization and the exempt status for federal income tax purposes:
☐ Has Not Changed During Preceding 12 Months
☐ Has Changed During Preceding 12 Months (Publisher must submit explanation of change with this statement)

PS Form 3526, September 2007 (Page 1 of 3 (Instructions Page 3)) PSN 7530-01-000-9931 PRIVACY NOTICE: See our Privacy policy in www.usps.com

---

13. Publication Title	14. Issue Date for Circulation Data Below
Infectious Disease Clinics of North America	September 2009

15. Extent and Nature of Circulation		Average No. Copies Each Issue During Preceding 12 Months	No. Copies of Single Issue Published Nearest to Filing Date
a. Total Number of Copies (Net press run)		1975	1800
b. Paid Circulation (By Mail and Outside the Mail)	(1) Mailed Outside-County Paid Subscriptions Stated on PS Form 3541. (Include paid distribution above nominal rate, advertiser's proof copies, and exchange copies)	1030	960
	(2) Mailed In-County Paid Subscriptions Stated on PS Form 3541 (Include paid distribution above nominal rate, advertiser's proof copies, and exchange copies)		
	(3) Paid Distribution Outside the Mails Including Sales Through Dealers and Carriers, Street Vendors, Counter Sales, and Other Paid Distribution Outside USPS®	308	311
	(4) Paid Distribution by Other Classes Mailed Through the USPS (e.g. First-Class Mail®)		
c. Total Paid Distribution (Sum of 15b (1), (2), (3), and (4))	▶	1338	1271
d. Free or Nominal Rate Distribution (By Mail and Outside the Mail)	(1) Free or Nominal Rate Outside-County Copies Included on PS Form 3541	78	79
	(2) Free or Nominal Rate In-County Copies Included on PS Form 3541		
	(3) Free or Nominal Rate Copies Mailed at Other Classes Through the USPS (e.g. First-Class Mail)		
	(4) Free or Nominal Rate Distribution Outside the Mail (Carriers or other means)		
e. Total Free or Nominal Rate Distribution (Sum of 15d (1), (2), (3) and (4))	▶	78	79
f. Total Distribution (Sum of 15c and 15e)	▶	1416	1350
g. Copies not Distributed—(See instructions to publishers #4 (page #3))	▶	559	450
h. Total (Sum of 15f and g)	▶	1975	1800
i. Percent Paid (15c divided by 15f times 100)		94.49%	94.15%

16. Publication of Statement of Ownership

☐ If the publication is a general publication, publication of this statement is required. Will be printed in the December 2009 issue of this publication. ☐ Publication not required

17. Signature and Title of Editor, Publisher, Business Manager, or Owner

[signature] Stephen R. Bushing – Subscription Services Coordinator

Date: September 15, 2009

I certify that all information furnished on this form is true and complete. I understand that anyone who furnishes false or misleading information on this form or who omits material or information requested on the form may be subject to criminal sanctions (including fines and imprisonment) and/or civil sanctions (including civil penalties).

PS Form 3526, September 2007 (Page 2 of 3)

Moving?

Make sure your subscription moves with you!

To notify us of your new address, find your **Clinics Account Number** (located on your mailing label above your name), and contact customer service at:

Email: journalscustomerservice-usa@elsevier.com

800-654-2452 (subscribers in the U.S. & Canada)
314-447-8871 (subscribers outside of the U.S. & Canada)

Fax number: 314-447-8029

Elsevier Health Sciences Division
Subscription Customer Service
3251 Riverport Lane
Maryland Heights, MO 63043

*To ensure uninterrupted delivery of your subscription, please notify us at least 4 weeks in advance of move.

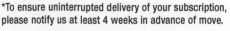

Printed and bound by CPI Group (UK) Ltd, Croydon, CR0 4YY

03/10/2024

01040447-0010